Informing Clinical Practice in Nephrology

Mohsen El Kossi • Arif Khwaja • Meguid El Nahas
Editors

Informing Clinical Practice in Nephrology

The Role of RCTs

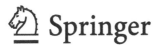 Springer

Editors
Mohsen El Kossi, MBBCh, MSc, MD, FRCP
Doncaster Royal Infirmary
Doncaster
UK

Arif Khwaja, FRCP, PhD
Sheffield Kidney Institute
Northern General Hospital
Sheffield
UK

Meguid El Nahas, MD, PhD, FRCP
Sheffield Kidney Institute
Northern General Hospital
Sheffield
UK

ISBN 978-3-319-34820-9   ISBN 978-3-319-10292-4   (eBook)
DOI 10.1007/978-3-319-10292-4

Springer Cham Heidelberg New York Dordrecht London
© Springer International Publishing Switzerland 2015
Softcover reprint of the hardcover 1st edition 2015

Printed on acid-free paper

Springer is part of Springer Science+Business Media (www.springer.com)

Preface

Nephrology practice has been informed over the last quarter of a century by a large number of clinical trials that translated animal experimentation findings into the bedside. These clinical trials have also informed and shaped the Nephrology Practice Guidelines worldwide.

However, a closer look at many of these clinical trials finds them wanting and reveals major flaws that make their conclusions challengeable and their subsequent impact of practice misguided. Consequently, our practice and guidelines have been shaped in some instances by clinical trials that are inconclusive at best and misleading in their conclusions and recommendations at worst.

This has prompted the editors of this monograph along with its publisher to call upon experts in the various fields of nephrology to undertake a thorough and critical appraisal and evaluation of the published clinical trials that have shaped our practice in recent times in general nephrology, dialysis, and transplantation. We have also included a critical appraisal template based on standard guidelines including the CONSORT statement to allow for a comparative evaluation of clinical trials within one area of nephrology and also across its different fields: General Nephrology, Dialysis, and Transplantation. Of note, the implementation of the Critical Appraisal template was left entirely to individual authors' evaluations.

Parameters	Yes	No	Comment
Validity			
Is the *Randomization* Procedure well described?	+1	−1	
Double *blinded*?	+2	−2	
Is the *sample size* calculation described/adequate?	+3	−3	
Does it have a hard primary *endpoint*?	+1	−1	
Is the endpoint surrogate?	−2	0	
Is the follow-up appropriate?	+1	−1	
Was there a *Bias*?	−2	+2	
Is the drop out >25 %?	−1	+1	
Is the analysis *ITT*?	+3	−3	
Utility/Usefulness			
Can the findings be generalized?	+1	−1	
Was the NNT <100?	+1	−1	
Score	...		

The critical appraisals of mostly randomized clinical trials (RCT) have revealed the strength but also the weakness of the published literature upon which we base our current practice.

We hope that the monograph will alert nephrologists worldwide to the value of published RCT and provide them with a most valuable reference that assists them in their understanding and evaluation of key publications in nephrology. This in turn should allow them to better judge the literature upon which they base their daily clinical practice and avoid misplaced and unfounded assumptions.

The quality of the clinical practice and health care we deliver as nephrologists depend to a large extent on the quality of the RCT and publications we base our knowledge and guidelines upon.

Abbreviations

AKI	Acute kidney injury
aAMR	Acute antibody-mediated rejection
ABPM	Ambulatory blood pressure monitoring
ADPKD	Autosomal dominant polycystic kidney disease
ALG	Anti-lymphocyte globulin
ATG	Anti-thymocyte globulin
ATP III	Adult Treatment Panel III
BUN	Blood urea nitrogen
CAC	Coronary artery calcification
cAMR	Chronic antibody-mediated rejection
CAPD	Continuous ambulatory peritoneal dialysis
CKD	Chronic kidney disease
CKD-MBD	Chronic kidney disease-mineral bone disorder
CMV	Cytomegalovirus
CNIs	Calcineurin inhibitors
CRP	C reactive protein
CsA	Cyclosporine A
CSWD	Corticosteroid withdrawal
CTT	Cholesterol treatment trialist
CVD	Cardiovascular disease
DM	Diabetes mellitus
DOPPS	Dialysis Outcomes and Practice Patterns Study
DSA	Donor-specific alloantibodies
DSM	Drug Safety and Monitoring
eGFR	Estimated glomerular filtration rate
Epo	Erythropoietin
ESAs	Erythropoiesis stimulating agents
ESRD	End stage renal disease
FGF23	Fibroblast growth factor 23
FSGS	Focal and segmental glomerulosclerosis
Hb	Hemoglobin
HD	Hemodialysis
HMG-CO	Hydroxymethylglutaryl-CoA
IDPN	Intradialytic parenteral nutrition
IFG	Impaired fasting glucose
ITT	Intention to treat
KDIGO	Kidney Disease Improving Global Outcomes
KDOQI	Kidney Disease Outcomes Quality Initiative
LDL	Low-density lipoprotein
MACE	Major adverse cardiovascular events
MAP	Mean arterial pressure
MCD	Minimal change disease

MI	Myocardial infarction
MMF	Mycophenolate mofetil
MN	Membranous nephropathy
MPGN	Membranoproliferative glomerulonephritis
mTOR	Mammalian target of rapamycin
ND-CKD	Nondialysis-dependent CKD
NNT	Number needed to treat
NODAT	New onset diabetes after transplant
NYHA	New York Heart Association
OL-HDF	Online hemodiafiltration
POC	Proof of concept
PP	Per protocol
PTLD	Post-transplant lymphoproliferative disease
RAAS	Renin-angiotensin-aldosterone system
RCT	Randomized controlled trial
RRT	Renal replacement therapy
SCC	Squamous cell carcinoma
SCD	Sudden cardiac death
SD	Standard deviation
TKV	Total kidney volume
UAER	Urine albumin excretion rate
VC	Vascular calcification

Contents

Contributors

Richard J. Baker, MB, BChir, PhD, FRCP Renal Unit, St. James's University Hospital, Leeds, West Yorkshire, UK

Aminu K. Bello, MBBS, MMedSci, PhD, FRCP, FASN Division of Nephrology and Immunology, Faculty of Medicine and Dentistry, University of Alberta, Edmonton, AB, Canada

Charles Chazot, MD NephroCare Tassin-Charcot, Lyon, France

Mark J. Courtney, MD, FRCPC Division of Nephrology and Immunology, Department of Medicine, University of Alberta, Edmonton, AB, Canada

Simon J Davies, BSc, MD, FRCP Department of Nephrology, University Hospital of North Staffordshire, Staffordshire, UK

Mohsen El Kossi, MBBCh, MSc, MD, FRCP Doncaster Renal Unit, Doncaster Royal Infirmary Hospital, Doncaster, UK

Meguid El Nahas, MD, PhD, FRCP Sheffield Kidney Institute, Global Kidney Academy, Sheffield, UK

Bo Feldt-Rasmussen, MD, DMSc Department of Nephrology, Rigshospitalet, University of Copenhagen, Copenhagen, Denmark

Richard J. Glassock, MD, MACP Department of Medicine, Geffen School of Medicine at UCLA, Laguna Niguel, CA, USA

Arif Khwaja, FRCP, PhD Northern General Hospital, Sheffield Kidney Institute, Sheffield, UK

Adeera Levin, BSc (Honours), MD, FRCPC, FACP Division of Nephrology, Department of Medicine, St. Paul's Hospital, University of British Columbia, Vancouver, BC, Canada

Khalid Mahdi, MBBS, MRCP Northern General Hospital, Sheffield Kidney Institute, Sheffield, South Yorkshire, UK

J. Okel Division of Nephrology and Immunology, Department of Medicine, University of Alberta, Edmonton, AB, Canada

Lionel Rostaing, MD, PhD Department of Nephrology, University Hospital of Toulouse, Toulouse, France

N. Shah Division of Nephrology and Immunology, Department of Medicine, University of Alberta, Edmonton, AB, Canada

Vimarsha G. Swami, BSc, MD Division of Nephrology and Immunology, Department of Medicine, University of Alberta, Edmonton, AB, Canada

Yangmin Zeng, MD Division of Nephrology, Department of Medicine, St. Paul's Hospital, University of British Columbia, Vancouver, BC, Canada

Autosomal Dominant Polycystic Kidney Disease (ADPKD) Clinical Trials: A Critical Appraisal

Vimarsha G. Swami, Julious Okel, Nikhil Shah, Mark J. Courtney, and Aminu K. Bello

Introduction

Autosomal dominant polycystic kidney disease (ADPKD) is the most common monogenic hereditary kidney disease in humans, occuring in 1 out of every 800–1,000 individuals, and is the cause of end-stage renal disease (ESRD) in 5–10 % of the prevalent patients on renal replacement therapy (RRT) worldwide [1]. The disease is characterized by the development, growth, and expansion of multiple renal cysts, leading to destruction of normal renal parenchyma, massively enlarged kidneys, and subsequent kidney function loss [2–4]. The natural course of ADPKD is often of progressive nature, eventually leading to ESRD in approximately 50 % of patients afflicted.

Despite extensive research over several decades, there has been no specific therapy for ADPKD that is effective in preventing or delaying disease progression. ADPKD is thus managed generically as in acquired chronic kidney disease

(CKD) by treating risk factors with an emphasis on blood pressure control and treatment of its specific complications (infections, hematuria, stones, etc.) [5]. A greater understanding of the underlying complex pathogenetic mechanisms over the last decades have led to a proliferation of clinical studies investigating the potential role of emerging therapeutic strategies such as somatostatin analogues, vasopressin antagonists, mammalian target of rapamycin (mTOR) inhibitors, and statins in modulating the course of ADPKD [6].

We performed an extensive literature review of these studies using search terms: "polycystic kidney, autosomal dominant" with subheadings "diet therapy, drug therapy, mortality, prevention and control, therapy." This search yielded 392 publications. Of these, 65 studies were relevant to drug management of ADPKD, but only randomized controlled trials (RCTs) were selected for appraisal (Fig. 1.1). Each study was appraised for validity and clinical utility based on a standardized scoring system based on method of randomization, study design, sample size, end points, follow-up, bias, dropout rates, and analytical approach.

We found 22 RCTs to date (11 June 2014) on ADPKD management (Table 1.1). Most (16 of 22) of the studies were published over the current decade (2010 and onwards), six were published in the last decade (2000–2009), and only one study was conducted prior to the year 2000, and this was a subgroup analysis from the modification of diet in renal disease (MDRD) study that comprised ADPKD patients in almost a quarter of its study population.

The trials fell within six therapeutic categories:

1. Blood pressure lowering medications – 7 trials
2. Low-protein diet – 1 trial
3. Statins – 3 trials
4. mTOR inhibitors – 6 trials
5. Vasopressin receptor antagonists – 1 trial
6. Somatostatin analogues – 4 trials

V.G. Swami, BSc, MD • J. Okel, MD
N. Shah, MD • M.J. Courtney, MD, FRCPC
Division of Nephrology and Immunology,
Department of Medicine, University of Alberta,
11-107 Clinical Science Building 11350 83 Ave,
Edmonton, AB T6G 2G3, Canada
e-mail: vimarsha@ualberta.ca; okel@ualberta.ca

A.K. Bello, MBBS, MMedSci, PhD, FRCP, FASN (✉)
Division of Nephrology and Immunology,
Department of Medicine, University of Alberta,
11-107 Clinical Science Building 11350 83 Ave,
Edmonton, AB T6G 2G3, Canada

Division of Nephrology and Immunology,
Faculty of Medicine and Dentistry,
University of Alberta,
11-107 Clinical Sciences Building,
Edmonton, AB T6G 2G3, Canada
e-mail: aminu1@ualberta.ca

M. El Kossi, A. Khwaja, and M. El Nahas (eds.), *Informing Clinical Practice in Nephrology: The Role of RCTs*,
DOI 10.1007/978-3-319-10292-4_1, © Springer International Publishing Switzerland 2015

MEDLINE SEARCH:
"Polycystic Kidney, Autosomal
dominant", Subheadings: "diet
therapy, drug therapy, mortality,
prevention & control, therapy"

396 studies

331 Excluded   Studies not relevant to therapeutic
                    management of Autosomal
                    dominant polycystic kidney disease

65 relevant
studies

45 Excluded   Not randomized controlled trials

22 Randomized
Controlled Trials
Included

Fig. 1.1 Flow-chart summary of literature search and study selection

Five major studies out of the total 22 published clinical trials were selected for a full appraisal based on their quality and rigorous methodological framework (Table 1.1). The remaining studies, which scored relatively poorly due to their small sample sizes, inadequate follow-up, suboptimal study designs, and/or lack of rigor in conduct, were not appraised in further details (Table 1.1).

Keywords: ADPKD, Clinical trials, Management, BP, Cysts growth, Novel agents

mTOR Inhibitors Trials

The inhibition of mTOR has proved to have antiproliferative effects in a number of experimental models and clinical disease characterized by dysregulated cell growth. One of the hypotheses behind the pathogenesis of ADPKD is that a dysregulation renal tubules proliferation leads to cystic dilatations. With that notion in mind, successful attempts have been made in experimental models of PKD to slow the progression of cystic expansion as well as the associated decline in kidney function by mTOR inhibition. This has led to a number of RCTs testing this hypothesis in humans with ADPKD.

Everolimus in patients with autosomal dominant polycystic kidney disease

Walz G, Budde K, Mannaa M, et al. N Engl J Med. 2010;363(9):830–40 [7]

Abstract

Background: Autosomal dominant polycystic kidney disease (ADPKD) is a slowly progressive hereditary disorder that usually leads to end-stage renal disease. Although the underlying gene mutations were identified several years ago, efficacious therapy to curtail cyst growth and prevent renal failure is not available. Experimental and observational studies suggest that the mammalian target of rapamycin (mTOR) pathway plays a critical role in cyst growth.

Methods: In this 2-year, double-blind trial, we randomly assigned 433 patients with ADPKD to receive either placebo or the mTOR inhibitor everolimus. The primary outcome was the change in total kidney volume, as measured on magnetic resonance imaging, at 12 and 24 months.

Results: Total kidney volume increased between baseline and 1 year by 102 ml in the everolimus group, versus 157 ml in the placebo group ($P=0.02$) and between baseline and 2 years by 230 and 301 ml, respectively ($P=0.06$). Cyst volume increased by 76 ml in the everolimus group and 98 ml in the placebo group after 1 year ($P=0.27$) and by 181 and 215 ml, respectively, after 2 years ($P=0.28$). Parenchymal volume increased by 26 ml in the everolimus group and 62 ml in the placebo group after 1 year ($P=0.003$) and by 56 and 93 ml, respectively, after 2 years ($P=0.11$). The mean decrement in the estimated glomerular filtration rate after 24 months was 8.9 ml per minute per 1.73 m^2 of body-surface area in the everolimus group versus 7.7 ml per minute in the placebo group ($P=0.15$). Drug-specific adverse events were more common in the everolimus group; the rate of infection was similar in the two groups.

Conclusions: Within the 2-year study period, as compared with placebo, everolimus slowed the increase in total kidney volume of patients with ADPKD but did not slow the progression of renal impairment.

Table 1.1 Summary of clinical appraisal scores for all the randomized controlled trials conducted in ADPKD

Trial No.	Intervention	Study with reference	Design	N	Intervention	Comparator	Follow-up	End points	Score %	Conclusions and comment
1	mTOR inhibitors	Stallone et al. [26]	Open label	55	Rapamycin + Ramipril	Ramipril alone	24 months	Total kidney volume, cyst volume, eGFR		Rapamycin reduced cyst volume Limited by: Open label – unblinded Short duration of follow-up Small sample size Use of surrogate end points
2	mTOR inhibitors	Soliman et al. [27]	Single blind, placebo controlled	16	Sirolimus + telmisartan	Telmisartan + placebo	24 months	Total kidney volume		Sirolimus slowed increase in total kidney volume in the first 6 months only Limited by: Lack of randomization Small sample size and inadequate power Surrogate end point
3	mTOR inhibitors	Walz et al. [7]	Double blind, placebo controlled	433	Everolimus	Placebo	24 months	Total kidney volume, cyst volume, parenchymal volume, eGFR	+13 %	See Appraisal
4	mTOR inhibitors	Serra et al. [11]	Open label	100	Sirolimus	No treatment	18 months	Total kidney volume, eGFR	+0 %	See Appraisal
5	mTOR inhibitors	Perico et al. [28]	Open label, crossover	21	Sirolimus	Conventional antihypertensives	6 months	Total kidney volume, cyst volume, eGFR		Sirolimus halted cyst growth and increased parenchymal volume Limited by: Open label and not blinded Small sample size and inadequate power Short follow-up period High dropout rates Use of surrogate end points
6	mTOR inhibitors	Braun et al. [29]	Open label	30	Rapamycin (low dose, standard dose)	Conventional anti-hypertensives	12 months	Total kidney volume, mGFR (iothalamate clearance)		Low-dose rapamycin increased mGFR Limited by: Open label and unblinded Small sample size and inadequate power Short duration of follow-up
7	Vasopression receptor antagonists	Torres et al. [13]	Double blind, placebo controlled	1,445	Tolvaptan	Placebo	36 months	Total kidney volume, eGFR	+62 %	See Appraisal
8	Somatostatin	Hogan et al. [30]	Double blind, placebo controlled	34	Octreotide	Placebo	12 months	Liver volume changes Total kidney volume, eGFR, quality of life		Octreotide slowed increase in total kidney volume Limited by: Study not powered to detect renal changes

(continued)

Table 1.1 (continued)

Trial No.	Intervention	Study with reference	Design	N	Intervention	Comparator	Follow-up	End points	Score %	Conclusions and comment
9	Somatostatin	Hogan et al. [31]	Open label	34	Octreotide	Placebo	12 months	Liver volume changes Total kidney volume, eGFR, quality of life		The previous benefit on total kidney volume was not sustained with an additional 1 year of treatment Limited by: As above, not primarily a kidney study
10	Somatostatin	Ruggenenti et al. [22]	Double blind, placebo controlled, crossover	14	Long-acting octreotide	Placebo	6 months	Total kidney volume, cyst volume, parenchymal volume, mGFR (iohexol clearance)		Octreotide slowed increase in total kidney volume and cyst volume No difference in mGFR Limited by: Very small sample size and inadequate power Follow-up period of 6 months may have been sufficient to measure health-related quality of life changes but not to detect changes in GFR
11	Somatostatin	van Keimpema et al. [32]	Double blind, placebo controlled	32	Long-acting lanreotide	Placebo	6 months	Primary end-point liver volume Total kidney volume, cyst volume, parenchymal volume, eGFR		Lanreotide slowed increase in total kidney volume Limited by: Primary end-point liver volume Study not powered to detect renal changes
12	Low-protein diet	Klahr et al. [33]	Unblinded	200	Low-protein diet	Normal protein diet	26 months	eGFR and mGFR (iothalamate)		In patients with GFR 13–24, low-protein diet slowed renal disease progression This is a subgroup analysis of the MDRD study, therefore not powered to detect changes in subgroups such as ADPKD At best hypothesis generating
13	Statin	Fassett et al. [19]	Open label	60	Pravastatin	No treatment	24 months	eGFR, urinary protein excretion		No changes with treatment Limited by: An open label trial which lends it to potential treatment bias during follow-up Small sample size and it is not clear whether the study sample had statistical power to answer the study question GFR not measured but estimated

#		Author	Design	N			Duration	Outcomes	%	Appraisal
14	Statin	van Dijk et al. [20]	Double blind, placebo controlled, crossover	10	Simvastatin	Placebo	4 weeks	iGFR (inulin clearance), effective renal plasma flow (PAH clearance)		Simvastatin increased renal plasma flow Limited by: The sample size was very small and power most likely to be inadequate This is a study primarily aimed at studying the functional and hemodynamic effects of statins in ADPKD
15	Statin	Cadnapaphornchai et al. [16]	Double blind, placebo controlled	110	Pravastatin + lisinopril	Placebo + lisinopril	36 months	HtTKV, UAE, LVMI	+73 %	See Appraisal
16	Anti-HTN	Nakamura et al. [34]	Unblinded	20	Telmisartan	Enalapril	12 months	BP, serum Cr, UAE		Telmisartan resulted in improved UAE Limited by: Open label trial which lends it to potential observer bias during follow-up Small sample size and it is not clear whether the sample had statistical power to answer the study question The use of surrogate end points further limits the clinical utility of the study findings; GFR not measured BP measured casually and not over 24 h; thus raising questions over accuracy of recordings
17	Anti-HTN	Ulusoy et al. [35]	Unblinded	32	Losartan	Ramipril	12 months	BP, GFR, LVMI		Both agents reduced BP and LVMI Limited by: Open label and unblended lending to observer bias Inadequate sample size to estimate impact on ADPKD progression Quality of BP measurements; BP measured casually and not over 24 h; thus raising questions over accuracy of recordings Method of CKD progression assessment; FGR not measured
18	Anti-HTN	Nutahara et al. [36]	Unblinded	49	Amlodipine	Candesartan	36 months	BP, creatinine clearance, UAE		Candesartan decreased UAE vs. amplodipine Limited by: Open label and unblinded lending to observer bias Inadequate sample size to detect changes in kidney function Quality of BP measurements; BP measured casually and not over 24 h; thus raising questions over accuracy of recordings GFR not measured

(continued)

Table 1.1 (continued)

Trial No.	Intervention	Study with reference	Design	N	Intervention	Comparator	Follow-up	End points	Score %	Conclusions and comment
19	Anti-HTN	Ecder et al. [37]	Unblinded	24	Enalapril	Amlodipine	60 months	Mean arterial pressure, creatinine clearance, ACR		Enalapril decreased UAE. Limited by: Open label and unblinded lending to observer bias; Inadequate sample size to detect changes in kidney function; Quality of BP measurements; BP measured casually and not over 24 h; thus raising questions over accuracy of recordings; GFR not measured
20	Anti-HTN	Zeltner et al. [38]	Double blind	46	Ramipril	Metoprolol	36 months	BP, eGFR, ACR, LVMI		No difference in outcomes between ramipril and metoprolol in ADPKD. Good BP control and monitoring (24 h ABPM) in both groups. Limited by: Small sample size and inadequate power to show functional differences; GFR was not measured
21	Anti-HTN	Schrier et al. [25]	Unblinded	75	BP target <120/80	BP target <135–140/85–90	84 months	LVMI, eGFR		Rigorous BP control decreased LVMI. Limited by: Unblinded study; Small sample size and inadequate power to detect renal functional changes; High dropout rates; GFR not measured; 24 h ABPM not recorded
22	Anti-HTN	van Dijk et al. [39]	Double blind, placebo controlled	104	Enalapril	Atenolol or placebo	36 months	mGFR (inulin)		Enalapril did not slow decline in mGFR vs. placebo or atenolol. GFR measured by inulin clearance. RPF measured by PAH clearance. Limited by: Small sample size and inadequate power to detect renal functional changes, especially in ADPKD with normal renal function at onset; 24 h ABPM not recorded

ACR urinary albumin to creatinine ratio, *ADPKD* adult polycystic kidney disease, *BP* blood pressure, *CKD* chronic kidney disease, *Cr* creatintine, *GFR* glomerular filtration rate, *eGFR* estimated GFR, *mGFR* measured GFR, *HTN* hypertension, *HtTKV* height-adjusted total kidney volume, *LVMI* left ventricular mass index, *mTOR* mammalian target of rapamycin

Critical Appraisal

Parameters	Yes	No	Comment
Validity			
Is the **randomization** procedure well described?		−1	Randomization was only described as 1:1 with the eligible patients assigned to either receive everolimus or placebo
Double **blinded**?	+2		Described as double blinded
Is the **sample size** calculation described/ adequate?	+3		$N = 433$; exceeded requirement of $N = 260$ to detect a 50 % relative reduction in annual increase in total kidney volume, 90 % power and two-sided significance of 4 %. The sampling allowed for dropout and was larger than estimated SD
Does it have a hard primary **end point**?		−1	The primary outcome was a change in kidney volume measured on MRI and secondary outcomes of changes in cyst sizes and parenchymal volume at months 12 and 24 and in renal function at month 24
Is the end-point surrogate?	−2		Surrogate end points only
Is the follow-up appropriate?		−1	24-month follow-up period was likely insufficient to show any impact on disease progression towards ESRD
Was there a **Bias**?	−1		Early CKD patients only, all Caucasians and of younger age extraction
Is the dropout >25 %?	−1		~35 %: largely due to side effects associated with everolimus, including leukopenia, thrombocytopenia, and hyperlipidemia
Is the analysis **ITT**?	+3		Analysis was based on the initial treatment intent
Utility/usefulness			
Can the findings be generalized?	+1		Included patients with stage I–III CKD and ADPKD diagnosed clinically or by MRI single kidney volume >1,000 mL only
Score		13 %	**Study with major limitations**

ADPKD adult polycystic kidney disease, *CKD* chronic kidney disease, *GFR* glomerular filtration rate, *ITT* intention to treat, *MRI* magnetic resonance imaging, *SD* standard deviation

Comments and Discussion

This trial by Walz et al. was a multicenter (patients were recruited from 24 academic centers in three countries – Germany, Austria, and France), double-blinded, placebo-controlled study aimed to assess the effect of everolimus in ADPKD progression (cyst growth). It was a 2-year trial and randomized 433 patients with ADPKD. Patients were given either everolimus 2.5 mg twice a day or placebo (control). Everolimus slowed the increase in total kidney volume (TKV) but not the decline in kidney function (worsening of eGFR) compared to placebo.

Despite its robust design and large sample size, the study has important limitations on several key fronts:

1. Limited generalizability: The study was focused on patients with early CKD (Stages 1–3), a group of patients with ADPKD that hardly progress. This coupled with the use of surrogate end points and the high incidence of everolimus adverse effects, and consequent high dropout rate of 35 % limits the application of these study findings to clinical practice. Further, the study was limited to younger patients with CKD (mean age of 44 years) and all whites. The implications of the study findings in patients with a more advanced disease, the elderly, and other racial backgrounds could not be ascertained.

2. Lack of concordance of structure and function. Although, observational data in patients with ADPKD have shown that cyst volume correlates well with the disease progression [8]; Chapman et al. [8] showed TKV to be a reasonable predictor of the risk of progression to stage 3 CKD over 8-year follow-up in ADPKD. However, TKV remains a surrogate end point and its prognostic value in this study of a 2-year follow-up is uncertain.

3. Limited follow-up period: The study follow-up period of 2 years is relatively short to detect significant decline in eGFR in ADPKD which may be slowly progressive over many years especially in the initial stages of the disease.

4. Poor measures of kidney function: eGFR formulas have been shown to underestimate values and decline in measured GFR in ADPKD, suggesting that eGFR may have limited utility in ADPKD [9, 10].

Sirolimus and kidney growth in autosomal dominant polycystic kidney disease.

Serra AL, Poster D, Kistler AD, et al. N Engl J Med. 2010;363(9):820–9 [11]

Abstract

Background: In autosomal dominant polycystic kidney disease (ADPKD), aberrant activation of the mammalian target of rapamycin (mTOR) pathway is associated with progressive kidney enlargement. The drug sirolimus suppresses mTOR signaling.

Methods: In this 18-month, open-label, randomized, controlled trial, we sought to determine whether sirolimus halts the growth in kidney volume among patients with ADPKD. We randomly assigned 100 patients between the ages of 18 and 40 years to receive either sirolimus (target dose, 2 mg daily) or standard care. All patients had an estimated creatinine clearance of at least 70 ml per minute. Serial magnetic resonance imaging was performed to measure the volume of polycystic kidneys. The primary outcome was total kidney volume at 18 months on blinded assessment. Secondary outcomes were the glomerular filtration rate and urinary albumin excretion rate at 18 months.

Results: At randomization, the median total kidney volume was 907 cm^3 (interquartile range, 577–1,330) in the sirolimus group and 1,003 cm^3 (interquartile range, 574–1,422) in the control group. The median increase over the 18-month period was 99 cm^3 (interquartile range, 43–173) in the sirolimus group and 97 cm^3 (interquartile range, 37–181) in the control group. At 18 months, the median total kidney volume in the sirolimus group was 102 % of that in the control group (95 % confidence interval, 99–105; $P=0.26$). The glomerular filtration rate did not differ significantly between the two groups; however, the urinary albumin excretion rate was higher in the sirolimus group.

Conclusion: In adults with ADPKD and early chronic kidney disease, 18 months of treatment with sirolimus did not halt polycystic kidney growth.

Critical Appraisal

Parameters	Yes	No	Comment
Validity			
Is the **randomization** procedure well described?	+1		Randomization list generated using a permuted block design
Double **blinded**?		−2	Open label, no placebo
Is the **sample size** calculation described/adequate?	+3		$N=100$; exceeded requirement of $N=80$ to detect a 50 % relative difference in annual increase in total kidney volume, 80 % power and two-sided alpha level of 0.05
Does it have a hard primary **end point**?		−1	The primary outcome was percent in change in total kidney volume. GFR and UAER at 18 months used as secondary outcomes
Is the end-point surrogate?		−2	Surrogate end points only
Is the follow-up appropriate?		−1	18-month follow-up period was likely insufficient to show effect of rapamycin on GFR; prognostic value of total kidney volume in a study of 24 year follow-up has not yet been established
Was there a **Bias**?		−1	Early CKD patients only, all Caucasians and of younger age extraction
Is the dropout >25 %?		+1	4 % (4/100 patients)

Parameters	Yes	No	Comment
Is the analysis **ITT**?	+3		Described as ITT
Utility/usefulness			
Can the findings be generalized?	+1		Patients age 18–40 with ADPKD (minimum 2 % increase in total kidney volume over a 6-month pre-study period) and early CKD with GFR >70
Are the findings easily translatable?		−1	Clinical translatability is limited by the lack of hard non-surrogate primary end points, short follow-up time, and small sample size
Was the NNT <100?		−1	Negative study
Score		0 %	**Study with major limitations**

ADPKD adult polycystic kidney disease, *CKD* chronic kidney disease, *GFR* glomerular filtration rate, *ITT* intention to treat, *UAER* urinary albumin excretion

Comments and Discussion

This is one of the few large randomized studies on the use of mTOR inhibitors in ADPKD, and the findings are mostly in agreement with the study by Walz et al. [7]. The key objective was to determine if rapamycin (sirolimus) would slow kidney cysts growth and reduce TKV. There was no clinically meaningful reduction in TKV irrespective of patients' demographics, level of kidney function, and/or albuminuria. Though not blinded, the methodology was strong with small dropout rate (<4 %) compared to the everolimus trial [7].

The study of Serra and colleagues has a number of limitations:

1. Lack of blinding always raises concern over a potential observer bias during follow-up.
2. The follow-up period of 18 months is relatively short to detect significant clinical outcomes in ADPKD, especially early in the course of the disease.
3. The use of surrogate end points instead of hard primary end points coupled with the study being done in early CKD stages (GFR >70 ml/min), in relatively young population (18–40 years), limits the application of study results to usual clinical practice.

The above limitations make any conclusion about the impact of sirolimus on the progression of ADPKD at best hypothetical.

Vasopressin V2 Receptor Antagonists Trial

The pathogenesis of ADPKD is thought to be related to a dysregulated growth of renal tubules cells. One of the hypotheses implicates ADH (vasopressin) and the related increase in intracellular cAMP in the pathogenesis of renal cysts proliferation and luminal fluid secretion. Experimental studies based on the suppression of vasopressin release by means of high water intake, genetic elimination of vasopressin, and vasopressin V2-receptor blockade [12] all seem to reduce the cyst burden and protect kidney function. This is the rationale behind the testing of this concept in patients with ADPKD.

TEMPO Trial

Tolvaptan in patients with autosomal dominant polycystic kidney disease.

Torres VE, Chapman AB, Devuyst O, Gansevoort RT, Grantham JJ, Higashihara E, Perrone RD, Krasa HB, Ouyang J, Czerwiec FS, TEMPO 3:4 Trial Investigators. N Engl J Med. 2012;367(25):2407–18 [13].

Abstract

Background: The course of autosomal dominant polycystic kidney disease (ADPKD) is often associated with pain, hypertension, and kidney failure. Preclinical studies indicated that vasopressin V(2)-receptor antagonists inhibit cyst growth and slow the decline of kidney function.

Methods: In this phase 3, multicenter, double-blind, placebo-controlled, 3-year trial, we randomly assigned 1,445 patients, 18–50 years of age, who had ADPKD with a total kidney volume of 750 ml or more and an estimated creatinine clearance of 60 ml per minute or more, in a 2:1 ratio to receive tolvaptan, a V(2)-receptor antagonist, at the highest of three twice-daily dose regimens that the patient found tolerable, or placebo. The primary outcome was the annual rate of change in the total kidney volume. Sequential secondary end points included a composite of time to clinical progression (defined as worsening kidney function, kidney pain, hypertension, and albuminuria) and rate of kidney-function decline.

Results: Over a 3-year period, the increase in total kidney volume in the tolvaptan group was 2.8 % per year (95 % confidence interval [CI], 2.5–3.1), versus 5.5 % per year in the placebo group (95 % CI, 5.1–6.0; $P < 0.001$). The composite end point favored tolvaptan over placebo (44 vs. 50 events per 100 follow-up years, $P = 0.01$), with lower rates of worsening kidney function (2 vs. 5 events per 100 person-years of follow-up, $P < 0.001$) and kidney pain (5 vs. 7 events per 100 person-years of follow-up, $P = 0.007$). Tolvaptan was associated with a slower decline in kidney function (reciprocal of the serum creatinine level, −2.61 [mg per milliliter] (−1) per year vs. −3.81 [mg per milliliter] (−1) per year; $P < 0.001$). There were fewer ADPKD-related adverse events in the tolvaptan group but more events related to aquaresis (excretion of electrolyte-free water) and hepatic adverse events unrelated to ADPKD, contributing to a higher discontinuation rate (23 %, vs. 14 % in the placebo group).

Conclusions: Tolvaptan, as compared with placebo, slowed the increase in total kidney volume and the decline in kidney function over a 3-year period in patients with ADPKD but was associated with a higher discontinuation rate, owing to adverse events.

Critical Appraisal

Parameters	Yes	No	Comment
Validity			
Is the randomization procedure well described?		−1	
Double **blinded**?	+2		Described as double blinded
Is the **sample size** calculation described/adequate?	+3		$N = 1{,}445$; exceeded requirement of $N = 600$ to detect a 20 % relative difference in total kidney volume, 85 % power and two-sided alpha level of 0.045
Does it have a hard primary **end point**?		−1	Change in total kidney volume, kidney function (reciprocal of serum creatinine) over 36 months
Is the end-point surrogate?	−2		Surrogate end points only
Is the follow-up appropriate?	+1		36-month follow-up period was sufficient to show effect of tolvaptan on renal function
Was there a **Bias**?		+2	No selection, performance, exclusion or detection biases
Is the dropout >25 %?		+1	20 % (288/1,445 patients)
Is the analysis **ITT**?	+3		Described as ITT
Utility/usefulness			
Can the findings be generalized?	+1		Patients age 18–50 with ADPKD (total kidney volume ≥750 mL) and early CKD with GFR >60
Was the NNT <100?		−1	Negative study
Score		62 %	

ADPKD adult polycystic kidney disease, *CKD* chronic kidney disease, *GFR* glomerular filtration rate, *ITT* intention to treat

Comments and Discussion

This study had strong methodological framework and represents the most important RCT on ADPKD to date focusing on a novel intervention. It was multicenter, double-blind, placebo-controlled, parallel-group trial of large sample size well powered to answer the study question, which was to assess efficacy and safety of tolvaptan in ADPKD. Tolvaptan slowed the increased in TKV and the decline in renal function over a 3-year period compared to placebo. It represents the only randomized control trial to date on utility of vasopressin receptor antagonists in ADPKD. It supports data from animal models of ADPKD, where vasopressin V2-receptor blockade was shown to inhibit cystogenesis [13]. Despite its strong methodological design, clinical translatability is limited due to important flaws in the study:

1. The use of changes in TKV as primary end point. While such changes may reflect subsequent or parallel changes in kidney function [8, 14], they remain surrogate to the true estimation of the decline of GFR or the incidence of ESRD. Furthermore, changes in TKV upon treatment with an agent that stimulates diuresis, and presumably the reduction of renal cysts, and kidney, urine content, cannot be equated with reduced cystogenesis.

2. Use of changes in the reciprocal of serum creatinine slope as a secondary end point for the progression of functional decline in ADPKD. Changes in serum creatinine levels, in a trial of an agent associated with changes in plasma volume due to excessive aquaresis as well as changes in fluid intake, are difficult to interpret.

3. Also the use of eGFR that seemed to agree with the changes in reciprocal of serum creatinine in this study underlies the concern about the inaccuracy of both related methods in measuring CKD progression (true/measured GFR) in ADPKD; eGFR has been shown to significantly underestimated CKD progression in ADPKD compared to measured GFR (mGFR) [9].

4. The study population included only patients with early CKD, >75 % with eGFR higher than 80 ml/min; CKD progression tends to be slow early in the course of ADPKD and accelerates considerably in later stages of renal dysfunction. Furthermore, a significant percentage of patients included in this study are likely to be non-progressive.

5. All the trial participants were required by design to increase their fluid intake in order to avoid dehydration, and it is very well known that increased water intake do suppress vasopressin-mediated cAMP generation and cystogenesis. The increased water intake on its own could have impacted on outcomes in the control group thus confounding the interpretation and possibly the power of the study.

Tolvaptan was associated with a high incidence of adverse events. This led to a high dropout rate of 20 % largely due to the side effects of tolvaptan, namely, an elevation of liver enzymes as well as aquaresis-related symptoms (thirst, polyuria). As a result of the incidence of liver injury, the US Food and Drug Administration (FDA) imposed limitations on tolvaptan use, namely, that the drug not be used in patients with underlying liver disease and that the maximal duration of tolvaptan therapy be 30 days in all other patients. This would preclude its use in a chronic condition such as ADPKD.

This study at best will be described as proof of concept indicating the potential of V2 receptor antagonism as a novel therapy in ADPKD. It is noteworthy that symptomatic pain relief was observed in patients treated with tolvaptan probably through a reduction in TKV.

Statins Trial

Statins are pleomorphic agents that have numerous cellular actions beyond the control of cellular lipids uptake and cholesterol blood levels. They have been shown to have anti-inflammatory as well as antiproliferative actions. The antiproliferative effects of statins may depend on underlying cellular transduction pathways modulation including the formation of intermediate metabolites of the mevalonate pathway, particularly the nonsterol isoprenoids, which appear to be essential in cell replication [15]. Consequently, statins have been shown to inhibit cystogenesis in experimental rodent models of ADPKD. This has been the basis of current RCTs on the impact of statins in patients with ADPKD.

Effect of pravastatin on total kidney volume, left ventricular mass index, and microalbuminuria in pediatric autosomal dominant polycystic kidney disease.

Cadnapaphornchai MA, George DM, McFann K, et al. Clin J Am Soc Nephrol. 2014;9(5):889–96 [16].

Abstract

Background and Objectives: In autosomal dominant polycystic kidney disease (ADPKD), progressive kidney cyst formation commonly leads to ESRD. Because important manifestations of ADPKD may be evident in childhood, early intervention may have the largest effect on long-term outcome. Statins are known to slow progressive nephropathy in animal models of ADPKD. This randomized double-blind placebo-controlled phase III clinical trial was conducted from 2007 to 2012 to assess the effect of pravastatin on height-corrected total kidney volume (HtTKV) and left ventricular mass index (LVMI) by magnetic resonance imaging (MRI) and urine microalbumin excretion (UAE) in children and young adults with ADPKD.

Designs, Setting, Participants, and Measurements: There were 110 pediatric participants with ADPKD and normal kidney function receiving lisinopril who were randomized to treatment with pravastatin or placebo for a 3-year period with evaluation at 0, 18, and 36 months. The primary outcome variable was a ≥ 20 % change in HtTKV, LVMI, or UAE over the study period.

Results: Ninety-one participants completed the 3-year study (83 %). Fewer participants receiving pravastatin achieved the primary end point compared with participants receiving placebo (69 % versus 88 %; $P=0.03$). This was due primarily to a lower proportion reaching the increase in HtTKV (46 % versus 68 %; $P=0.03$), with similar findings observed between study groups for LVMI (25 % versus 38 %; $P=0.18$) and UAE (47 % versus 39 %; $P=0.50$). The percent change in HtTKV adjusted for age, sex, and hypertension status over the 3-year period was significantly decreased with pravastatin (23 % ± 3 % versus 31 % ± 3 %; $P=0.02$).

Conclusions: Pravastatin is an effective agent to slow progression of structural kidney disease in children and young adults with ADPKD. These findings support a role for early intervention with pravastatin in this condition.

Critical Appraisal

Parameters	Yes	No	Comment
Validity			
Is the **randomization** procedure well described?		+1	Randomization method along with trial design given in [17]
Double **blinded**?	+2		Described as double blinded
Is the **sample size** calculation described/adequate?	+3		N=110; exceeded requirement of N=100 to detect a 30 % relative difference in the number of subjects reaching the primary end point, 80 % power and significance 0.05
Does it have a hard primary **end point**?		−1	Defined as ≥20 % increase in height-adjusted total kidney volume (HtTKV), left ventricular mass index (LVMI), or urinary albumin excretion (UAE)
Is the end-point surrogate?	−2		Surrogate end points only
Is the follow-up appropriate?	+1		36-month follow-up period was sufficient to show effect of statin on primary end points
Was there a **Bias**?		+2	There was a small randomization bias as far as the placebo group had a significantly better renal function (lower serum creatinine) at the onset
Is the dropout >25 %?		+1	17 % (19/110 patients)
Is the analysis **ITT**?	+3		
Utility/usefulness			
Can the findings be generalized?	+1		Pediatric patients age 8–22 with ADPKD and normal renal function receiving lisinopril as far as changes in TKV is concerned
Score		73 %	

ADPKD adult polycystic kidney disease, *ITT* intention to treat

Comments and Discussion

This double-blind, placebo-controlled phase III randomized controlled trial represents one of the few trials on pediatric ADPKD. The trial was based on the premise that experimental and clinical data from observational studies are suggestive of the role of statin in showing promise in some experimental models of ADPKD in rodents as well as ameliorating endothelial dysfunction and its known impact on CVD [15].

In this study, pravastatin reduced the rate of kidney enlargement, with lower progression to the end point of ≥20 % increase in height-adjusted TKV even after adjustment for age, sex, and hypertension status. Though this study represents the most robust ADPKD-specific statin trial to date, it still has notable limitations:

1. The use of surrogate renal end points (height-adjusted TKV) and microalbuminuria are not hard end points that invariably predict the incidence of ESRD in ADPKD.
2. The validity of using composite, and somewhat unrelated, end points without clear weighing has been questioned [18].
3. The study of children with ADPKD and essentially normal renal function (GFR >80 ml/min) limits the application of study results to usual clinical practice. Also, ADPKD is not invariably progressive at this stage of CKD; progression rate has not been predetermined before randomization.

Of notes previous studies of statin treatment in ADPKD were largely inconclusive due to methodological flaws [19, 20].

Somatostatin Analogue (Octerotide) Trial

A role has been postulated for GH and its second messenger insulin-like growth factor-1 (IGF-1) in the pathogenesis of ADPKD. Somatostatin has the capacity to inhibit GH release but also to inhibit adenyl cyclase and post-cAMP events that have also been implicated in cystogenesis. Preclinical animal experimentation showed a beneficial effect of somatostatin analogues in ADPKD. A number of clinical trials have since been reported.

ALADIN Study
Lancet. 2013 Nov 2;382(9903):1485–95. doi: 10.1016/S0140-6736(13)61407-5. Epub 2013 Aug 21.

Effect of long-acting somatostatin analogue on kidney and cyst growth in autosomal dominant polycystic kidney disease (ALADIN): a randomized, placebo-controlled, multicenter trial.

Caroli A, Perico N, Perna A, Antiga L, Brambilla P, Pisani A, Visciano B, Imbriaco M, Messa P, Cerutti R, Dugo M, Cancian L, Buongiorno E, De Pascalis A, Gaspari F, Carrara F, Rubis N, Prandini S, Remuzzi A, Remuzzi G, Ruggenenti P; ALADIN study group. [21]

Abstract
Background: Autosomal dominant polycystic kidney disease slowly progresses to end-stage renal disease and has no effective therapy. A pilot study suggested that the somatostatin analogue octreotide long-acting release (LAR) could be

nephroprotective in this context. We aimed to assess the effect of 3 years of octreotide-LAR treatment on kidney and cyst growth and renal function decline in participants with this disorder.

Methods: We did an academic, multicenter, randomized, single-blind, placebo-controlled, parallel-group trial in five hospitals in Italy. Adult (>18 years) patients with estimated glomerular filtration rate (GFR) of 40 mL/min per 1.73 m(2) or higher were randomly assigned (central allocation by phone with a computerized list, 1:1 ratio, stratified by center, block size four and eight) to 3-year treatment with two 20 mg intramuscular injections of octreotide-LAR ($n=40$) or 0.9 % sodium chloride solution ($n=39$) every 28 days. Study physicians and nurses were aware of the allocated group; participants and outcome assessors were masked to allocation. The primary end point was change in total kidney volume (TKV), measured by MRI, at 1-year and 3-year follow-up. Analyses were by modified intention to treat. This study is registered with ClinicalTrials.gov, NCT00309283.

Findings: Recruitment was between April 27, 2006, and May 12, 2008. 38 patients in the octreotide-LAR group and 37 patients in the placebo group had evaluable MRI scans at 1-year follow-up; at this timepoint, mean TKV increased significantly less in the octreotide-LAR group (46.2 mL, SE 18.2) compared with the placebo group (143.7 mL, 26.0; $p=0.032$). 35 patients in each group had evaluable MRI scans at 3-year follow-up; at this timepoint, mean TKV increase in the octreotide-LAR group (220.1 mL, 49.1) was numerically smaller than in the placebo group (454.3 mL, 80.8), but the difference was not significant ($p=0.25$). 37 (92.5 %) participants in the octreotide-LAR group and 32 (82.1 %) in the placebo group had at least one adverse event ($p=0.16$). Participants with serious adverse events were similarly distributed in the two treatment groups. However, four cases of cholelithiasis or acute cholecystitis occurred in the octreotide-LAR group and were probably treatment related.

Interpretation: These findings provide the background for large randomized controlled trials to test the protective effect of somatostatin analogues against renal function loss and progression to end-stage kidney disease.

Funding: Polycystic Kidney Disease Foundation

Critical Appraisal

Parameters	Yes	No	Comment
Validity			
Is the **randomization** procedure well described?	+1		After baseline assessment, central randomization by telephone was used to allocate study participants, in a 1:1 ratio, to 3-year octreotide LAR or placebo, according to a computer-generated randomization list
Double **blinded**?		−2	Investigators aware of allocation

Parameters	Yes	No	Comment
Is the **sample size** calculation described/ adequate?		−3	Sample size was estimated for the main prespecified outcome variable, absolute TKV change, assuming a two group t-test (two sided) of the difference between octreotide LAR and placebo
			40 participants were randomly assigned to octreotide LAR and 39 to placebo
			Sample size likely to be too small to have adequate power; see number required in TEMPO study
Does it have a hard primary **end point**?		−1	The primary end point was change in TKV, as measured by MRI, at 1-year and 3-year follow-up. Secondary end points were changes in TCV and GFR, and safety variables, including vital signs, clinical laboratory tests, and adverse events
Is the end-point surrogate?	−2		TKV as a surrogate for ADPKD progression
			Changes in eGFR = secondary end points, thus not powered to evaluate
Is the follow-up appropriate?	+1		1 and 3 years
Was there a **Bias**?	−2		Unblinded thus generating potential for observer bias
Is the dropout >25 %?		+1	
Is the analysis **ITT**?		−3	Not mentioned
Utility/usefulness			
Can the findings be generalized?		−1	
Was the NNT <100?			Not applicable as study negative at 3 years with no statistical difference in TKV between groups
Score	**0 %**		Inconclusive study due to the limitations highlighted above

ADPKD adult polycystic kidney disease, *TKV* total kidney volume

Comments and Discussion

The ALADIN study is at best a phase 2, proof of concept (POC), study. It is therefore hypothesis generating and not conclusive.

It has major limitations including:

1. The study is unblinded, thus subject to investigators' potential bias.
2. The study has a very small sample size unlikely to be sufficient to detect meaningful changes in TKV or renal function. 35–40 patients per group compared to the TEMPO study, with a similar primary end point of TKV measured by MRI, where 1,445 patients were randomized [13].

3. TKV has to be considered a surrogate, soft, end point, for ADPKD progression as GFR was not measured in this study. This suspicion is reinforced by the impact of the intervention at 1 year, but no longer significant statistically at 3 years. This was also supported by a study from the same group where changes in TKV and size upon treatment with octreotide were not accompanied in the short term with parallel renal functional changes (measured GFR) [22].

Conclusion

The negative ALADIN study is at best hypothesis generating, that somatostatin analogues are ineffective in ADPKD, and at worst inconclusive. Other studies on somatostatin analogues in ADPKD are mostly flawed or don't address ADPKD progression as the primary end point and are shown in Table 1.1.

General Discussion

We note that there are inherent challenges in organizing clinical trials in CKD, especially for an ADPKD-specific population. First, ADPKD is rare in adults affecting roughly 0.1 % of the population, with only 2,144 patients started on RRT annually in the United States [23]. While it may be relatively simpler to recruit large sample sizes for trials on hypertension, heart disease, or even CKD, organizing large-scale trials on an ADPKD-specific population are more challenging [4]. Also, the natural history of patients in an ADPKD cohort can vary greatly based on factors such as genotype, smoking, blood pressure control, and patient demographics. Further, ADPKD can be complicated by coexisting kidney diseases. It can be difficult to control all these factors adequately in a large-scale trial. Finally, the surrogate end points eGFR and TKV are perhaps the most commonly used end points in ADPKD studies to date. eGFR has been shown to underestimate true GFR in ADPKD [9]. Though TKV shows promise as a predictor of progression of CKD, its prognostic value in studies of limited follow-up time has not yet been explored [8]. While progression to ESRD and cardiovascular events are ideal hard end points, this may be difficult to achieve in such a rare disease with slow progression over decades. In the meanwhile, the use of surrogate end points such as changes in TKV over a long observation time requires validatory studies with measured GFR to ascertain their predictability at different stages of ADPKD. So far most published studies on the evaluation of kidney function and its progression of ADPKD have been to a large extent inconclusive due to the abovementioned limitations (Table 1.1) [5, 7, 11, 13, 16, 19, 20, 22, 24–39].

Blood pressure control remains the cornerstone in management of CKD including ADPKD. It also serves to limit the CVD complications associated with this condition. Whether intensive BP control has advantages over standard target levels is uncertain as shown by the study of Schrier and colleagues [25]. Also whether the inhibition of the renin-angiotensin-aldosterone-system (RAAS) offers therapeutic advantages over other class of antihypertensive agents is debatable [39] in spite of the hypothetical role of this system in the pathogenesis and progression of ADPKD [40]. The on-going large, double-blinded, placebo-controlled HALT-PKD trials [41] may soon provide stronger RCT evidence to define the role of RAAS inhibition in ADPKD.

Other interventions such as mTOR inhibition, somatostatin analogues, as well as statins cannot be recommended for the reasons highlighted in this review.

These should remain in the domain of clinical investigations and not be prescribed to patients with ADPKD.

Summary and Recommendations

In summary, the key issues on the interpretation and application of clinical trials in ADPKD include:

1. Lack of conformity with the standards of conducting and reporting clinical trials. Of all the 22 trials appraised, majority have not met our standard appraisal criteria and were not in conformity with the required standard of clinical trials (e.g., the CONSORT statement).
2. ADPKD being a rare disease, it is imperative to focus intervention trials on patients at higher risk of CKD progression. They warrant further identification.
3. For the reason mentioned in [4], more emphasis should be put on progressive and advanced ADPKD rather than intervening in those with ADPKD and normal renal function where the progression pattern is likely to be heterogeneous and unpredictable. Establishing those with a significant pretreatment progression rate may allow for more effective interventions and conclusive RCTs with a smaller patients' number.
4. Lack of well-validated end points and overreliance on surrogate outcomes such as total kidney volume (TKV) or cyst volume (CV) may be a major issue in ADPKD trials. The use of TKV as the gold standard for evaluation of ADPKD progression has been propelled by the development of the concept of MRI-measured TKV and its acceptability as a marker of disease progression in clinical trials, this without due consideration of significant intra- and interobserver variability of these MRI-based measurements. Also, the predictability of these measurements for the progression of ADPKD to ESRD is poorly established. Their validation need to be urgently ascertained if they are to continue to be used in drug intervention trials and not prove misleading.

5. TKV or cyst volume estimations in studies where the variability of urine output is affected by diuresis or aquaresis may confound their interpretation as the amount of residual urine within the kidneys and cysts may be a major confounder. The estimation of parenchymal kidney volume may be more helpful in such instances.

6. eGFR should not be used as it has been shown to significantly underestimate mGFR progression/decline in CKD including ADPKD.

7. Creatinine-based estimations of ADPKD progression may also be confounded by the fact that changes in tubular secretion of creatinine can be affected by interventions preserving renal tubular structure and minimizing tubular cystogenesis.

Conclusions

We are still far from the promised land of development of effective interventions for ADPKD. There is a long list of potential treatments (calcimimetics, roscovitine, triptolide, glucosylceramide inhibitors, sorafenib, thiazolidinediones, potassium channel blockers, HDAC inhibitors, and metformin [4, 42]) arising from a wealth of preclinical studies over the last several decades showing efficacy of these agents in animals. Overreliance on rodents models of PKD that may not fully be representative of human ADPKD may have encouraged misplaced enthusiasm. Clinical studies aiming to translate these findings from basic research in humans have so far been disappointing.

References

1. Wuthrich RP, Serra AL, Kistler AD. Autosomal dominant polycystic kidney disease: new treatment options and how to test their efficacy. Kidney Blood Press Res. 2009;32(5):380–7.
2. Schrier RW, Brosnahan G, Cadnapaphornchai MA, et al. Predictors of autosomal dominant polycystic kidney disease progression. J Am Soc Nephrol. 2014. doi:10.1681/ASN.2013111184.
3. Ravichandran K, Edelstein CL. Polycystic kidney disease: a case of suppressed autophagy? Semin Nephrol. 2014;34(1):27–33.
4. Mahnensmith RL. Novel treatments of autosomal dominant polycystic kidney disease. Clin J Am Soc Nephrol. 2014;9(5):831–6. doi:10.2215/CJN.02480314; 10.2215/CJN.02480314.
5. Czarnecki PG, Steinman TI. Polycystic kidney disease: new horizons and therapeutic frontiers. Minerva Urol Nefrol. 2013;65(1):61–8.
6. Chang MY, Ong AC. New treatments for autosomal dominant polycystic kidney disease. Br J Clin Pharmacol. 2013;76(4):524–35.
7. Walz G, Budde K, Mannaa M, et al. Everolimus in patients with autosomal dominant polycystic kidney disease. N Engl J Med. 2010;363(9):830–40.
8. Chapman AB, Bost JE, Torres VE, et al. Kidney volume and functional outcomes in autosomal dominant polycystic kidney disease. Clin J Am Soc Nephrol. 2012;7(3):479–86.
9. Ruggenenti P, Gaspari F, Cannata A, et al. Measuring and estimating GFR and treatment effect in ADPKD patients: results and implications of a longitudinal cohort study. PLoS One [Electronic Resource]. 2012;7(2):e32533.
10. Rosansky SJ, Glassock RJ. Is a decline in estimated GFR an appropriate surrogate end point for renoprotection drug trials? Kidney Int. 2014;85(4):723–7. doi: 10.1038/ki.2013.506; 10.1038/ki.2013.506.
11. Serra AL, Poster D, Kistler AD, et al. Sirolimus and kidney growth in autosomal dominant polycystic kidney disease. N Engl J Med. 2010;363(9):820–9.
12. Meijer E, Gansevoort RT, de Jong PE, et al. Therapeutic potential of vasopressin V2 receptor antagonist in a mouse model for autosomal dominant polycystic kidney disease: optimal timing and dosing of the drug. Nephrol Dial Transplant. 2011;26(8):2445–53.
13. Torres VE, Chapman AB, Devuyst O, Gansevoort RT, Grantham JJ, Higashihara E, Perrone RD, Krasa HB, Ouyang J, Czerwiec FS, TEMPO 3:4 Trial Investigators. Tolvaptan in patients with autosomal dominant polycystic kidney disease. N Engl J Med. 2012;367(25):2407–18.
14. Grantham JJ, Torres VE, Chapman AB, et al. Volume progression in polycystic kidney disease. N Engl J Med. 2006;354:2122–30.
15. Oda H, Keane WF. Recent advances in statins and the kidney. Kidney Int Suppl. 1999;71:S2–5.
16. Cadnapaphornchai MA, George DM, McFann K, et al. Effect of pravastatin on total kidney volume, left ventricular mass index, and microalbuminuria in pediatric autosomal dominant polycystic kidney disease. Clin J Am Soc Nephrol. 2014;9(5):889–96.
17. Cadnapaphornchai MA, George DM, Masoumi A, McFann K, Strain JD, Schrier RW. Effect of statin therapy on disease progression in pediatric ADPKD: design and baseline characteristics of participants. Contemp Clin Trials. 2011;32(3):437–45. doi:10.1016/j.cct.2011.01.008. Epub 2011 Jan 23.
18. Ferreira-Gonzalez I, Permanyer-Miralda G, Domingo-Salvany A, et al. Problems with the use of composite end points in cardiovascular trials: systematic review of randomised controlled trials. BMJ. 2007;334(7597):786.
19. Fassett RG, Coombes JS, Packham D, Fairley KF, Kincaid-Smith P. Effect of pravastatin on kidney function and urinary protein excretion in autosomal dominant polycystic kidney disease. Scand J Urol Nephrol. 2010;44(1):56–61. http://www.bmj.com/content/334/7597/786.
20. van Dijk MA, Kamper AM, van Veen S, Souverijn JH, Blauw GJ. Effect of simvastatin on renal function in autosomal dominant polycystic kidney disease. Nephrol Dial Transplant. 2001;16(11):2152–7.
21. Caroli A, Perico N, Perna A, Antiga L, Brambilla P, Pisani A, Visciano B, Imbriaco M, Messa P, Cerutti R, Dugo M, Cancian L, Buongiorno E, De Pascalis A, Gaspari F, Carrara F, Rubis N, Prandini S, Remuzzi A, Remuzzi G, Ruggenenti P, ALADIN Study Group. Effect of longacting somatostatin analogue on kidney and cyst growth in autosomal dominant polycystic kidney disease (ALADIN): a randomised, placebo-controlled, multicentre trial. Lancet. 2013;382(9903):1485–95.
22. Ruggenenti P, Remuzzi A, Ondei P, et al. Safety and efficacy of long-acting somatostatin treatment in autosomal-dominant polycystic kidney disease. Kidney Int. 2005;68(1):206–16.
23. Torres VE, Harris PC, Pirson Y. Autosomal dominant polycystic kidney disease. Lancet. 2007;369(9569):1287–301.
24. Patch C, Charlton J, Roderick PJ, Gulliford MC. Use of antihypertensive medications and mortality of patients with autosomal dominant polycystic kidney disease: a population-based study. Am J Kidney Dis. 2011;57(6):856–62.
25. Schrier R, McFann K, Johnson A, et al. Cardiac and renal effects of standard versus rigorous blood pressure control in

autosomal-dominant polycystic kidney disease: results of a seven-year prospective randomized study. J Am Soc Nephrol. 2002;13(7):1733–9.

26. Stallone G, Infante B, Grandaliano G, et al. Rapamycin for treatment of type I autosomal dominant polycystic kidney disease (RAPYD-study): a randomized, controlled study. Nephrol Dial Transplant. 2012;27(9):3560–7.

27. Soliman A, Zamil S, Lotfy A, Ismail E. Sirolimus produced S-shaped effect on adult polycystic kidneys after 2-year treatment. Transplant Proc. 2012;44(10):2936–9.

28. Perico N, Antiga L, Caroli A, et al. Sirolimus therapy to halt the progression of ADPKD. J Am Soc Nephrol. 2010;21(6):1031–40.

29. Braun WE, Schold JD, Stephany BR, Spirko RA, Herts BR. Low-dose rapamycin (sirolimus) effects in autosomal dominant polycystic kidney disease: an open-label randomized controlled pilot study. Clin J Am Soc Nephrol. 2014;9(5):881–8.

30. Hogan MC, Masyuk TV, Page LJ, et al. Randomized clinical trial of long-acting somatostatin for autosomal dominant polycystic kidney and liver disease. J Am Soc Nephrol. 2010;21(6):1052–61.

31. Hogan MC, Masyuk TV, Page L, et al. Somatostatin analog therapy for severe polycystic liver disease: results after 2 years. Nephrol Dial Transplant. 2012;27(9):3532–9.

32. van Keimpema L, Nevens F, Vanslembrouck R, et al. Lanreotide reduces the volume of polycystic liver: a randomized, double-blind, placebo-controlled trial. Gastroenterology. 2009;137(5):1661–8.e1-2.

33. Klahr S, Breyer JA, Beck GJ, et al. Dietary protein restriction, blood pressure control, and the progression of polycystic kidney disease. Modification of diet in renal disease study group. J Am Soc Nephrol. 1995;5(12):2037–47.

34. Nakamura T, Sato E, Fujiwara N, et al. Changes in urinary albumin excretion, inflammatory and oxidative stress markers in ADPKD patients with hypertension. Am J Med Sci. 2012;343(1):46–51.

35. Ulusoy S, Ozkan G, Orem C, Kaynar K, Kosucu P, Kiris A. A comparison of the effects of ramipril and losartan on blood pressure control and left ventricle hypertrophy in patients with autosomal dominant polycystic kidney disease. Ren Fail. 2010;32(8):913–7.

36. Nutahara K, Higashihara E, Horie S, et al. Calcium channel blocker versus angiotensin II receptor blocker in autosomal dominant polycystic kidney disease. Nephron. 2005;99(1):18–23.

37. Ecder T, Chapman AB, Brosnahan GM, Edelstein CL, Johnson AM, Schrier RW. Effect of antihypertensive therapy on renal function and urinary albumin excretion in hypertensive patients with autosomal dominant polycystic kidney disease. Am J Kidney Dis. 2000;35(3):427–32.

38. Zeltner R, Poliak R, Stiasny B, Schmieder RE, Schulze BD. Renal and cardiac effects of antihypertensive treatment with ramipril vs metoprolol in autosomal dominant polycystic kidney disease. Nephrol Dial Transplant. 2008;23(2):573–9.

39. van Dijk MA, Breuning MH, Duiser R, van Es LA, Westendorp RG. No effect of enalapril on progression in autosomal dominant polycystic kidney disease. Nephrol Dial Transplant. 2003;18(11):2314–20.

40. Tkachenko O, Helal I, Shchekochikhin D, Schrier RW. Renin-angiotensin-aldosterone system in autosomal dominant polycystic kidney disease. Curr Hypertens Rev. 2013;9(1):12–20.

41. Torres VE, Chapman AB, Perrone RD, et al. Analysis of baseline parameters in the HALT polycystic kidney disease trials. Kidney Int. 2012;81(6):577–85.

42. Chang MY, Ong AC. Mechanism-based therapeutics for autosomal dominant polycystic kidney disease: recent progress and future prospects. Nephron. 2012;120(1):25–34.

Lupus Nephritis Clinical Trials: A Critical Appraisal

Richard J. Glassock

Introduction

The interest in finding effective and safe treatments for lupus nephritis (LN) has been both long standing and intense [1]. Achieving this goal has been very frustrating since no new treatment has been approved by regulatory authorities for the treatment of LN in over 50 years. Nevertheless, many randomized clinical trials have been designed and executed, and some have been instrumental in altering the landscape of "off-label" management of LN, particularly in severe proliferative forms. It is generally believed that combinations of high-dose anti-inflammatory glucocorticoids and some type of immunosuppressive agents are required for adequate control of LN that will delay or prevent its progression to ESRD and ameliorate the consequences of marked proteinuria (nephrotic syndrome) while at the same time reducing the burden of extrarenal manifestations of systemic lupus erythematosus (e.g., arthritis, dermatitis, serositis, and hematological/neurological disturbances). But LN is in all likelihood not due to a single pathogenic process, and it can present with diverse clinical and pathological features [2]. Relapses of clinically active disease are common and difficult to predict. The value of intermediate outcomes (surrogates) for prediction of hard endpoints (such as ESRD) has been difficult to prove, since the occurrence of these endpoints is often delayed by 5 or more years from the apparent onset of disease, with contemporary regimens. Adverse events consequent to treatment are common and occasionally fatal, further confounding the execution and interpretation of studies. This heterogeneity, unpredictability, and susceptibility to complicating diseases has hampered the conduct of LN randomized clinical trials.

Finding suitable surrogate endpoints for trial design has been a challenge. Nevertheless, progress has occurred and several treatment regimens are now generally regarded as effective and reasonably safe for management of severe proliferative LN. The situation for treatment of the pure membranous LN is much less certain [3].

Trial #1

Austin HA, Klippel JH, Balow J, le Riche NGH, Steinberg AD, Plotz PH, Decker JL. Therapy of Lupus Nephritis: Controlled trial of prednisone and cytotoxic drugs. N Engl J Med. 1986;314:614–19

Abstract

We evaluated renal function in 107 patients with active lupus nephritis who participated in long-term randomized therapeutic trials (median follow-up, 7 years). For patients taking oral prednisone alone, the probability of renal failure began to increase substantially after 5 years of observation. Renal function was better preserved in patients who received various cytotoxic drug therapies, but the difference was statistically significant only for intravenous cyclophosphamide plus low-dose prednisone as compared with high-dose prednisone alone ($P=0.027$). The advantage of treatment with intravenous cyclophosphamide over oral prednisone alone was particularly apparent in the high-risk subgroup of patients who had chronic histological changes on renal biopsy at study entry. Patients treated with intravenous cyclophosphamide have not experienced hemorrhagic cystitis, cancer, or a disproportionate number of major infections. We conclude that, as compared with high-dose oral prednisone alone, treatment of lupus glomerulonephritis with intravenous cyclophosphamide reduces the risk of end-stage renal failure with few serious complications.

R.J. Glassock, MD, MACP
Department of Medicine,
Geffen School of Medicine at UCLA,
8 Bethany, Laguna Niguel 92677, CA, USA
e-mail: glassock@cox.net

Critical Appraisal

Parameters	Yes	No	Comment
Validity			
Is the **randomization** procedure well described?	+1		Random from masked card sequence
Double **blinded**?		−2	Open label
Is the **sample size** calculation described/adequate?		−3	No power calculation
Does it have a hard primary **endpoint**?	+1		Probability of renal failure (ESRD) censored for death
Is the endpoint surrogate?		+2	
Is the follow-up appropriate?	+1		Followed for more than 65 months
Was there a **Bias**?		−1	Ancestry not stated; unequal distribution of pathological classes
Is the dropout >25 %?		+1	
Is the analysis **ITT**?		−3	Kaplan-Meier; censored
Utility/usefulness			
Can the findings be generalized?	0		Not applicable to A-A
Was the NNT <100?	+1		
Score	**0 %**		

Summary and Discussion

This is the "granddaddy" of RCT in LN and it had a profound impact on clinical practice despite its several flaws. The studies were carried out over many years (1969–1981) and incorporated several randomized protocols. One of the comparator groups (oral prednisone only) was a historical rather than concurrent control. The number of subjects randomized to each regimen was small (prednisone only=28; oral azathioprine (AZA)=19; oral cyclophosphamide (CYC)=18; oral AZA+oral CYC=22; IV CYC=20). The distribution of glomerular lesion among the groups was not equal. 5/20 (25 %) assigned to IV CYC had membranous LN, 5/29 (17 %) assigned to the oral prednisone group had membranous LN, and 1/18 (6 %) assigned to the oral CYC group had membranous LN. Altogether 78/107 (73 %) subjects had proliferative LN and 16/107 (15 %) had membranous LN. Over the course of follow-up (varying from 65 to 126 months for those developing ESRD), a total of 23/107 (21 %) developed ESRD and only 4 subjects were lost to follow up. In the prednisone only category, 10/28 developed ESRD (36 %) whereas only 1/20 (5 %) of those assigned to IV CYC developed ESRD—a significant difference. On the other hand, 6/40 (15 %) of patients assigned to oral CYC or AZA+CYC developed ESRD, a value which was not significant. An outcome of ESRD or doubling of baseline serum creatinine occurred in 24/38 (63 %) of the prednisone only treated group compared with 13/ 46 (28 %) in the oral CYC or oral AZA+CYC group and 5/21 (24 %) in the IV CYC group. The difference in outcomes between the assigned treatment groups did not become apparent until at least 5–7 years had elapsed, at which time only 78/107 randomized patients had been followed. Among the 72 subjects deemed to be at high risk of ESRD at randomization (chronic lesions in renal biopsy), the only comparison that achieved statistical significance was the IV CYC group versus the oral prednisone group, but the study was underpowered to examine similar comparisons with the other treatment groups. Adverse events were common in all groups but of differing character— major infections were seen in 25 % of the oral prednisone only group but only in 10 % of the IV CYC group. But premature ovarian failure was seen in 71 % of the oral CYC group and in 45 % of the IV CYC group, and hemorrhagic cystitis was seen in about 15 % of those who received oral CYC but none of the IV CYC-treated patient group. Deaths (n=13) were equally divided between the groups.

Conclusions

This seminal study, although quite seriously flawed by contemporary standards, did support the view that high-dose prednisone alone strategies were inadequate and unsafe for management of severe proliferative LN. At best, this study was hypothesis generating that a regimen of intermittent IV CYC (in high dosage) was superior (in efficacy or safety) to other immunosuppressive regimens, including oral CYC+prednisone. Subsequent randomized, controlled trials, conducted by the NIH group, showed that intermittent IV CYC is superior to intermittent IV methylprednisolone in treatment of severe LN [4] and that IV methylprednisolone added to IV cyclophosphamide has greater short- and long-term efficacy at no increase toxicity compared with high-dose IV CYC plus oral steroids [5, 6]. In addition, longer-term treatment with IV CYC (monthly for 6 months and then quarterly for an additional 2 years) reduced relapse rates but had no beneficial effect on renal function decline compared with shorter courses of IV CYC (monthly for 6 months) in severe LN (4). These additional studies, published between 1992 and 2001 and generally of moderate quality, tended to solidify the opinion that intermittent IV CYC plus intermittent IV methyl prednisolone was the "standard of care" in severe lupus nephritis, despite the lack of any comparisons to other regimens, such as oral CYC. In fact, there has never been an adequately powered RCT directly comparing a daily oral CYC+prednisone regimen to an intermittent IV CYC+prednisone regimen in severe LN for efficacy (hard endpoint of ESRD) and safety.

Trial #2

Chan TM, LI FK, Tang CS, Wong RW, Fang GX, Ji YL, Lau CS, Wong AK, Tong MK, Chan KW, Lai KN. Efficacy of mycophenolate mofetil in patients with diffuse proliferative lupus nephritis: Hong Kong-Guangzhou Nephrology Study Group. N Engl J Med. 2000;343:1156–62

Abstract

Background: The combination of cyclophosphamide and prednisolone is effective for the treatment of severe lupus nephritis but has serious adverse effects. Whether mycophenolate mofetil can be substituted for cyclophosphamide is not known.

Methods: In 42 patients with diffuse proliferative lupus nephritis, we compared the efficacy and side effects of a regimen of prednisolone and mycophenolate mofetil given for 12 months with those of a regimen of prednisolone and cyclophosphamide given for 6 months, followed by prednisolone and azathioprine for 6 months. Complete remission was defined as a value for urinary protein excretion that was less than 0.3 g per 24 h, with normal urinary sediment, a normal serum albumin concentration, and values for serum creatinine and creatinine clearance that were no more than 15 % above the baseline values. Partial remission was defined as a value for urinary protein excretion that was between 0.3 and 2.9 g per 24 h, with a serum albumin concentration of at least 30 g per liter.

Results: Eighty-one percent of the 21 patients treated with mycophenolate mofetil and prednisolone (group 1) had a complete remission, and 14 % had a partial remission, as compared with 76 and 14 %, respectively, of the 21 patients treated with cyclophosphamide and prednisolone followed by azathioprine and prednisolone (group 2). The improvements in the degree of proteinuria and the serum albumin and creatinine concentrations were similar in the two groups. One patient in each group discontinued treatment because of side effects. Infections were noted in 19 % of the patients in group 1 and in 33 % of those in group 2 ($P=0.29$). Other adverse effects occurred only in group 2; they included amenorrhea (in 23 % of the patients), hair loss (19 %), leukopenia (10 %), and death (10 %). The rates of relapse were 15 and 11 %, respectively.

Conclusions: For the treatment of diffuse proliferative lupus nephritis, the combination of mycophenolate mofetil and prednisolone is as effective as a regimen of cyclophosphamide and prednisolone followed by azathioprine and prednisolone but is less toxic.

Critical Appraisal

Parameters	Yes	No	Comment
Validity			
Is the **randomization** procedure well described?		−1	Not well described
Double **blinded**?		−2	Open label
Is the **sample size** calculation described/ adequate?		−3	No power calculation
Does it have a hard primary **endpoint**?		−1	Complete remission (urine protein <300 mg/day) with normal serum albumin concentration, normal urinary sediment, and stable renal function as the endpoints. Not possible to have a hard endpoint due to infrequency of events
Is the endpoint surrogate?	−1		
Is the follow-up appropriate?	0		12 months only
Was there a **Bias**?		+1	Chinese subjects only
Is the dropout >25 %?		+1	
Is the analysis **ITT**?	−3		
Utility/usefulness			
Can the findings be generalized?	0		Not to Caucasians or A-A
Was the NNT <100?	+1		
Score	**0 %**		

Summary and Discussion

This was a very influential trial, despite its several weaknesses. The number of randomized subjects is small ($n=42$) and the follow-up short (12 months). Randomized patients had class IV or class V plus IV LN, and baseline renal function was normal or only slightly reduced. Most patients had nephrotic syndrome, with serological as well as histological activity of disease, but only moderate evidence of chronicity. The dose of MMF was 2.0 g/day for 6 months and then 1.0 g/day for the remaining 6 months. The comparator arm received 2.5 mg/kg/day of oral CYC for 6 months and then 1.5 mg/kg/day of oral azathioprine (AZA). After 12 months, AZA was replaced with MMF, and AZA dosage was reduced to 1 mg/kg/day in the comparator arm. The primary endpoint at 12 months was a complete remission of abnormal urinary findings plus stable renal function, as assessed by serum creatinine alone (not by measured GFR). Possible effects of steroids on creatinine generation were not considered, but both arms of the trial received similar doses of prednisone (about 0.8 mg/kg initially and then tapering doses over 6 months).

Complete remission developed in 81 % of the MMF group and in 76 % of the oral CYC group at 12 months, and treatment failure and relapse rates were similar in the two arms (about 10–20 %), but the study is likely to be underpowered to show a difference. Adverse events were common (19–33 %), slightly more in the CYC group, but not significant (again underpowered to examine safety).

Conclusions

This study is primarily hypothesis generating and does not establish efficacy or safety of MMF, in the dosage described, compared with a sequential oral CYC + AZA regimen. The lowering of the dosage of MMF at 6 months may have contributed to the findings suggestive of equivalence of oral MMF to a sequential oral CYC + AZA regimen for LN. The study cannot be generalized to Caucasians or African-American with severe LN. A follow-up study at 5 years with a "hard endpoint" of doubling of serum creatinine showed similar results (6.3 % in MMF and 10.0 % in the CYC + AZA groups), but hospitalizations for serious infections were lower in the MMF group [7]. The study was underpowered to examine ESRD rates.

Trial #3

Houssiau FA, Vasconcelos C, D'Cruz D, Sebastiani GD, Garrido EER, Danieli MG, Abramovicz D, Blockmans D, Mathieu A, Direskeneli H, Galeazzi M, Gul A, Levy Y, Petera P, Popovic R, Petrovic R, Sinico RA, Cattaneo R, Font J, Depresseux G, Cosyns JP, Cervera R. Immunosuppressive therapy in lupus nephritis: the Euro-Lupus Nephritis Trial, a randomized trial of low-dose versus high dose intravenous cyclophosphamide. Arthritis Rheum. 2002;46:2121–31

Abstract

Objective: Glomerulonephritis is a severe manifestation of systemic lupus erythematosus (SLE) that is usually treated with an extended course of intravenous (IV) cyclophospha-mide (CYC). Given the side effects of this regimen, we evaluated the efficacy and the toxicity of a course of low-dose IV CYC prescribed as a remission-inducing treatment, followed by azathioprine (AZA) as a remission-maintaining treatment.

Methods: In this multicenter, prospective clinical trial (the Euro-Lupus Nephritis Trial [ELNT]), we randomly assigned 90 SLE patients with proliferative glomerulone-phritis to a high-dose IV CYC regimen (6 monthly pulses and 2 quarterly pulses; doses increased according to the white blood cell count nadir) or a low-dose IV CYC regimen (6 fortnightly pulses at a fixed dose of 500 mg), each of which was followed by AZA. Intent-to-treat analyses were performed.

Results: Follow-up continued for a median of 41.3 months in the low-dose group and 41 months in the high-dose group. Sixteen percent of those in the low-dose group and 20 % of those in the high-dose group experienced treatment failure (not statistically significant by Kaplan-Meier analysis). Levels of serum creatinine, albumin, C3, and 24-h urinary protein and the disease activity scores significantly improved in both groups during the first year of follow-up. Renal remission was achieved in 71 % of the low-dose group and 54 % of the high-dose group (not statistically significant). Renal flares were noted in 27 % of the low-dose group and 29 % of the high-dose group. Although episodes of severe infection were more than twice as frequent in the high-dose group, the difference was not statistically significant.

Conclusion: The data from the ELNT indicate that in European SLE patients with proliferative lupus nephritis, a remission-inducing regimen of low-dose IV CYC (cumulative dose 3 g) followed by AZA achieves clinical results comparable with those obtained with a high-dose regimen.

Critical Appraisal

Parameters	Yes	No	Comment
Validity			
Is the **randomization** procedure well described?		−1	Not well described
Double **blinded**?		−2	Open label
Is the **sample size** calculation described/ adequate?		−3	No power calculation
Does it have a hard primary **endpoint**?	+1		Treatment failure including relapse and serum creatinine—GFR not measured
Is the endpoint surrogate?		+1	
Is the follow-up appropriate?	+1		Followed for more than 40 months
Was there a **Bias**?		+1	No African-Americans
Is the dropout >25 %?		+1	
Is the analysis **ITT**?	+3		
Utility/usefulness			
Can the findings be generalized?	0		Except for A-A
Was the NNT <100?	+1		
Score	**19 %**		

Summary and Discussion

This study introduced a new "twist" on the use of IV CYC regimens in proliferative LN—that of a lower-dose shorter duration treatment, with consolidation of remission with AZA rather than continued quarterly IV CYC dosing, now known as the "Euro-Lupus regimen" (6 IV CYC pulses at 500 mg each every 2 weeks and then 2 mg/kg/day of AZA starting 2 weeks after the last IV CYC dose). The sample size ($n=90$) was reasonable, but the study may have been underpowered to show a true difference between the two treatment groups. Renal remission was high in both groups (54 % in the high-dose group, equivalent to the NIH protocol group (see Trial #1), and 71 % in the Euro-Lupus protocol group). Rates of treatment failures and adverse events were equivalent in both groups, but the study was underpowered to examine safety in both groups. Steroid dosage did not differ, blunting arguments that a serum creatinine-based endpoint might be biased by muscle loss due to steroids.

Conclusions

Although plausibly underpowered to examine the main endpoints, this study did promote a conversion from the then commonly used high-dose, prolonged CYC regimen of the NIH to one involving lower IV CYC dosage over shorter intervals combined with AZA consolidation (maintenance). A 10-year follow-up cohort analysis of 84 patients from the original study showed equivalent "hard" outcomes for the two groups (doubling of serum creatinine), 14 % in the Euro-Lupus protocol group and 11 % in the NIH protocol group [8]. Due to the ancestry of the randomized patients, this protocol cannot be assumed to be effective in African-Americans, Asians, or Hispanics or in membranous LN.

Trial #4

Contreras G, Pardo V, Leclrecq B, Lenz O, Tozman E, ONan P, Roth D. Sequential therapies for proliferative lupus nephritis. N Engl J Med. 2004;350:971–80

Abstract

Background: Long-term therapy with cyclophosphamide enhances renal survival in patients with proliferative lupus nephritis; however, the beneficial effect of cyclophosphamide must be weighed against its considerable toxic effects.

Methods: Fifty-nine patients with lupus nephritis (12 in World Health Organization class III, 46 in class IV, and 1 in class Vb) received induction therapy consisting of a maximum of 7 monthly boluses of intravenous cyclophosphamide (0.5–1.0 g per square meter of body surface area) plus corticosteroids. Subsequently, the patients were randomly assigned to one of three maintenance therapies: quarterly intravenous injections of cyclophosphamide, oral azathioprine (1–3 mg per kilogram of body weight per day), or oral mycophenolate mofetil (500–3,000 mg per day) for 1–3 years. The baseline characteristics of the three groups were similar, with the exception that the chronicity index was 1.9 points lower in the cyclophosphamide group than in the mycophenolate mofetil group ($P=0.009$).

Results: During maintenance therapy, five patients died (four in the cyclophosphamide group and one in the mycophenolate mofetil group), and chronic renal failure developed in five (three in the cyclophosphamide group and one each in the azathioprine and mycophenolate mofetil groups). The 72-month event-free survival rate for the composite endpoint of death or chronic renal failure was higher in the mycophenolate mofetil and azathioprine groups than in the cyclophosphamide group ($P=0.05$ and $P=0.009$, respectively). The rate of relapse-free survival was higher in the mycophenolate mofetil group than in the cyclophosphamide group ($P=0.02$). The incidence of hospitalization, amenorrhea, infections, nausea, and vomiting was significantly lower in the mycophenolate mofetil and azathioprine groups than in the cyclophosphamide group.

Conclusions: For patients with proliferative lupus nephritis, short-term therapy with intravenous cyclophosphamide followed by maintenance therapy with mycophenolate mofetil or azathioprine appears to be more efficacious and safer than long-term therapy with intravenous cyclophosphamide.

Critical Appraisal

Parameters	Yes	No	Comment
Validity			
Is the **randomization** procedure well described?		+1	Sealed enveloped—stratified by ancestry
Double **blinded**?	0		Open label; masking not attempted
Is the **sample size** calculation described/adequate?	+3		
Does it have a hard primary **endpoint**?	+1		Composite—patient and renal survival
Is the endpoint surrogate?		+2	
Is the follow-up appropriate?	+1		72 months for composite endpoint
Was there a **Bias**?		+1	Low chronicity score at baseline in the CYC group
Is the dropout >25 %?		+1	
Is the analysis **ITT**?		−3	
Utility/usefulness			
Can the findings be generalized?	+1		
Was the NNT <100?	+1		
Score	**50 %**		

Summary and Discussion

This study is one of the first to examine the issue of maintenance regimens for the avoidance of relapse and renal failure after "induction" therapy—in this case with the NIH IV CYC regimen. The randomization step, after induction therapy, minimized the risk of bias. Remission status and intensity of induction therapy were equivalent in the three maintenance arms at the time of randomization. About 80 % of the subjects were in complete or partial remission at the time they were randomized to the maintenance regimens (continued IV CYC, MMF, or AZA for 1–3 years). Renal function was normal or near normal in all groups at randomization. Steroid dosage was approximately equal in the three groups post randomization.

The results were striking. Maintenance therapy with IV CYC performed poorly by all criteria with event-free survival (composite endpoint) at <50 % in 5 years of follow-up, versus 85–90 % in the AZA and MMF groups. This was driven mainly by patient survival, as the cumulative rate of renal survival was comparable in the three groups—74 % for IV CYC group, 80 % in the AZA group, and 95 % in the MMF group. Relapse-free interval was highest for the MMF group and lowest for the IV CYC group and intermediate for the AZA group. Hospitalization rates were higher for IV CYC. 55 of the 59 randomized subjects were African-Americans or Hispanics, which precluded any comparison of the results between Caucasian and non-Caucasian subjects.

Conclusions

This well-done trial provided a "death knell" for maintenance therapy with IV CYC (or oral CYC for that matter as well) in proliferative LN after completion of "induction" therapy, at least in African-Americans and Hispanics. From then on, it was a contest between MMF and AZA (see below).

Trial #5

Ginzler EM, Dooley MA, Aranow C, Kim MY, Buyon J, Merrill JT, Petri M, Gilkeson GS, Wallace DJ, Weisman MH, Appel GB. Mycophenolate mofetil or intravenous cyclophosphamide for lupus nephritis. N Engl J Med. 2005;353:2219–28

Abstract

Background: Since anecdotal series and small, prospective, controlled trials suggest that mycophenolate mofetil may be effective for treating lupus nephritis, larger trials are desirable.

Methods: We conducted a 24-week randomized, open-label, noninferiority trial comparing oral mycophenolate mofetil (initial dose, 1,000 mg per day, increased to 3,000 mg per day) with monthly intravenous cyclophosphamide (0.5 g per square meter of body surface area, increased to 1.0 g per square meter) as induction therapy for active lupus nephritis. A change to the alternative regimen was allowed at 12 weeks in patients who did not have an early response. The study protocol specified adjunctive care and the use and tapering of corticosteroids. The primary endpoint was complete remission at 24 weeks (normalization of abnormal renal measurements and maintenance of baseline normal measurements). A secondary endpoint was partial remission at 24 weeks.

Results: Of 140 patients recruited, 71 were randomly assigned to receive mycophenolate mofetil and 69 were randomly assigned to receive cyclophosphamide. At 12 weeks, 56 patients receiving mycophenolate mofetil and 42 receiving cyclophosphamide had satisfactory early responses. In the intention-to-treat analysis, 16 of the 71 patients (22.5 %) receiving mycophenolate mofetil and 4 of the 69 patients receiving cyclophosphamide (5.8 %) had complete remission, for an absolute difference of 16.7 percentage points (95 % confidence interval, 5.6–27.9 percentage points; $P=0.005$), meeting the prespecified criteria for noninferiority and demonstrating the superiority of mycophenolate mofetil to cyclophosphamide. Partial remission occurred in 21 of the 71 patients (29.6 %) and 17 of the 69 patients (24.6 %), respectively ($P=0.51$). Three patients assigned to cyclophosphamide died, two during protocol therapy. Fewer severe infections and hospitalizations but more diarrhea cases occurred among those receiving mycophenolate.

Conclusions: In this 24-week trial, mycophenolate mofetil was more effective than intravenous cyclophosphamide in inducing remission of lupus nephritis and had a more favorable safety profile.

Critical Analysis

Parameters	Yes	No	Comment
Validity			
Is the **randomization** procedure well described?	+1		
Double **blinded**?		−1	Open label—but an oral vs. IV comparison
Is the **sample size** calculation described/ adequate?	+3		No power calculation
Does it have a hard primary **endpoint**?		−1	Complete remission at 6 months. Not possible to have a hard endpoint due to infrequency of events
Is the endpoint surrogate?	−1		See above
Is the follow-up appropriate?	+1		Followed to relapse

Parameters	Yes	No	Comment
Was there a **Bias**?		+1	High crossover rates
Is the dropout >25 %?	−1		Discontinue in 21 % of MMF and 36 % in IV CYC
Is the analysis **ITT**?	+3		
Utility/usefulness			
Can the findings be generalized?	+1		
Was the NNT <100?	N/A		Comparator, noninferiority trial
Score	**40 %**		

Summary and Discussion

This large trial ($n=140$) was designed as a noninferiority, open-label trial with an endpoint of complete remission (stable normal serum creatinine levels, normal protein excretion, and a normal urine sediment) at 6 months. Importantly, crossover to other treatment was allowed at 3 months if treatment failed. A total of 6 patients (8 %) assigned to MMF crossed over to IV CYC therapy at 3 months, and 12 patients (18 %) assigned to IV CYC crossed over to MMF therapy at 3 months. A complete remission at 6 months was seen in 29 % of the MMF group who received MMF for the entire period. This contrasts to only 10 % of the IV CYC group that received IV CYC for the entire period. The complete + partial remission rate at 6 months was 52 % in the MMF group and 30 % in the IV CYC group by ITT analysis. African-Americans and Hispanics comprised 107/140 (76 %) of the randomized patients. About 45 % had nephrotic syndrome at entry, and most patients had normal or near normal renal function at baseline. A total of 27/140 (20 %) had "pure" membranous LN. The dose of MMF was 2.0 g/day initially, and this was advanced to a maximum of 3.0 g/day. IV CYC was given in monthly pulses according to the NIH protocol. Steroid exposure was similar in both groups. Adverse events, especially serious infections, were more common with IV CYC.

Conclusions

This reasonably well-done study provided moderately strong evidence for superiority of MMF over IV CYC (at least in the doses administered) for induction treatment of moderate to severe LN. Whether MMF induction treatment will ultimately lead to better long-term outcomes in LN was not tested in this short-term study. The ancestral distribution (mostly A-A or Hispanics) generates the hypothesis that Caucasians may be more responsive to IV CYC and non-Caucasians may be more responsive to MMF [9, 10]. This hypothesis has not yet been formally tested in an RCT.

Trial #6

Moroni G, Doria A, Mosca M, Alberighi OD, Ferraccioli G, Todesco S, Manno C, Altieri P, Ferrara R, Greco S, Ponticelli C. A randomized pilot trial comparing cyclosporine and azathioprine for maintenance therapy in diffuse proliferative lupus nephritis over 4 years. Clin J Am Soc Nephrol. 2006;1:925–32

Abstract

There is no agreement about the best maintenance treatment for patients with diffuse lupus nephritis. This multicenter, randomized trial compared the safety and efficacy of cyclosporine and azathioprine. Seventy-five patients with diffuse proliferative lupus were given three intravenous methylprednisolone pulses followed by prednisone and oral cyclophosphamide for a median of 90 day. Subsequently, patients were randomly assigned either to cyclosporine or to azathioprine for 2 years (core study). Treatment continued for up to 4 years (follow-up study). The primary outcome measure was the incidence of disease flares. Secondary endpoints were in daily proteinuria, creatinine clearance, and adverse effects. Seven flares occurred in the cyclosporine group, and eight occurred in the azathioprine group. At the end of the core study, mean proteinuria decreased from 2.8 ± 3.57 to 0.4 ± 0.85 g/day ($P<0.0001$) in the cyclosporine group and from 2.2 ± 1.94 to 0.5 ± 0.78 g/day ($P<0.0002$) in the azathioprine group. After 4 years, mean proteinuria was 0.2 ± 0.24 and 0.3 ± 0.33 g/day, respectively. At the end of the core study and completion of the follow-up, creatinine clearance and BP levels did not change significantly from baseline in either group. Five of the 36 patients who were receiving cyclosporine and four of the 33 who were receiving azathioprine stopped the treatment because of adverse effects. For patients with diffuse proliferative lupus nephritis, azathioprine or cyclosporine combined with corticosteroids demonstrated equal efficacy in the prevention of flares.

Critical Appraisal

Parameters	Yes	No	Comment
Validity			
Is the **randomization** procedure well described?	+1		
Double **blinded**?		−2	Open label
Is the **sample size** calculation described/ adequate?		−3	Pilot study only— sample size selected only on feasibility considerations. Probably underpowered. No power calculation

Parameters	Yes	No	Comment
Does it have a hard primary **endpoint**?		−1	Renal relapses (flares) are the endpoint. Not possible to have a hard endpoint due to infrequency of events
Is the endpoint surrogate?	−2		
Is the follow-up appropriate?	+1		4 years, probably adequate for endpoint
Was there a **Bias**?		+2	
Is the dropout >25 %?		+1	
Is the analysis **ITT**?	+3		
Utility/usefulness			
Can the findings be generalized?	+1		? Not to A-A
Was the NNT <100?	+1		
Score	**13 %**		Pilot trial, not confirmatory trial

Summary and Discussion

This pilot trial is primarily hypothesis generating due to its design. Nevertheless, it does point in the direction of approximately equal efficacy for avoidance of relapses with CsA (in low and tapering dosage) compared to AZA (at 2 mg/kg/day, tapered to 1 mg/kg/day in stable patients). Randomization to the two arms of the trial occurred at an early point in the induction therapy (3 months of oral CYC+oral and IV methylprednisolone). Disease flares were relatively uncommon in both groups (7/36 in CsA [20 %] and 8/33 [24 %] in AZA at 4 years). Creatinine clearance tended (nonsignificantly) to be higher in the AZA group during follow-up, but proteinuria was approximately equal in the two groups during follow-up. Adverse events were equal and generally mild. No patient died or developed ESRD.

Conclusions

This trial needs confirmation in a properly designed well-powered trial to confirm the results. It provides only weak evidence for the possibility of equivalent benefits for CsA compared with AZA maintenance therapy for the promotion of prolonged relapse-free interval in diffuse proliferative LN following induction therapy with oral CYC and steroids. Other pilot trials comparing CSA or Tacrolimus to IV CYC (or MMF) for induction of remission in LN have been encouraging as well [11–13], but larger trials with longer follow-up are needed to more fully evaluate the efficacy and safety of protocols of treatment of proliferative LN involving usage of calcineurin inhibitors (CNI) for initial induction of remission. The KDIGO guidelines do not currently recommend CNI for initial remission induction [3].

Trial #7

Appel GB, Contreras G, Dooley MA, Ginzler EM, Isenberg D, Jayne D, Li LS, Mysler E, Sanchez-Guerrero J, Solomons N, Wofsy D; Aspreva Lupus Management Study Group. Mycophenolate mofetil versus cyclophosphamide for induction treated of lupus nephritis. J Am Soc Nephrol. 2009;20:1103–12

Abstract

Recent studies have suggested that mycophenolate mofetil (MMF) may offer advantages over intravenous cyclophosphamide (IV CYC) for the treatment of lupus nephritis, but these therapies have not been compared in an international randomized, controlled trial. Here, we report the comparison of MMF and IV CYC as induction treatments for active lupus nephritis in a multinational, two-phase (induction and maintenance) study. We randomly assigned 370 patients with class III to V lupus nephritis to open-label MMF (target dosage 3 g/day) or IV CYC (0.5–1.0 g/m^2 in monthly pulses) in a 24-week induction study. Both groups received prednisone, tapered from a maximum starting dosage of 60 mg/day. The primary endpoint was a prespecified decrease in urine protein to creatinine ratio and stabilization or improvement in serum creatinine. Secondary endpoints included complete renal remission, systemic disease activity and damage, and safety. Overall, we did not detect a significantly different response rate between the two groups: 104 (56.2 %) of the 185 patients responded to MMF compared with 98 (53.0 %) of the 185 patients who responded to IV CYC. Secondary endpoints were also similar between treatment groups. There were nine deaths in the MMF group and five in the IV CYC group. We did not detect significant differences between the MMF and IV CYC groups with regard to rates of adverse events, serious adverse events, or infections. Although most patients in both treatment groups experienced clinical improvement, the study did not meet its primary objective of showing that MMF was superior to IV CYC as an induction treatment for lupus nephritis.

Critical Appraisal

Parameters	Yes	No	Comment
Validity			
Is the **randomization** procedure well described?	+1		Well described
Double **blinded**?		−1	Open label; compares oral vs. an IV regimen
Is the **sample size** calculation described/ adequate?	+3		Large study; well-powered

Parameters	Yes	No	Comment
Does it have a hard primary **endpoint**?		−1	Renal response (CR + PR). Not possible to have a hard endpoint due to infrequency of events
Is the endpoint surrogate?	−1		
Is the follow-up appropriate?	0		For the endpoint at 6 months
Was there a **Bias**?		+2	
Is the dropout >25 %?		+1	
Is the analysis **ITT**?	+3		
Utility/usefulness			
Can the findings be generalized?	+1		Diverse ancestral population
Was the NNT <100?	N/A		Comparator trial
Score	**53 %**		

Summary and Discussion

Although this large, multisite, international, RCT, designed with a superiority format, did not achieve its primary objective, it suggested that the two approaches to induction of remission (IV CYC + steroids and oral MMF + steroids) are quite similar in efficacy, at least after 6 months of treatment. The sample size (n = 370) and ancestral diversity of the randomized subject are the strengths of the study. At baseline, 26 % of the subjects had eGFR <60 ml/min/1.73 m^2 and urine protein averaged 4.1 g/dL. Only 16 % of the subjects had "pure" membranous LN. The primary endpoint was "renal response" defined as a decrease in urine protein to creatinine ratio (UPCR) to <3.0 gm/gm if nephrotic-range proteinuria (UPCR ≥ 3.0 gm/gm) was present at randomization *or* a decline in UPCR of ≥50 % from baseline values if the initial UPCR was <3.0 gm/gm *and* the occurrence of a stabilization (±25 %) or improvement of serum creatinine. Changes in urine sediment were *not* used to define "renal response." Complete remission, which did include urine sediment, was a secondary endpoint.

At the end of the study (6 months), 56 % of the MMF and 53 of the IV CYC groups had developed a "renal response" and were then re-randomized to a maintenance of remission trial comparing MMF to AZA (see Trial #9 below). The "renal response" rate seemed higher in the non-Caucasian, non-Hispanic, or non-Asian group. Complete remissions were uncommon in both groups at 6 months (8.6 % in MMF group and 8.1 % in IV CYC group). Adverse events were more common in the IV CYC group (mainly infections). Withdrawals due to adverse events were more common in the MMF group. There were 9 deaths in the MMF group (7 in Asians) and 5 in the IV CYC (2 in Asians) group.

Conclusions

This well-designed and conducted landmark trial, even though it did not meet its primary objective, still had an influence on medical practice. No longer would physicians have to exclusively rely on protocols involving CYC for initial (induction) management of moderately severe LN. Due to study design, no statement can be made about long-term efficacy (or safety) of the MMF or CYC regimens employed. In addition, it remains uncertain if the induction periods had been extended to 12 months instead of 6 months and whether the results would have been different. The analysis of an interaction of ancestry or treatment response requires confirmation in a properly designed and well-powered prospective trial.

Trial #8

Bao H, Liu ZH, Xie HL, Hu WX, Zhang HT, Li LS. Successful treatment of Class V + IV lupus nephritis with multi-target therapy. J Am Soc Nephrol. 2008;19:2001–10

Abstract

Treatment of class V + IV lupus nephritis remains unsatisfactory despite the progress made in the treatment of diffuse proliferative lupus nephritis. In this prospective study, 40 patients with class V + IV lupus nephritis were randomly assigned to induction therapy with mycophenolate mofetil, tacrolimus, and steroids (multitarget therapy) or intravenous cyclophosphamide (IV CYC). Patients were treated for 6 months unless complete remission was not achieved, in which case treatment was extended to 9 months. An intention-to-treat analysis revealed a higher rate of complete remission with multitarget therapy at both 6 and 9 months (50 and 65 %, respectively) than with IV CYC (5 and 15 %, respectively). At 6 months, eight (40 %) patients in each group experienced partial remission, and at 9 months, six (30 %) patients receiving multitarget therapy and eight (40 %) patients receiving IV CYC experienced partial remission. There were no deaths during this study. Most adverse events were less frequent in the multitarget therapy group. Calcineurin inhibitor nephrotoxicity was not observed, but three patients developed new-onset hypertension with multitarget therapy. In conclusion, multitarget therapy is superior to IV CYC for inducing complete remission of class V + IV lupus nephritis and is well tolerated.

Critical Appraisal

Parameters	Yes	No	Comment
Validity			
Is the **randomization** procedure well described?	+1		
Double **blinded**?		−2	Open label
Is the **sample size** calculation described/ adequate?	+2		N = 40

Parameters	Yes	No	Comment
Does it have a hard primary **endpoint**?		−1	Complete remission (including urine sediment). Not possible to evaluate hard endpoint due to infrequency of events
Is the endpoint surrogate?	−1		
Is the follow-up appropriate?	0		6–9 months
Was there a **Bias**?		+2	
Is the dropout >25 %?		+1	
Is the analysis **ITT**?	+3		All patients followed to relapse
Utility/usefulness			
Can the findings be generalized?	0		Only to Asians with class V+IV LN
Was the NNT <100?	N/A		Comparator trial
Score	**33 %**		

Summary and Discussion

This reasonably well-done trial compared IV CYC + steroid induction treatment with a "cocktail" of MMF, tacrolimus, and steroids ("multitarget therapy") in a small group of Chinese patients with a form of LN generally regarded as having a particularly poor outcome [14]. The primary endpoint was complete remission (CR; including urine sediment exams) at 6–9 months. Strikingly, the CRT rate was 65 % in the "multitarget" therapy group and only 15 % in the IV CYC group. Partial remissions were about equal at 9 months in the two groups: 30 % in the "multitarget" therapy group and 40 % in the IV CYC group. Ninety-five percent of the patients in the multitarget therapy group had a "renal response" at 9 months compared with about 55 % in the IV CYC group (see also Trial #7 for comparison purposes). Unfortunately, the trial design did not include comparison groups treated with MMF + steroids or tacrolimus + steroids, so uncertainties remain regarding the efficacy of components of the "multitarget" regimen in this group of patients with LN. In Trial #7 (see above), the frequency of the class V+IV lesion is uncertain. No deaths were recorded, and evidence of nephrotoxicity of the "multitarget" therapy was not found on repeat renal biopsies.

Conclusions

This trial raises the possibility that specific combination regimens might be indicated for specific renal pathologies in diffuse proliferative LN. The proof of this concept will require further RCT comparing "multitarget" therapy to MMF or tacrolimus (or cyclosporine) + steroids separately in this subset of LN [15, 16]. The results of this trial cannot be generalized to patients of non-Asian ancestry.

Trial #9

Austin HA 3rd, Illei GG, Braun MJ, Balow JE. **Randomized, controlled trial of prednisone, cyclophosphamide and cyclosporine in lupus membranous nephropathy. J Am Soc Nephrol. 2009;20:901–11**

Abstract

Patients with lupus membranous nephropathy (LMN) are at substantial long-term risk for morbidity and mortality associated with protracted nephrotic syndrome, including ESRD. The optimal treatment for this condition is controversial. Forty-two patients with LMN participated in a randomized, controlled trial to compare adjunctive immunosuppressive drugs with prednisone alone. Adjunctive regimens included either cyclosporine (CsA) for 11 months or alternate-month intravenous pulse cyclophosphamide (IV CYC) for six doses; the control group received alternate-day prednisone alone. Median proteinuria was 5.4 g/day (range 2.7–15.4 g/day). We assessed the primary outcome, time to remission of proteinuria during the 12-month protocol, by univariate survival analysis. At 1 year, the cumulative probability of remission was 27 % with prednisone, 60 % with IV CYC, and 83 % with CsA. Although both IV CYC and CsA were more effective than prednisone in inducing remissions of proteinuria, relapse of nephrotic syndrome occurred significantly more often after completion of CsA than after IV CYC. By multivariate survival analysis, treatment with prednisone and high-grade proteinuria (>5 g/day) but not race or ethnicity was independently associated with a decreased probability of remission. Adverse effects during the 12-month protocol included insulin-requiring diabetes (one with prednisone and two with CsA), pneumonia (one with prednisone and two with CsA), and localized herpes zoster (two with IV CYC). In conclusion, regimens containing CsA or IV CYC are each more effective than prednisone alone in inducing remission of proteinuria among patients with LMN.

Critical Analysis

Parameters	Yes	No	Comment
Validity			
Is the **randomization** procedure well described?	+1		7 patients not randomized to CsA due to concerns of toxicity
Double **blinded**?		−2	Open label
Is the **sample size** calculation described/ adequate?		−3	No power calculation; possibly underpowered

Parameters	Yes	No	Comment
Does it have a hard primary **endpoint**?		−1	Time to remission and frequency of sustained remission with prednisone as control. Not possible to have a hard endpoint due to infrequency of events
Is the endpoint surrogate?	−2		
Is the follow-up appropriate?	0		Followed for more than 12 months—too short for a renal function endpoint
Was there a **Bias**?		0	Possible in randomization
Is the dropout >25 %?		+1	
Is the analysis **ITT**?		−2	Cumulative relapse-free survival
Utility/usefulness			
Can the findings be generalized?	+1		
Was the NNT <100?	+0		Comparative
Score	**0 %**		

Summary and Discussion

This is the only RCT in "pure" membranous LN—it is flawed due to small sample size ($n=42$), thus possibly underpowered. The patient characteristics were balanced at the time of entry, but patients were not randomized to CsA if there were concerns of toxicity ($n=7$), so the groups were of unequal size. RAS inhibition treatment was stable during the post-randomization period. At 1 year of observation, the cumulative likelihood of remission was 27 % with prednisone (control), 60 % with IV CYC, and 83 % with CsA. Relapses were common after stopping CsA. Adverse events were not common. There were no deaths.

Conclusions

This trial is primarily hypothesis generating rather than confirmatory. The lack of an MMF treatment arm is a weakness. It cannot test the efficacy of any regimen on ESRD outcomes. Optimal treatment of membranous LN is still uncertain.

Trial #10

Houssiau FA, D'Cruz D, Sangle S, Remy P, Vasconcelos C, Petrovic R, Fiehn C, de Ramon Garrido E, Gilboe IM, Tektonidou M, Blockmans D, Ravelingien I, le Guern V, Depresseux G, Guillevin L, Cervera R; MAINTAIN Nephritis Trial Group. Azathioprine versus mycophenolate mofetil for long-term immunosuppression in lupus nephritis: results from the MAINTAIN Nephritis Trial. Ann Rheum Dis. 2010;69:2083–9.

Abstract

Background: Long-term immunosuppressive treatment does not efficiently prevent relapses of lupus nephritis (LN). This investigator-initiated randomized trial tested whether mycophenolate mofetil (MMF) was superior to azathioprine (AZA) as maintenance treatment.

Methods: A total of 105 patients with proliferative LN were included. All received three daily intravenous pulses of 750 mg methylprednisolone, followed by oral glucocorticoids and six fortnightly intravenous pulses of 500 mg cyclophosphamide. Based on randomization performed at baseline, AZA (target dose, 2 mg/kg/day) or MMF (target dose, 2 g/day) was given at week 12. Analyses were by intent to treat. Time to renal flare was the primary endpoint. Mean (SD) follow-up of the intent-to-treat population was 48 (14) months.

Results: The baseline clinical, biological, and pathological characteristics of patients allocated to AZA or MMF did not differ. Renal flares were observed in 13 (25 %) AZA-treated and 10 (19 %) MMF-treated patients. Time to renal flare, to severe systemic flare, to benign flare, and to renal remission did not statistically differ. Over a 3-year period, 24-h proteinuria, serum creatinine, serum albumin, serum C3, hemoglobin, and global disease activity scores improved similarly in both groups. Doubling of serum creatinine occurred in four AZA-treated and three MMF-treated patients. Adverse events did not differ between the groups except for hematological cytopenias, which were statistically more frequent in the AZA group ($p=0.03$) but led only one patient to drop out.

Conclusions: Fewer renal flares were observed in patients receiving MMF, but the difference did not reach statistical significance.

Critical Appraisal

Parameters	Yes	No	Comment
Validity			
Is the **randomization** procedure well described?	+1		
Double **blinded**?		−1	Open label; masking not easily done
Is the **sample size** calculation described/adequate?	+3		
Does it have a hard primary **endpoint**?		−1	Time to flare is the endpoint. Not possible to have a hard endpoint due to infrequency of events

Parameters	Yes	No	Comment
Is the endpoint surrogate?	−2		
Is the follow-up appropriate?	+1		Followed for 48 months
Was there a **Bias**?		+2	No A-A
Is the dropout >25 %?		+1	
Is the analysis **ITT**?	+3		
Utility/usefulness			
Can the findings be generalized?	0		Not to A-A
Was the NNT <100?	+1		
Score	**50 %**		

Summary and Discussion

This is a well-done trial evaluating an intermediate end-point in LN—prevention of renal flares (relapses; both nephritic [increase in serum creatinine] and nephrotic [increase in proteinuria] in character) by maintenance therapy with either AZA (2 mg/kg/day) or MMF (targeted at 2.0 g/day). Randomization occurred at 3 months after initial induction treatment with the Euro-Lupus regimen (see Trial #4) irrespective of remission status (see also Trial #12 below). The trial was designed to test superiority of MMF over AZA.

Renal flares occurred in 25 % of AZA-treated and 19 % of MMF-treated subjects (NS), and the type of flare did not differ between the treatment groups. Adverse events were not different except for the increased cytopenia in AZA-treated subjects. A weakness is that pharmacokinetic studies were not performed, raising possible issues about inadequate dosing, especially for MMF.

Conclusions

This study supports the view that AZA and MMF are equivalent for preventing relapses in moderately severe LN following induction therapy with IV CYC, irrespective of the remission status at the time maintenance therapy is begun.

Pharmacokinetic (PK) studies are needed to be sure that this is not due to dosing/absorption/clearance variations.

Trial #12

Dooley MA, Jayne D, Ginzler EM, Isenberg D, Olsen NJ, Wofsy D, Eitner F, Appel GB, Contreras G, Lisk L, Solomons N; ALMS Group. Mycophenolate versus azathioprine as maintenance therapy for lupus nephritis. N Engl J Med. 2011;365:1886–95.

Abstract

Background: Maintenance therapy, often with azathioprine or mycophenolate mofetil, is required to consolidate remission and prevent relapse after the initial control of lupus nephritis.

Methods: We carried out a 36-month, randomized, double-blind, double-dummy, phase 3 study comparing oral mycophenolate mofetil (2 g per day) and oral azathioprine (2 mg per kilogram of body weight per day), plus placebo in each group, in patients who met response criteria during a 6-month induction trial. The study group underwent repeat randomization in a 1:1 ratio. Up to 10 mg of prednisone per day or its equivalent was permitted. The primary efficacy endpoint was the time to treatment failure, which was defined as death, end-stage renal disease, doubling of the serum creatinine level, renal flare, or rescue therapy for lupus nephritis. Secondary assessments included the time to the individual components of treatment failure and adverse events.

Results: A total of 227 patients were randomly assigned to maintenance treatment (116 to mycophenolate mofetil and 111 to azathioprine). Mycophenolate mofetil was superior to azathioprine with respect to the primary endpoint, time to treatment failure (hazard ratio, 0.44; 95 % confidence interval, 0.25–0.77; $P=0.003$), and time to renal flare and time to rescue therapy (hazard ratio, <1.00; $P<0.05$). Observed rates of treatment failure were 16.4 % (19 of 116 patients) in the mycophenolate mofetil group and 32.4 % (36 of 111) in the azathioprine group. Adverse events, most commonly minor infections and gastrointestinal disorders, occurred in more than 95 % of the patients in both groups ($P=0.68$). Serious adverse events occurred in 33.3 % of patients in the azathioprine group and in 23.5 % of those in the mycophenolate mofetil group ($P=0.11$), and the rate of withdrawal due to adverse events was higher with azathioprine than with mycophenolate mofetil (39.6 % vs. 25.2 %, $P=0.02$).

Conclusions: Mycophenolate mofetil was superior to azathioprine in maintaining a renal response to treatment and in preventing relapse in patients with lupus nephritis who had a response to induction therapy.

Critical Appraisal

Parameters	Yes	No	Comment
Validity			
Is the **randomization** procedure well described?	+1		Random from sealed envelops
Double **blinded**?	+2		
Is the **sample size** calculation described/ adequate?	+3		

Parameters	Yes	No	Comment
Does it have a hard primary **endpoint**?		0	Composite endpoint of death, ESRD, 2x Sc r, renal flares, or rescue therapy for LN
Is the endpoint surrogate?	0		
Is the follow-up appropriate?	+1		36 months' follow-up
Was there a **Bias**?		+2	
Is the dropout >25 %?		+1	
Is the analysis **ITT**?	+3		
Utility/usefulness			
Can the findings be generalized?	+1		
Was the NNT <100?	+1		
Score	**94 %**		

Summary and Discussion

This well-done trial provides evidence bearing on the choice of agent for prevention of relapses following induction of moderately severe LN. This study differs from that described in Trial #11 in that patients received either MMF or IV CYC for induction, and all subjects were in remission (complete or partial) at the time (6 months after the start of induction therapy, they were re-randomized to receive AZA (2 mg/day) or MMF (2 g/day)) (see also Trial #7). The endpoint was a complex composite ("treatment failure") of death, ESRD, doubling of serum creatinine, renal flare, or rescue therapy for LN. Observed rates of treatment failure were 16.4 % for MMF and 32.4 % for AZA. Serious adverse events were only slightly increased in the AZA group compared with the MMF group, but withdrawals due to adverse events were higher in the AZA group than in the MMF group. Time to ESRD or time to doubling of serum creatinine was not statistically different between the two groups ($p=0.07$). Among those receiving MMF for maintenance therapy, treatment failure occurred in 4.7 % of those induced by IV CYC and 10.1 % of those receiving MMF for induction. Among those receiving AZA for maintenance therapy, treatment failure occurred in 14.5 % of those receiving IV CYC for induction and 20.1 % in those receiving MMF for induction. An MMF induction/maintenance regimen was only moderately better than an IV CYC/AZA induction/maintenance regimen (30 % improvement of endpoint), but this could not be formally tested due to limited power. MMF showed better results across the spectrum of ancestries. No pharmacokinetic (PK) studies were performed.

Conclusions

This well-done study suggests strongly that MMF may be the preferred maintenance regimen in LN when a complete or partial remission has been obtained with induction therapy, particularly when MMF was used as the induction of remission agent. It leaves open the question as to when to start "maintenance" therapy and whether attaining a remission prior to the onset of maintenance therapy is crucial for optimum results. The long-term impact of these regimens of ESRD remains uncertain. Whether dosing of patients guided by PK studies would improve the outcomes of MMF or AZA management of post-induction therapy of LN has not been adequately tested.

Trial #13

Rovin BH, Furie R, Latinis K, Looney RJ, Fervenza FC, Sanchez-Guerrero J, Maciuca R, Zhang D, Garg JP, Brunetta P, Appel G; LUNAR Investigator Group. Efficacy and safety of rituximab in patients with active proliferative lupus nephritis: the Lupus Nephritis Assessment with Rituximab study. Arthritis Rheum. 2012;64:1215–26.

Abstract

Objective: To evaluate the efficacy and safety of rituximab in a randomized, double-blind, placebo-controlled phase III trial in patients with lupus nephritis treated concomitantly with mycophenolate mofetil (MMF) and corticosteroids

Methods: Patients ($n=144$) with class III or class IV lupus nephritis were randomized 1:1 to receive rituximab (1,000 mg) or placebo on days 1, 15, 168, and 182. The primary endpoint was renal response status at week 52.

Results: Rituximab depleted peripheral CD19+ B cells in 71 of 72 patients. The overall (complete and partial) renal response rates were 45.8 % among the 72 patients receiving placebo and 56.9 % among the 72 patients receiving rituximab ($P=0.18$); partial responses accounted for most of the difference. The primary endpoint (superior response rate with rituximab) was not achieved. Eight placebo-treated patients and no rituximab-treated patients required cyclophosphamide rescue therapy through week 52. Statistically significant improvements in serum complements C3 and C4 and anti-double-stranded DNA (anti-dsDNA) levels were observed among patients treated with rituximab. In both treatment groups, a reduction in anti-dsDNA levels greater than the median reduction was associated with reduced proteinuria. The rates of serious adverse events, including infections, were similar in both groups. Neutropenia, leukopenia, and hypotension occurred more frequently in the rituximab group.

Conclusion: Although rituximab therapy led to more responders and greater reductions in anti-dsDNA and C3/C4 levels, it did not improve clinical outcomes after 1 year of treatment. The combination of rituximab and MMF and corticosteroids did not result in any new or unexpected safety signals.

Critical Appraisal

Parameters	Yes	No	Comment
Validity			
Is the **randomization** procedure well described?		−1	Not well described
Double **blinded**?	+2		Placebo controlled with MMF as background therapy
Is the **sample size** calculation described/ adequate?	+3		144 patients randomized
Does it have a hard primary **endpoint**?		−1	Composite renal response (RR) endpoint at 1 year (CR/NR, NoRR). Hard endpoints not possible due to infrequency
Is the endpoint surrogate?	−1		
Is the follow-up appropriate?	0		Only 12 months' follow-up
Was there a **Bias**?		+1	Differing duration of LN prior to treatment assignment
Is the dropout >25 %?		+1	
Is the analysis **ITT**?	+3		
Utility/usefulness			
Can the findings be generalized?	+1		
Was the NNT <100?	N/A		Comparator study
Score	**53 %**		

Summary and Discussion

This is the first real RCT of biological modulation of LN with a chimeric anti-CD20 monoclonal antibody (rituximab) as an add-on therapy to MMF+steroids for the induction of remission in LN, designed as a superiority trial, and it disappointingly failed to meet its objectives. It followed on a similarly negative RCT of rituximab as an add-on therapy to steroids for symptomatic systemic lupus without nephritis (EXPLORER) [17]. The primary endpoint of renal response occurred in 57 % of the rituximab arm and in 46 % of the placebo despite improvement in serology (anti-dsDNA antibody and serum complement levels). The reason(s) for failure is (are) unknown, but cannot be traced to inadequate depletion of circulating B19+ cells. Perhaps the slight differences in duration of LN prior to randomization or the endpoints used were involved in the negative nature of the study. Also, an unrecognized interaction with the background therapy

(MMF and steroids) is always possible. It is noteworthy that 8 placebo-treated patients required rescue therapy but no rituximab patients. Partial remissions occurred in only 15 % of the placebo arm and 31 % of the rituximab arm, and renal responses developed in 70 % of African-Americans in the rituximab arm versus 45 % in the placebo arm, both non-primary events and mainly hypothesis generating. Except for infusion reactions attributed to the active drug, adverse events were approximately equal in the two groups. There were 2 deaths in the rituximab group and none in the placebo group.

Conclusions

This is a well-powered and carefully conducted but negative study that provides no support for the use of rituximab as an add-on therapy to MMF+steroid for the induction of remissions.

Whether rituximab will have more beneficial effects on refractory or relapsing cases, as suggested by observational studies, or will allow for persistence of stable remission without maintenance steroids or immunosuppressive agents (MMF or AZA) is unknown but worthy of testing in an RCT. Other novel agents have also failed in trials of LN. Abetimus sodium, a novel B-cell tolerogen, did not show any effectiveness in reducing the frequency of renal flares in LN [18]. Abatacept, a CTLA4-Ig fusion protein, failed to show efficacy for complete remission in LN [19]. The latter failure has been attributed to the choice of endpoints in the trial [20]. Belimumab, an anti-Blys or BAFF monoclonal antibody, has shown modest efficacy on SLE, but insufficient numbers of subjects were enrolled in the pivotal trial to demonstrate any effectiveness in LN, but post hoc analyses of the data have been encouraging [21]. A pivotal trial comparing belimumab+standard of care (MMF or IV CYC+steroid) versus placebo+standard of care is in progress (NCT #01639339, GlaxoSmithKline). The results of this trial are eagerly anticipated. Many more trials of biological agents as immune modulators are under active investigation in LN [22].

Perspectives

Viewed through the lens of randomized clinical trials, much progress has been made in the treatment of lupus nephritis over the past three decades. Trial design has been strengthened, and larger studies with more sharply defined endpoints have been conducted. Parallel improvements in our understanding of the complex and heterogeneous pathogenesis of SLE and LN have encouraged the development of more "targeted" immunomodulatory therapies. Nevertheless, no new drug has been approved by the US Food and Drug Administration for LN in over 50 years. In addition to the comprehensive KDIGO analysis mentioned in the Introduction [3], several systematic reviews and meta-analyses of various regimens used in LN have appeared in recent years [23–25] and a review of the status of treatment of severe lupus nephritis has been published [26].

In my opinion, the field has been held back by the difficulty in determining "patient-centered," clinically meaningful endpoints that are broadly applicable to diverse treatment regimens and that can be adapted to economical study design over feasible time periods of observation. Rigorous testing of new (as well as old) biomarkers to improve the precision and accuracy of prognostication will be vitally necessary for the field of therapy of LN to proceed to the successful development of approved new products.

References

1. KDIGO clinical practice guidelines for glomerulonephritis. Kidney Int Suppl. 2012;2:221–32.
2. Glassock RJ. The treatment of severe proliferative lupus nephritis. In: Lewis EJ, Schwartz MM, Korbet SM, Chan DTK, editors. Lupus nephritis. 2nd ed. Oxford: Oxford University Press; 2011. p. 281–316.
3. Austin III HA, Illei GG, Balow JE. Lupus membranous nephropathy. In: Lewis EJ, Schwartz MM, Korbet SM, Chan DTK, editors. Lupus nephritis. 2nd ed. Oxford: Oxford University Press; 2011. p. 169–98.
4. Boumpas DT, Austin 3rd HA, Vaughn EM, Klippel JH, Steinberg AD, Yarboro CH, et al. Controlled trial of pulse methylprednisolone versus two regimens of pulse cyclophosphamide in severe lupus nephritis. Lancet. 1992;340:741–5.
5. Gourley MF, Austin 3rd HA, Scott D, Yarboro CH, Vaughan EM, Muir J, et al. Methylprednisolone and cyclophosphamide, alone or in combination, in patients with lupus nephritis. A randomized, controlled trial. Ann Intern Med. 1996;125:549–57.
6. Illei GG, Austin HA, Crane M, Collins L, Gourley MF, Yarboro CH, et al. Combination therapy with pulse cyclophosphamide plus pulse methylprednisolone improves long-term renal outcome without adding toxicity in patients with lupus nephritis. Ann Intern Med. 2001;135:248–57.
7. Chan TM, Tse KC, Tang CS, Mok MY, Li FK, Hong Kong Nephrology Study Group. Long-term study of mycophenolate mofetil as continuous induction and maintenance treatment for diffuse proliferative lupus nephritis. J Am Soc Nephrol. 2005;16:1076–84.
8. Houssiau FA, Vasconcelos C, D'Cruz D, Sebastiani GD, de Ramon Garrido E, Danieli MG, et al. The 10-year follow-up data of the Euro-Lupus Nephritis Trial comparing low-dose and high-dose intravenous cyclophosphamide. Ann Rheum Dis. 2010;69:61–4.
9. Isenberg D, Appel GB, Contreras G, Dooley MA, Ginzler EM, Jayne D, et al. Influence of race/ethnicity on response to lupus nephritis treatment: the ALMS study. Rheumatology (Oxford). 2010;49:128–40.
10. Mohan S, Radhakrishnan J. Geographical variation in the response of lupus nephritis to mycophenolate mofetil induction therapy. Clin Nephrol. 2011;75:233–41.
11. Yang M, Li M, He W, Wang B, Gu Y. Calcineurin inhibitors may be a reasonable alternative to cyclophosphamide in the induction treatment of active lupus nephritis: a systematic review and meta-analysis. Exp Ther Med. 2014;7:1663–70.
12. Li X, Ren H, Zhang Q, Zhang W, Wu X, Xu Y, et al. Mycophenolate mofetil or tacrolimus compared with intravenous cyclophosphamide in the induction treatment for active lupus nephritis. Nephrol Dial Transplant. 2012;27:1467–72.
13. Tanaka H, Watanabe S, Aizawa-Yashiro T, Oki E, Kumagai N, Tsuruga K, et al. Long-term tacrolimus-based immunosuppressive treatment for young patients with lupus nephritis: a prospective study in daily clinical practice. Nephron Clin Pract. 2012;121:c165–73.
14. Najafi CC, Korbet SM, Lewis EJ, Schwartz MM, Reichlin M, Evans J, et al. Significance of histologic patterns of glomerular injury upon long-term prognosis in severe lupus glomerulonephritis. Kidney Int. 2001;59:2156–63.
15. Glassock RJ. Multitarget therapy of lupus nephritis: base hit or home run? J Am Soc Nephrol. 2008;19:1842–4.
16. Kurasawa T, Nagasawa H, Nishi E, Takei H, Okuyama A, Kondo T, et al. Successful treatment of class IV+V lupus nephritis with combination therapy of high-dose corticosteroids, tacrolimus and intravenous cyclophosphamide. Intern Med. 2013;52:1125–30.
17. Merrill JT, Neuwelt CM, Wallace DJ, Shanahan JC, Latinis KM, Oates JC, et al. Efficacy and safety of rituximab in moderately-to-severely active systemic lupus erythematosus: the randomized, double-blind, phase II/III systemic lupus erythematosus evaluation of rituximab trial. Arthritis Rheum. 2010;62:222–33.
18. Cardiel MH, Tumlin JA, Furie RA, Wallace DJ, Joh T, Linnik MD, et al. Abetimus sodium for renal flare in systemic lupus erythematosus: results of a randomized, controlled phase III trial. Arthritis Rheum. 2008;58:2470–80.
19. Furie R, Nicholls K, Cheng TT, Houssiau F, Burgos-Vargas R, Chen SL, et al. Efficacy and safety of abatacept in lupus nephritis: a twelve-month, randomized, double-blind study. Arthritis Rheum. 2014;66:379–89.
20. Wofsy D, Hillson JL, Diamond B. Abatacept for lupus nephritis: alternative definitions of complete response support conflicting conclusions. Arthritis Rheum. 2012;64:3660–5.
21. Dooley MA, Houssiau F, Aranow C, D'Cruz DP, Askanase A, Roth DA, et al. Effect of belimumab treatment on renal outcomes: results from the phase 3 belimumab clinical trials in patients with SLE. Lupus. 2013;22:63–72.
22. Rovin BH, Parikh SV. Lupus nephritis: the evolving role of novel therapeutics. Am J Kidney Dis. 2014;63:677–90.
23. Rovin BH. Lupus nephritis: guidelines for lupus nephritis–more recommendations than data? Nat Rev Nephrol. 2012;8:620–1.
24. Hogan J, Appel GB. Update on the treatment of lupus nephritis. Curr Opin Nephrol Hypertens. 2013;22:224–30.
25. Tian SY, Feldman BM, Beyene J, Brown PE, Uleryk EM, Silverman ED. Immunosuppressive therapies for the induction treatment of proliferative lupus nephritis: a systematic review and network metaanalysis. J Rheumatol. 2014;41(10):1998–2007.
26. Chan TM. Treatment of severe lupus nephritis: the new horizon. Nat Rev Nephrol. 2015;11(1):46–61.

ANCA-Associated Glomerulonephritis Clinical Trials: A Critical Appraisal

Khalid Mahdi and Arif Khwaja

Background

Antineutrophil cytoplasmic antibodies (ANCA) were first described in 1982 in patients with pauci-immune glomerulonephritis. Since then, circulating ANCA has been recognized in a range of small vessel vasculitides collectively as ANCA-associated vasculitis (AAV). AAV encompasses a number of clinical syndromes including granulomatosis with polyangitis (GPA formerly known as Wegener's granulomatosis), microscopic polyangitis (MPA), and Churg-Strauss syndrome (CSS). Proteinase 3 (PR3)-ANCA is strongly associated with patients with GPA, while myeloperoxidase (MPO)-ANCA occurs more frequently in MPA.

AAV has an estimated annual incidence of 20 per million and a prevalence of over 200 per million of the population. Although clinical phenotypes vary between the different syndromes, AAV predominantly affects microscopic blood vessels within the respiratory tract and the kidneys – the European Vasculitis Study Group (EUVAS) has further subclassified AAV by the extent and severity of organ involvement [1].

Both genetic and environmental factors contribute to the etiology of AAV, and adoptive transfer experiments involving murine ANCA indicate that ANCA is directly pathogenic in animal models [2]. Furthermore, there is emerging evidence that molecular mimicry with microbial antigens contributes to ANCA formation, and while traditionally AAV has been thought of as being mediated by antibody production through autoreactive B cells, there is increasing evidence that autoreactive T cells play an important role in disease pathogenesis via antigen presentation, co-stimulation, and production of proinflammatory cytokines.

Prior to introduction of immunosuppressive therapy, AAV was invariably fatal with 93 % of patients dying within 2 years as a result of renal or respiratory disease [3]. Five-year survival rates now approach 80 %, thanks to the introduction of glucocorticoid therapy, cyclophosphamide, and more recently rituximab together with adjunctive therapies including plasma exchange and dialysis. In the 1990s, cyclophosphamide combined with glucocorticoids became the "gold-standard" therapy for AAV. This was based largely on observational data from the National Institutes of Health and it is worth noting that the use of cyclophosphamide as an induction agent in AAV was never tested in a randomized controlled trial until relatively recently [4]. Despite the apparent success in therapy, treatment-related toxicity (e.g., leukopenia, sepsis) is now a major cause of early mortality and up to 50 % of patients relapse within 5 years despite ongoing immunosuppression.

In this chapter we will critically review the key randomized controlled trials that have shaped contemporary clinical practice in the management of AAV evaluating studies for induction and maintenance of remission (see Table 3.1). We have included both positive and negative outcome studies that inform clinical practice.

Induction Studies

Trial 1: RAVE

Publication: Rituximab versus cyclophosphamide for ANCA-associated vasculitis

Authors: Stone JH, Merkel PA, Spiera R, Seo P, Langford CA, Hoffman GS, Kallenberg CG, St Clair EW, Turkiewicz A, Tchao NK, Webber L, Ding L, Sejismundo LP, Mieras K, Weitzenkamp D, Ikle D, Seyfert-Margolis V, Mueller M, Brunetta P, Allen NB, Fervenza FC, Geetha D, Keogh KA, Kissin EY, Monach PA, Peikert T, Stegeman C, Ytterberg SR, Specks U, and RAVE-ITN Research Group

Reference: *N Engl J Med*. 2010 Jul 15;363(3):221–32

K. Mahdi, MBBS, MRCP • A. Khwaja, FRCP, PhD (✉)
Sheffield Kidney Institute, Northern General Hospital,
Herries Road, Sheffield, UK
e-mail: khalid.mahdi@gmail.com; arif.khwaja@sth.nhs.uk

M. El Kossi, A. Khwaja, and M. El Nahas (eds.), *Informing Clinical Practice in Nephrology: The Role of RCTs*,
DOI 10.1007/978-3-319-10292-4_3, © Springer International Publishing Switzerland 2015

Table 3.1 Overview of key trials in renal vasculitis

Study	Induction or maintenance	Agents used	Key comments
RAVE	Induction	Rituximab vs. cyclophosphamide	Rituximab was not inferior to cyclophosphamide in induction of remission and may be more effective than cyclophosphamide in relapsing disease. Excludes patients with severe kidney disease
CYCLOPS	Induction	Pulse cyclophosphamide vs. daily oral cyclophosphamide	Less cumulative dose and lower rates of leukopenia in the pulse group compared with daily oral cyclophosphamide with no difference in time to remission. Underpowered study therefore of limited utility
NORAM	Induction	Cyclophosphamide vs. methotrexate	Methotrexate was non-inferior to cyclophosphamide in remission rates in early AAV. It was less effective in extensive disease. Early withdrawal of treatment in both arms was associated with high relapse rate. Limited applicability to those with significant kidney disease
RITUXIVAS	Induction	Rituximab vs. cyclophosphamide	Rituximab-based regimen was not superior to cyclophosphamide in achieving remission and had similar rate of adverse events. Small trial. Highlights the fact that the role of rituximab in severe disease is not known
Plasma exchange in focal necrotizing glomerulonephritis without anti-GBM antibodies	Induction	Plasma exchange vs. no plasma exchange	Higher rate of recovery of renal function in dialysis-dependent patients when treated with plasma exchange and immunosuppression compared to treatment with immunosuppression alone. Small, single-center, unblinded study with no clear power calculations for cohorts who were dialysis dependent
MEPEX	Induction	Plasma exchange vs. high-dose methyl prednisolone	Plasma exchange improved renal survival in patients with AAV and serum creatinine >500 μmol/L when compared to high-dose methyl prednisolone. However, there was no difference in ESRD or dialysis rates at 3 years
RAVE maintenance study	Maintenance	Rituximab vs. cyclophosphamide + azathioprine	Rituximab was non-inferior to conventional therapy with cyclophosphamide and azathioprine in maintaining remission. This was a steroid withdrawal study, so efficacy of rituximab in those maintained on long-term, low-dose steroids not clear
CYCAZAREM	Maintenance	Azathioprine vs. cyclophosphamide	Azathioprine was as effective as cyclophosphamide in maintaining remission
WEGENT	Maintenance	Azathioprine vs. methotrexate	Methotrexate was not safer than azathioprine as a maintenance therapy
IMPROVE	Maintenance	Mycophenolate vs. azathioprine	Higher relapse rates with mycophenolate compared to azathioprine

Abstract

Background: Cyclophosphamide and glucocorticoids have been the cornerstone of remission-induction therapy for severe antineutrophil cytoplasmic antibody (ANCA)-associated vasculitis for 40 years. Uncontrolled studies suggest that rituximab is effective and may be safer than a cyclophosphamide-based regimen.

Methods: We conducted a multicenter, randomized, double-blind, double-dummy, non-inferiority trial of rituximab (375 mg/m^2 of body surface area per week for 4 weeks) as compared with cyclophosphamide (2 mg/kg of body weight per day) for remission-induction. Glucocorticoids were tapered off; the primary end point was remission of disease without the use of prednisone at 6 months.

Results: Nine centers enrolled 197 ANCA-positive patients with either Wegener's granulomatosis or microscopic polyangiitis. Baseline disease activity, organ involvement, and the proportion of patients with relapsing disease were similar in the two treatment groups. Sixty-three patients in the rituximab group (64 %) reached the primary end point, as compared with 52 patients in the control group (53 %), a result that met the criterion for non-inferiority ($P < 0.001$). The rituximab-based regimen was more efficacious than the cyclophosphamide-based regimen for inducing remission of relapsing disease; 34 of 51 patients in the rituximab group (67 %) as compared with 21 of 50 patients in the control group (42 %) reached the primary end point ($P = 0.01$). Rituximab was also as effective as cyclophosphamide in the treatment of patients with major renal disease or alveolar hemorrhage. There were no significant differences between the treatment groups with respect to rates of adverse events.

Conclusions: Rituximab therapy was not inferior to daily cyclophosphamide treatment for induction of remission in severe ANCA-associated vasculitis and may be superior in relapsing disease (funded by the National Institute of Allergy and Infectious Diseases, Genentech, and Biogen; ClinicalTrials.gov number, NCT00104299).

Critical Appraisal

Parameters	Yes	No	Comment
Validity			
Is the **Randomization** Procedure well described?	+1		
Double **blinded**?	+2		Randomized, double-blind, double-dummy, non-inferiority study
Is the **sample size** calculation described/adequate?	+3		Sample size based on assumption that 70 % of both groups would have disease remission at 6 months after discontinuation of prednisone at 6 months
Does it have a hard primary **end point**?	+1		Birmingham Vasculitis Activity Score for Wegener's granulomatosis (BVAS/WG) of 0 and successful completion of steroid taper at 6 months
Is the end point surrogate?		0	
Is the follow-up appropriate?	1		Data at 6 months presented which is inadequate when evaluating long-term effects of therapy but the specific end point here was short-term induction
Was there a **Bias**?		+2	
Is the dropout >25 %?		+1	
Is the analysis **ITT**?	+3		
Utility/usefulness			
Can the findings be generalized?	+1		Yes although only 66 % of patients in both limbs had kidney involvement
Are the findings easily translatable?	+1		Yes though the steroid-free taper may not reflect routine clinical practice
Was the NNT <100?			Not applicable as this was a non-inferiority study; however, the treatment difference of 11 % met the prespecified criteria for non-inferiority
Score	**100 %**		

Comment

RAVE is a well-conducted landmark study that clearly establishes the efficacy of rituximab (B cell depleting, chimeric, monoclonal antibody that targets CD20 on B cells) as induction therapy in AAV. The control group received what would be regarded as standard induction therapy of cyclophosphamide (2 mg/kg) combined with glucocorticoids. Rituximab was administered as four doses of 375 mg/m^2/week. In addition to the demonstrated non-inferiority with cyclophosphamide, rituximab was superior to cyclophosphamide in a prespecified analysis of patients who had relapsing disease at baseline. There was no difference in hospitalization and death in the two groups.

However, nephrologists need to be aware of salient features of the study design and population when deciding to utilize the drug. Firstly, patients with significant kidney disease (serum creatinine >4 mg/dl) or those with severe alveolar hemorrhage were excluded from the study. Indeed, 34 % of patients in both groups had no kidney involvement at all and kidney function was reasonably preserved in both groups at baseline though significantly worse in the rituximab group (estimated creatinine clearance 53.8±29.8 ml/min vs. 68.9±41.6 ml/min; $P=0.04$). Thus, the positive findings of the study are not applicable to those patients with severe AAV that nephrologists often manage. A further critically important feature of the study is the forced steroid taper such that by 5 months, all patients who had a remission without disease flares had discontinued glucocorticoids. This early discontinuation of steroids may well have driven up the event rate in the control group and may well explain why the remission rate in RAVE were lower than in other studies of AAV. However, given the well-documented toxicity associated with glucocorticoids, RAVE demonstrates that steroid-free therapy with adjunctive rituximab is an achievable therapeutic paradigm in AAV. The maintenance data from RAVE is discussed later in this chapter, but it is worth noting that the RAVE study provided the basis for the FDA granting approval to rituximab as a licensed therapy in AAV – to date the only licensed agent for AAV.

Trial 2: CYCLOPS

Publication: Pulse versus daily oral cyclophosphamide for induction of remission in antineutrophil cytoplasmic antibody-associated vasculitis: a randomized trial

Authors: de Groot K, Harper L, Jayne DR, Flores Suarez LF, Gregorini G, Gross WL, Luqmani R, Pusey CD, Rasmussen N, Sinico RA, Tesar V, Vanhille P, Westman K, Savage CO, and EUVAS (European Vasculitis Study Group)

Reference: *Ann Inn Med*. 2009 May 19;150(10):670–80

Abstract

Background: Current therapies for antineutrophil cytoplasmic antibody (ANCA)-associated vasculitis are limited by toxicity.

Objective: To compare pulse cyclophosphamide with daily oral cyclophosphamide for induction of remission.

Design: Randomized, controlled trial. Random assignments were computer generated; allocation was concealed by faxing centralized treatment assignment to providers at the time of enrollment. Patients, investigators, and assessors of outcomes were not blinded to assignment.

Setting: 42 centers in 12 European countries.

Patients: 149 patients who had newly diagnosed generalized ANCA-associated vasculitis with renal involvement but not immediately life-threatening disease.

Intervention: Pulse cyclophosphamide, 15 mg/kg every 2–3 weeks (76 patients), or daily oral cyclophosphamide, 2 mg/kg/day (73 patients), plus prednisolone.

Measurement: Time to remission (primary outcome): change in renal function, adverse events, and cumulative dose of cyclophosphamide (secondary outcomes)

Results: Groups did not differ in time to remission (hazard ratio, 1.098 [95 % CI, 0.78–1.55]; $P = 0.59$) or proportion of patients who achieved remission at 9 months (88.1 % vs. 87.7 %). Thirteen patients in the pulse group and six in the daily oral group achieved remission by 9 months and subsequently had relapse. Absolute cumulative cyclophosphamide dose in the daily oral group was greater than that in the pulse group (15.9 g [interquartile range, 11–22.5 g] vs. 8.2 g [interquartile range, 5.95–10.55 g]; $P < 0.001$). The pulse group had a lower rate of leukopenia (hazard ratio, 0.41 [CI, 0.23–0.71]).

Limitations: The study was not powered to detect a difference in relapse rates between the two groups. Duration of follow-up was limited.

Conclusion: The pulse cyclophosphamide regimen induced remission of ANCA-associated vasculitis as well as the daily oral regimen at a reduced cumulative cyclophosphamide dose and caused fewer cases of leukopenia.

Critical Appraisal

Parameters	Yes	No	Comment
Validity			
Is the **Randomization** Procedure well described?	+1		Computer-generated randomization
Double **blinded**?		−2	Open label
Is the **sample size** calculation described/adequate?		−3	Sample size based on ability to recruit patients and budgeting rather than statistical calculation
Does it have a hard primary **end point**?	+1		Time to remission

Parameters	Yes	No	Comment
Is the end point surrogate?		0	
Is the follow-up appropriate?	+1		Duration of follow-up limited – of 18 months
Was there a **Bias**?		+2	
Is the dropout >25 %?		+1	
Is the analysis **ITT**?	+3		
Utility/usefulness			
Can the findings be generalized?	+1		Although the study wasn't powered to detect differences in relapse rates
Are the findings easily translatable?	+1		
Was the NNT <100?		−1	No difference in primary outcome – time to remission. However, there was a 19 % risk reduction in leukopenia
Score	29 %		CYCLOPS is an underpowered study, and therefore, its results are inconclusive

Comments

Intravenous cyclophosphamide is often used as standard therapy over oral cyclophosphamide both in AAV and in lupus nephritis on the grounds that it is safer, with less total drug exposure and a reduced risk of life-threatening leukopenia. To some extent, this study supports the notion of intravenous cyclophosphamide being safer than oral cyclophosphamide – the time to remission is not significantly different in both groups, but there is a 19 % reduction in leukopenia in the intravenous-dosed group. However, it is important to note that the cumulative dose exposure of cyclophosphamide was significantly lower in the intravenous group versus the oral group (8.2 g vs. 15.9 g $p < 0.001$) which suggests that the total drug exposure is what is important in minimizing leukopenia rather than the actual mode of administration.

Other significant limitations include the fact the study wasn't powered to detect differences in relapse between the two groups which is clearly a major issue when trying to evaluate the clinical utility of the study. Indeed, there was a higher number of relapses in the intravenous group and these concerns were borne out by a retrospective analysis of long-term outcomes of 148 patients in the study which showed a significantly lower risk of relapse in the daily oral cyclophosphamide group compared to pulsed cyclophosphamide (HR = 0.50, 95 % CI 0.26–0.93; $p = 0.029$) although this was not associated in any difference in mortality [5].

Therefore, it is the total dose exposure to cyclophosphamide that seems to be critical rather than the mode or frequency of drug delivery. The higher the total dose exposure, the increased the chance of relapse-free disease, but the price of this is a significantly higher risk of leukopenia.

Trial 3: NORAM

Publication: Randomized trial of cyclophosphamide versus methotrexate for the induction of remission in early systemic antineutrophil cytoplasmic antibody-associated vasculitis

Authors: de Groot K, Ramussen N, Bacon PA, Tervaert JW, Feighery C, Gregorini G, Gross WL, Luqmani R, and Jayne DR

Reference: *Arthritis Rheum* 2005 Aug;52(8):2461–9

Abstract

Objective: Standard therapy for antineutrophil cytoplasmic antibody-associated systemic vasculitis (AASV) with cyclophosphamide (CYC) and prednisolone is limited by toxicity. This unblinded, prospective, randomized, controlled trial was undertaken to determine whether methotrexate (MTX) could replace CYC in the early treatment of AASV.

Methods: Patients with newly diagnosed AASV, with serum creatinine levels <150 µmol/L and without critical organ manifestations of disease, were randomized to receive either standard oral CYC, 2 mg/kg/day, or oral MTX, 20–25 mg/week; both groups received the same prednisolone regimen. All drug treatments were gradually tapered and withdrawn by 12 months. Follow-up continued to 18 months. The primary end point was the remission rate at 6 months (non-inferiority testing).

Results: One hundred patients were recruited from 26 European centers; 51 patients were randomized to the MTX group and 49 to the CYC group. At 6 months, the remission rate in patients treated with MTX (89.8 %) was not inferior to that in patients treated with CYC (93.5 %) ($P=0.041$). In the MTX group, remission was delayed among patients with more extensive disease ($P=0.04$) or pulmonary involvement ($P=0.03$). Relapse rates at 18 months were 69.5 % in the MTX group and 46.5 % in the CYC group; the median time from remission to relapse was 13 and 15 months, respectively ($P=0.023$, log rank test). Two patients from each group died. Adverse events (mean 0.87 episodes/patient) included leukopenia, which was less frequent in the MTX versus the CYC group ($P=0.012$), and liver dysfunction, which was more frequent in the MTX group ($P=0.036$).

Conclusion: MTX can replace CYC for initial treatment of early AASV. The MTX regimen used in the present study was less effective for induction of remission in patients with extensive disease and pulmonary involvement and was associated with more relapses than the CYC regimen after termination of treatment. The high relapse rates in both treatment arms support the practice of continuation of immunosuppressive treatment beyond 12 months.

Critical Appraisal

Parameters	Yes	No	Comment
Validity			
Is the **Randomization** Procedure well described?	+1		
Double **blinded**?		−2	Unblinded
Is the **sample size** calculation described/ adequate?	+3		Non-inferiority of methotrexate versus cyclophosphamide was calculated assuming a remission rate of 92 % after 6 months cyclophosphamide therapy
Does it have a hard primary **end point**?	+1		Induction of remission at 6 months using BVAS
Is the end point surrogate?		0	
Is the follow-up appropriate?	+1		
Was there a **Bias**?		+2	
Is the dropout >25 %?		+1	
Is the analysis **ITT**?	+3		
Utility/usefulness			
Can the findings be generalized?		−1	Only to patients with well-preserved kidney function. Serum creatinine at baseline (0.96 mg/ dl) in both groups. Withdrawal of immunosuppression at 12 months not representative of current practice
Are the findings easily translatable?	+1		
Was the NNT <100?			Not applicable as this was a non-inferiority study
Score	**62.5 %**		

Comments

This unblinded RCT compares the use of methotrexate (15–25 mg/week till month 10) to cyclophosphamide in early AAV (2 mg/kg/day for 3–6 months) with tapering and withdrawal of all immunosuppression (including steroids) by 12 months. In terms of the primary end point of remission at 6 months, there was no significant difference between the two groups with 89.8 % of the methotrexate group and 93.5 % of the cyclophosphamide group achieving remission. However, nephrologists need to be aware of important caveats to the study. Firstly, the study was not blinded and therefore, unblinded BVAS scoring could introduce a significant source of bias. Furthermore, only around 30 % of both groups had microscopic hematuria and the median creatinine at baseline was 0.96 mg/dl indicating that most patients in the study did not have kidney involvement. Furthermore, those with evidence of significant disease as measured by Disease Extent Index had a significantly longer time to remission with methotrexate than with cyclophosphamide as did those with pulmonary involvement. An important aspect of this study is that all immunosuppression was withdrawn at 12 months and such early withdrawal of therapy is not representative of standard, contemporary practice. However, such a design allowed important observations to be made about the risk of relapse after successful induction therapy. Relapse rates were high in both groups – 46.5 % in the cyclophosphamide group vs. 69.5 % in the methotrexate group. Thus, while data from NORAM could justify the use of methotrexate as induction therapy in AAV in those with limited, predominantly non-nephrological disease, perhaps its most important impact has been to highlight the dangers of early withdrawal of immunosuppressive therapy at 12 months.

Trial 4: RITUXIVAS

Publication: Rituximab versus cyclophosphamide in ANCA-associated renal vasculitis

Authors: Jones RB, Tervaert JW, Hauser T, Luqmani R, Morgan MD, Peh CA, Savage CO, Segelmark M, Tesar V, van Paassen P, Walsh D, Walsh M, Westman K, Jayne DR, and European Vasculitis Study Group

Reference: *N Engl J Med*. 2010;363(3):211

Abstract

Background: Cyclophosphamide induction regimens for antineutrophil cytoplasmic antibody (ANCA)-associated vasculitis are effective in 70–90 % of patients, but they are associated with high rates of death and adverse events. Treatment with rituximab has led to remission rates of 80–90 % among patients with refractory ANCA-associated vasculitis and may be safer than cyclophosphamide regimens.

Methods: We compared rituximab with cyclophosphamide as induction therapy in ANCA-associated vasculitis. We randomly assigned, in a 3:1 ratio, 44 patients with newly diagnosed ANCA-associated vasculitis and renal involvement to a standard glucocorticoid regimen plus either rituximab at a dose of 375 mg/m^2 of body surface area per week for 4 weeks, with two intravenous cyclophosphamide pulses (33 patients, the rituximab group), or intravenous cyclophosphamide for 3–6 months followed by azathioprine (11 patients, the control group). Primary end points were sustained remission rates at 12 months and severe adverse events.

Results: The median age was 68 years, and the glomerular filtration rate (GFR) was 18 ml/min/1.73 m^2 of body surface area. A total of 25 patients in the rituximab group (76 %) and 9 patients in the control group (82 %) had a sustained remission ($P=0.68$). Severe adverse events occurred in 14 patients in the rituximab group (42 %) and 4 patients in the control group (36 %) ($P=0.77$). Six of the 33 patients in the rituximab group (18 %) and 2 of the 11 patients in the control group (18 %) died ($P=1.00$). The median increase in the GFR between 0 and 12 months was 19 ml per minute in the rituximab group and 15 ml per minute in the control group ($P=0.14$).

Conclusions: A rituximab-based regimen was not superior to standard intravenous cyclophosphamide for severe ANCA-associated vasculitis. Sustained remission rates were high in both groups, and the rituximab-based regimen was not associated with reductions in early severe adverse events (funded by Cambridge University Hospitals National Health Service Foundation Trust and F. Hoffmann-La Roche; Current Controlled Trials number, ISRCTN28528813).

Critical Appraisal

Parameters	Yes	No	Comment
Validity			
Is the **Randomization** Procedure well described?	+1		
Double **blinded**?		−2	Open label
Is the **sample size** calculation described/ adequate?	+3		This is a small phase II study that was designed to test the hypothesis that rituximab improves remission rates in patients with significant kidney disease. Although the sample size calculation is adequately described, a larger phase III study would be required to fully evaluate this hypothesis
Does it have a hard primary **end point**?	+1		Sustained remission using BVAS and serious adverse events
Is the end point surrogate?		0	
Is the follow-up appropriate?	+1		12-month data – appropriate for a phase II exploratory
Was there a **Bias**?	−2		The randomization ratio was 3:1 between rituximab and the control arms. This meant that there were differences in baseline characteristics of the two populations which could have impacted on results particularly given the sample size. In particular, there were differences in ANCA pattern and median eGFR at baseline between the two groups

Parameters	Yes	No	Comment
Is the dropout >25 %?		+1	
Is the analysis ITT?	+3		
Utility/usefulness			
Can the findings be generalized?	+1		
Are the findings easily translatable?	+1		Yes though the steroid-free taper may not reflect routine clinical practice in all centers
Was the NNT <100?		−1	No difference between rituximab and control group
Score	**41 %**		

Comments

While the RAVE study clearly established that rituximab has disease-modifying activity in patients with AAV, RITUXIVAS attempted to address the efficacy and safety of rituximab in patients with severe kidney disease. It was effectively a phase 2 exploratory study and as such was unable to clearly answer the question it set out to address. There are two features in particular about the study design which may have masked an effect. Those randomized to rituximab also received two doses of IV cyclophosphamide and this may have driven up the adverse event rate in the rituximab group. Therefore, it's difficult to tease out what effects are due to cyclophosphamide and those due to rituximab. Furthermore, patients were randomized in a ratio of 3:1 between rituximab and cyclophosphamide, with a relatively small sample size of 44 subjects. With such a small sample size, there is a much higher risk of results being skewed by "outlier" data. Indeed, there were potentially significant, confounding differences in the baseline characteristics of the two groups. The baseline eGFR was 20 ml/min/1.73 m² in the rituximab group versus 12 ml/min/1.72 m² in the control group. Furthermore, the pattern of AAV was different with 55 % of the rituximab group having GPA compared to only 36 % of the control group. In summary, RITUXIVAS highlights the need for larger controlled studies in AAV patients with significant kidney disease and as yet, the role of rituximab in such patients is not well defined.

Trial 5: Plasma Exchange in Focal Necrotizing Glomerulonephritis Without Anti-GBM Antibodies

Publication: Plasma exchange in focal necrotizing glomerulonephritis without anti-GBM antibodies

Authors: Pusey CD, Rees AJ, Evans DJ, Peters K, and Lockwood CM

Reference: *Kidney Int.* 1991 Oct;40(4):757–63

Abstract

To determine whether plasma exchange was of additional benefit in patients treated with oral immunosuppressive drugs for focal necrotizing glomerulonephritis (without anti-GBM antibodies), we performed a randomized controlled trial with stratification for renal function on entry. Forty-eight cases were analyzed, 25 in the treatment group (plasma exchange, prednisolone, cyclophosphamide, and azathioprine) and 23 in the control group (drug therapy only). There was no difference in outcome in patients presenting with serum creatinine less than 500 µmol/L ($N=17$) or greater than 500 µmol/L but not on dialysis ($N=12$), all but one of whom had improved by 4 weeks. However, patients who were initially dialysis dependent ($N=19$) were more likely to have recovered renal function ($P=0.041$) if treated with plasma exchange as well as drugs (10 of 11) rather than with drugs alone (3 of 8). Long-term follow-up showed that improvement in renal function was generally maintained. The results of this trial confirm that focal necrotizing glomerulonephritis related to systemic vasculitis responds well to immunosuppressive drugs when treatment is started early and suggest that plasma exchange is of additional benefit in dialysis-dependent cases.

Critical Appraisal

Parameters	Yes	No	Comment
Validity			
Is the **Randomization** Procedure well described?	+1		
Double **blinded**?		−2	There was no sham plasma exchange group though clearly difficult to obtain ethical approval for invasive, sham interventions
Is the **sample size** calculation described/ adequate?		−3	No clear description of whether study powered to detect differences between subgroups
Does it have a hard primary **end point**?	+1		Dialysis independence and improvement in serum creatinine. The latter was defined as a fall of serum creatinine of greater than 25 % in those not on dialysis and dialysis independence in those who presented with dialysis dependence
Is the end point surrogate?		0	
Is the follow-up appropriate?	+1		12 months
Was there a **Bias**?		+2	
Is the dropout >25 %?		+1	

Parameters	Yes	No	Comment
Is the analysis **ITT**?		−3	No comment made as to whether analysis was ITT, but all patients enrolled completed treatment to randomized arms
Utility/usefulness			
Can the findings be generalized?	+1		
Are the findings easily translatable?	+1		
Was the NNT <100?	+1		
Score	**5.8 %**		

Comments

This landmark study from the Hammersmith Hospital, London, transformed the management of AAV at the time and was used to justify the use of plasma exchange (PEx) in patients with AAV who were dialysis dependent. The headline figures are indeed impressive with 10/11 of the dialysis-dependent patients recovering kidney functions while only 3/8 of the drug-only treatment doing so. For all other patients, PEx showed no benefit. However, what is striking about this single-center study is the relatively small number of patients (19) who were dialysis dependent and there were no power calculations to demonstrate whether the study was adequately powered to detect significant differences in the subgroup of patients who were dialysis dependent. Yet at the time of publication, there was little evidence to guide the management of AAV and this study provided a rationale for the use of PEx in patients with AAV and severe kidney disease.

Trial 6: MEPEX

Publication: Randomized trial of plasma exchange or high-dosage methylprednisolone as adjunctive therapy for severe renal vasculitis

Authors: Jayne DR, Gaskin G, Rasmussen N, Abramowicz D, Ferrario F, Guillevin L, Mirapeix E, Savage CO, Sinico RA, Stegeman CA, Westman KW, van der Woude FJ, de Lind van Wijngaarden RA, Pusey CD, and European Vasculitis Study Group

Reference: *J Am Soc Nephrol*. 2007 Jul;18(7):2180–8

Abstract

Systemic vasculitis associated with autoantibodies to neutrophil cytoplasmic antigens (ANCA) is the most frequent cause of rapidly progressive glomerulonephritis. Renal failure at presentation carries an increased risk for ESRD and death despite immunosuppressive therapy. This study investigated whether the addition of plasma exchange was more effective than intravenous methylprednisolone in the achievement of renal recovery in those who presented with a serum creatinine >500 μmol/L (5.8 mg/dl). A total of 137 patients with a new diagnosis of ANCA-associated systemic vasculitis confirmed by renal biopsy and serum creatinine >500 μmol/L (5.8 mg/dl) were randomly assigned to receive seven plasma exchanges ($n=70$) or 3,000 mg of intravenous methylprednisolone ($n=67$). Both groups received oral cyclophosphamide and oral prednisolone. The primary end point was dialysis independence at 3 months. Secondary end points included renal and patient survival at 1 year and severe adverse event rates. At 3 months, 33 (49 %) of 67 after intravenous methylprednisolone compared with 48 (69 %) or 70 after plasma exchange were alive and independent of dialysis (95 % confidence interval for the difference 18–35 %; $P=0.02$). As compared with intravenous methylprednisolone, plasma exchange was associated with a reduction in risk for progression to ESRD of 24 % (95 % confidence interval 6.1–41 %), from 43 to 19 %, at 12 months. Patient survival and severe adverse event rates at 1 year were 51 (76 %) of 67 and 32 of 67 (48 %) in the intravenous methylprednisolone group and 51 (73 %) of 70 and 35 of (50 %) 70 in the plasma exchange group, respectively. Plasma exchange increased the rate of renal recovery in ANCA-associated systemic vasculitis that presented with renal failure when compared with intravenous methylprednisolone. Patient survival and severe adverse event rates were similar in both groups.

Critical Appraisal

Parameters	Yes	No	Comment
Validity			
Is the **Randomization** Procedure well described?	+1		
Double **blinded**?		−2	There was no sham plasma exchange group though clearly difficult to obtain ethical approval for invasive, sham interventions
Is the **sample size** calculation described/ adequate?	+3		The sample size was based on a predicted renal recovery rate of 50 % with methylprednisolone and the study was designed to detect an increase in recovery rate of >20 % in the plasma exchange group

Parameters	Yes	No	Comment
Does it have a hard primary **end point**?	+1		Dialysis independence at 3 months
Is the end point surrogate?		0	
Is the follow-up appropriate?	+1		Short follow-up but appropriate for primary end point
Was there a **Bias**?		+2	
Is the dropout >25 %?		+1	
Is the analysis ITT?	+3		
Utility/usefulness			
Can the findings be generalized?	+1		
Are the findings easily translatable?	+1		Yes though doesn't answer whether plasma exchange combined with high-dose methylprednisolone confers an additional advantage
Was the NNT <100?	+1		20 % absolute risk reduction with an NNT of 5
Score	76 %		

Comments

Despite the shortcomings in the Hammersmith study, PEx became standard practice in the management of dialysis-dependent AAV. However, it wasn't until 2007 that the MEPEX study was able to more robustly define the place of PEx in the acute management of AAV. MEPEX established the superiority of PEx over intravenous high-dose methylprednisolone (MP) as part of induction therapy in patients with AAV who have severe kidney involvement. However, a number of concerns have been expressed about the study. Firstly, the PEx regime varied between centers. In addition, the trial doesn't address the issue of whether PEx would be of additional value used in conjunction with MP – rather, it shows that PEx with oral steroids is superior to MP. This is a valid concern though given the high rates of sepsis in AAV, many have argued that steroid minimization should be a key goal in AAV. Finally, it is clear that while PEx improves renal recovery at 3 months, the long-term benefits are marginal [6]. Although there were reduced rates of end-stage renal disease (ESRD) at 1 year (19 % in PEx group vs. 43 % in the MP group), at 3 years, there was no significant difference in the combined end point of death and ESRD (58 % in the PEx group vs. 68 % in those receiving MP). Thus, the initial reduction in dialysis dependence with PEx does not translate into improved long-term outcomes. This

was in part driven by the high rate of sepsis-related death (over 30 %) which may reflect the higher cumulative dose exposure to cyclophosphamide with the oral regime used and also the frailty of the MEPEX cohort who had a median age of 66 years. In summary, MEPEX supports the rationale to use PEx in AAV patients with severe kidney disease at presentation to reduce dialysis dependence at 3 and 12 months, but this does not translate improved long-term outcomes.

Maintenance Studies

Trial 1: RAVE Maintenance Study

Publication: Efficacy of remission-induction regimes for ANCA-associated vasculitis
  Authors: Specks U, Merkel PA, Seo P, Spiera R, Langford CA, Hoffman GS, Kallenberg CG, St Clair EW, Fessler BJ, Ding L, Viviano L, Tchao NK, Phippard DJ, Asare AL, Lim N, Ikle D, Jepson B, Brunetta P, Allen NB, Fervenza FC, Geetha D, Keogh K, Kissin EY, Monach PA, Peikert T, Stegeman C, Ytterberg SR, Mueller M, Sejismundo LP, Mieras K, Stone JH, and RAVE-ITN Research Group
  Reference: N Engl J Med. 2013 Aug 1;369(5):417–27

Abstract
Background: The 18-month efficacy of a single course of rituximab as compared with conventional immunosuppression with cyclophosphamide followed by azathioprine in patients with severe (organ-threatening) antineutrophil cytoplasmic antibody (ANCA)-associated vasculitis is unknown.

Methods: In a multicenter, randomized, double-blind, double-dummy, non-inferiority trial, we compared rituximab (375 mg/m^2 of body surface area administered once a week for 4 weeks) followed by placebo with cyclophosphamide administered for 3–6 months followed by azathioprine for 12–15 months. The primary outcome measure was complete remission of disease by 6 months, with the remission maintained through 18 months.

Results: A total of 197 patients were enrolled. As reported previously, 64 % of the patients in the rituximab group, as compared with 53 % of the patients in the cyclophosphamide-azathioprine group, had a complete remission by 6 months. At 12 and 18 months, 48 and 39 %, respectively, of the patients in the rituximab group had maintained the complete remissions, as compared with 39 and 33 %, respectively, in the comparison group. Rituximab met the prespecified criteria for non-inferiority ($P < 0.001$, with a non-inferiority margin of 20 %). There was no significant difference between the groups in any efficacy measure, including the duration of complete remission and the frequency or severity of relapses.

Among the 101 patients who had relapsing disease at baseline, rituximab was superior to conventional immunosuppression at 6 months ($P=0.01$) and at 12 months ($P=0.009$) but not at 18 months ($P=0.06$), at which time most patients in the rituximab group had reconstituted B cells. There was no significant between-group difference in adverse events.

Conclusions: In patients with severe ANCA-associated vasculitis, a single course of rituximab was as effective as continuous conventional immunosuppressive therapy for the induction and maintenance of remissions over the course of 18 months (funded by the National Institute of Allergy and Infectious Diseases and others; RAVE ClinicalTrials.gov number, NCT00104299).

Critical Appraisal

Parameters	Yes	No	Comment
Validity			
Is the Randomization Procedure well described?	+1		
Double **blinded**?	+2		
Is the **sample size** calculation described/adequate?	+3		
Does it have a hard primary **end point**?	+1		Complete remission of disease by 6 months through 18 months
Is the end point surrogate?		0	
Is the follow-up appropriate?	+1		18 months
Was there a **Bias**?		+2	No
Is the dropout >25 %?	−1		Patients who flared between 6 and 18 months were either dropped from the study or switched to nonstudy treatment or open-label rituximab
Is the analysis **ITT**?	+3		
Utility/usefulness			
Can the findings be generalized?	+1		
Are the findings easily translatable?	+1		
Was the NNT <100?			Not applicable as this study testing the non-inferiority of rituximab to cyclophosphamide + azathioprine
Score	**87.5 %**		

Comments

This study was a follow on from the RAVE induction study and demonstrated at 18 months, a single course of rituximab combined with glucocorticoids (for 6 months) was not inferior to 18 months of conventional treatment with cyclophosphamide induction and azathioprine maintenance. However, it is worth pointing out that only 39 and 33 % of the rituximab group and cyclophosphamide-azathioprine group, respectively, were in complete remission at 18 months. Interestingly, significant B cell depletion occurred in both groups and while rises in ANCA titer did not predict relapse, flare of disease was uncommon in those who were ANCA negative and B cell deplete.

The results of RAVE as already discussed are not applicable to those with severe renal disease or alveolar hemorrhage. It does however suggest that repeated courses of rituximab alone can be used to maintain remission in AAV. However, given the protocol-mandated steroid withdrawal, it is not clear whether rituximab is more efficacious, safer, or cost-effective in maintaining remission than a standard regime consisting of combined azathioprine and low-dose steroids. The MAINRITSAN trial (Clinicaltrials.gov NCT00748644) and the RITAZAREM trial (Clinicaltrials.gov NCT0169767) are both currently exploring the role of preemptive rituximab in comparison to azathioprine for maintaining remission.

Trial 2: CYCAZAREM

Publication: A randomized trial of maintenance therapy for vasculitis associated with antineutrophil cytoplasmic autoantibodies.

Authors: Jayne D, Rasmussen N, Andrassy K, Bacon P, Tervaert JW, Dadoniené J, Ekstrand A, Gaskin G, Gregorini G, de Groot K, Gross W, Hagen EC, Mirapeix E, Pettersson E, Siegert C, Sinico A, Tesar V, Westman K, Pusey C. European Vasculitis Study Group.

Reference: *N Engl J Med*. 2003 Jul 3;349(1):36–44

Abstract

Background: The primary systemic vasculitides usually associated with autoantibodies to neutrophil cytoplasmic antigens include Wegener's granulomatosis and microscopic polyangiitis. We investigated whether exposure to cyclophosphamide in patients with generalized vasculitis could be reduced by substitution of azathioprine at remission.

Methods: We studied patients with a new diagnosis of generalized vasculitis and a serum creatinine concentration of 5.7 mg/dl (500 µmol/L) or less. All patients received at least 3 months of therapy with oral cyclophosphamide and prednisolone. After remission, patients were randomly assigned to continued cyclophosphamide therapy (1.5 mg/kg of body weight per day) or a substitute regimen of azathioprine (2 mg/kg/day). Both groups continued to receive prednisolone and were followed for 18 months from study entry. Relapse was the primary end point.

Results: Of 155 patients studied, 144 (93 %) entered remission and were randomly assigned to azathioprine (71 patients) or continued cyclophosphamide (73 patients). There were eight deaths (5 %), seven of them during the first 3 months. Eleven relapses occurred in the azathioprine group (15.5 %), and 10 occurred in the cyclophosphamide group (13.7 %, $P=0.65$). Severe adverse events occurred in 15 patients during the induction phase (10 %), in 8 patients in the azathioprine group during the remission phase (11 %), and in 7 patients in the cyclophosphamide group during the remission phase (10 %, $P=0.94$ for the comparison between groups during the remission phase). The relapse rate was lower among the patients with microscopic polyangiitis than among those with Wegener's granulomatosis ($P=0.03$).

Conclusions: In patients with generalized vasculitis, the withdrawal of cyclophosphamide and the substitution of azathioprine after remission did not increase the rate of relapse. Thus, the duration of exposure to cyclophosphamide may be safely reduced.

Critical Appraisal

Parameters	Yes	No	Comment
Validity			
Is the **Randomization** Procedure well described?	+1		
Double **blinded**?		−2	
Is the **sample size** calculation described/adequate?	+3		Designed to detect an increase in relapse rate of more than 20 %
Does it have a hard primary **end point**?	+1		Relapse – defined using BVAS and determined by investigator with retrospective validation by independent observer
Is the end point surrogate?		0	
Is the follow-up appropriate?	+1		18 months
Was there a **Bias**?		+2	Although remission and relapse rates determined by investigator, there were no significant differences in BVAS scoring and lab variables
Is the dropout >25 %?		+1	

Parameters	Yes	No	Comment
Is the analysis **ITT**?		−3	Not explicitly stated in methodology
Utility/usefulness			
Can the findings be generalized?	+1		
Are the findings easily translatable?	+1		
Was the NNT <100?			Not applicable as this study is testing the non-inferiority of cyclophosphamide to azathioprine
Score	37.5 %		

Comments

This important study clearly demonstrated no difference in the efficacy of cyclophosphamide and azathioprine in maintaining remission. Interestingly, despite expectations, there was no significant difference in adverse events between the two groups though one might have expected a higher risk of sepsis and neutropenia in the cyclophosphamide group. This may well have been due to the closer monitoring patients receive in randomized controlled trials as "real-world" experience suggests that azathioprine is associated with significantly less toxicity than cyclophosphamide. In summary, this study significantly impacted on practice by demonstrating azathioprine could be used to minimize cyclophosphamide exposure once remission had been obtained.

Trial 3: WEGENT

Publication: Azathioprine or methotrexate for ANCA-associated vasculitis

Authors: Pagnoux C, Mahr A, Hamidou MA, Boffa JJ, Ruivard M, Ducroix JP, Kyndt X, Lifermann F, Papo T, Lambert M, Le Noach J, Khellaf M, Merrien D, Puéchal X, Vinzio S, Cohen P, Mouthon L, Cordier JF, Guillevin L, and French Vasculitis Study Group

Reference: *N Engl J Med*. 2008 Dec 25;359(26):2790–803

Abstract

Background: Current standard therapy for Wegener's granulomatosis and microscopic polyangiitis combines corticosteroids and cyclophosphamide to induce remission, followed by a less toxic immunosuppressant such as azathioprine or methotrexate for maintenance therapy. However, azathioprine and methotrexate have not been compared with regard to safety and efficacy.

Methods: In this prospective, open-label, multicenter trial, we randomly assigned patients with Wegener's granulomatosis or microscopic polyangiitis who entered remission with intravenous cyclophosphamide and corticosteroids to receive oral azathioprine (at a dose of 2.0 mg/kg of body weight per day) or methotrexate (at a dose of 0.3 mg/kg/week, progressively increased to 25 mg/week) for 12 months. The primary end point was an adverse event requiring discontinuation of the study drug or causing death; the sample size was calculated on the basis of the primary hypothesis that methotrexate would be less toxic than azathioprine. The secondary end points were severe adverse events and relapse.

Results: Among 159 eligible patients, 126 (79 %) had a remission, were randomly assigned to receive a study drug in two groups of 63 patients each, and were followed for a mean (+/− SD) period of 29 ± 13 months. Adverse events occurred in 29 azathioprine recipients and 35 methotrexate recipients ($P=0.29$); grade 3 or 4 events occurred in 5 patients in the azathioprine group and 11 patients in the methotrexate group ($P=0.11$). The primary end point was reached in 7 patients who received azathioprine as compared with 12 patients who received methotrexate ($P=0.21$), with a corresponding hazard ratio for methotrexate of 1.65 (95 % confidence interval, 0.65–4.18; $P=0.29$). There was one death in the methotrexate group. Twenty-three patients who received azathioprine and 21 patients who received methotrexate had a relapse ($P=0.71$); 73 % of these patients had a relapse after discontinuation of the study drug.

Conclusions: These results do not support the primary hypothesis that methotrexate is safer than azathioprine. The two agents appear to be similar alternatives for maintenance therapy in patients with Wegener's granulomatosis and microscopic polyangiitis after initial remission (ClinicalTrials.gov number, NCT00349674).

Critical Appraisal

Parameters	Yes	No	Comment
Validity			
Is the **Randomization Procedure** well described?	+1		
Double **blinded**?		−2	Open label
Is the **sample size** calculation described/adequate?	+3		Based on hypothesis that methotrexate would have a lower adverse event rate than azathioprine
Does it have a hard primary **end point**?	+1		Adverse event leading to death or discontinuation of drug
Is the end point surrogate?		0	
Is the follow-up appropriate?	+1		29 ± 13 months

Parameters	Yes	No	Comment
Was there a **Bias**?		+2	
Is the dropout >25 %?		+1	
Is the analysis **ITT**?	+3		
Utility/usefulness			
Can the findings be generalized?	+1		
Are the findings easily translatable?	+1		
Was the NNT <100?			Not applicable as the adverse event rate was similar in both groups
Score	**75 %**		

Comments

This study was based on the hypothesis that methotrexate would be safer and better tolerated than azathioprine in maintaining patients with AAV in remission after they had received a cyclophosphamide-glucocorticoid induction regime. Of note, just under 50 % of patients had kidney involvement at baseline and the median creatinine at randomization was between 1.4 and 1.52 mg/dl in both groups, and therefore, the results of the study are highly relevant to nephrologists. While the study failed to show that methotrexate was safer than azathioprine, it demonstrates that methotrexate is a perfectly acceptable alternative to azathioprine to maintain patients in AAV in remission with a similar relapse rate, though of course care should be exercised in dosing methotrexate in patients with impaired kidney function.

Trial 4: IMPROVE

Publication: Mycophenolate vs. azathioprine for remission maintenance in antineutrophil cytoplasmic antibody-associated vasculitis

Authors: Hiemstra TF, Walsh M, Mahr A, Savage CO, de Groot K, Harper L, Hauser T, Neumann I, Tesar V, Wissing KM, Pagnoux C, Schmitt W, Jayne DR, and European Vasculitis Study Group (EUVAS)

Reference: *JAMA*. 2010 Dec 1;304(21):2381–8

Abstract

Context: Current remission maintenance therapies for antineutrophil cytoplasmic antibody (ANCA)-associated vasculitis (AAV) are limited by partial efficacy and toxicity.

Objective: To compare the effects of mycophenolate mofetil with azathioprine on the prevention of relapses in patients with AAV.

Design, Setting, and Participants: Open-label randomized controlled trial, International Mycophenolate Mofetil Protocol to Reduce Outbreaks of Vasculitides (IMPROVE), to test the hypothesis that mycophenolate mofetil is more effective than azathioprine for preventing relapses in AAV. The trial was conducted at 42 centers in 11 European countries between April 2002 and January 2009 (42-month study). Eligible patients had newly diagnosed AAV (Wegener's granulomatosis or microscopic polyangiitis) and were aged 18–75 years at diagnosis.

Interventions: Patients were randomly assigned to azathioprine (starting at 2 mg/kg/day) or mycophenolate mofetil (starting at 2,000 mg/day) after induction of remission with cyclophosphamide and prednisolone.

Main Outcome Measures: The primary end point was relapse-free survival, which was assessed using a Cox proportional hazards model. The secondary end points were Vasculitis Damage Index, estimated glomerular filtration rate, and proteinuria.

Results: A total of 156 patients were assigned to azathioprine ($n=80$) or mycophenolate mofetil ($n=76$) and were followed up for a median of 39 months (interquartile range, 0.66–53.6 months). All patients were retained in the analysis by intention to treat. Relapses were more common in the mycophenolate mofetil group (42/76 patients) compared with the azathioprine group (30/80 patients), with an unadjusted hazard ratio (HR) for mycophenolate mofetil of 1.69 (95 % confidence interval [CI], 1.06–2.70; $P=.03$). Severe adverse events did not differ significantly between groups. There were 22 severe adverse events in 13 patients (16 %) in the azathioprine group and there were 8 severe adverse events in 8 patients (7.5 %) in the mycophenolate mofetil group (HR, 0.53 [95 % CI, 0.23–1.18]; $P=.12$). The secondary outcomes of Vasculitis Damage Index, estimated glomerular filtration rate, and proteinuria did not differ significantly between groups.

Conclusions: Among patients with AAV, mycophenolate mofetil was less effective than azathioprine for maintaining disease remission. Both treatments had similar adverse event rates.

Critical Appraisal

Parameters	Yes	No	Comment
Validity			
Is the **Randomization** Procedure well described?	+1		
Double **blinded**?		−2	Open label
Is the **sample size** calculation described/adequate?	+3		Powered to detect a reduction in relapses of 50 % by MMF

Parameters	Yes	No	Comment
Does it have a hard primary **end point**?	+1		Relapse-free survival as defined by BVAS scoring
Is the end point surrogate?		0	
Is the follow-up appropriate?	+1		39 months
Was there a **Bias**?		+2	
Is the dropout >25 %?		+1	
Is the analysis **ITT**?	+3		
Utility/usefulness			
Can the findings be generalized?	+1		
Are the findings easily translatable?	+1		
Was the NNT <100?			Not applicable as study designed to evaluate whether MMF could reduce relapse rate
Score	**75 %**		

Comments

As a result of its successful use in kidney transplantation and lupus nephritis [7], there was considerable interest in seeing whether mycophenolate mofetil (MMF) could reduce the risk of relapse in AAV particularly after a promising data from small pilot studies. MMF inhibits the inosine-monophosphate dehydrogenase DNA synthesis pathway and is a relatively lymphocyte-specific immunosuppressive therapy and therefore may be expected to be more effective in AAV than azathioprine. However, IMPROVE clearly demonstrates that MMF is actually inferior to azathioprine in maintaining remission in AAV with a significantly higher relapse rate. Furthermore, the trial is particularly relevant to nephrologists as patients had significant kidney disease with a median creatinine at baseline of between 2.7 and 2.9 mg/dl. IMPROVE establishes that there is no role for MMF as first-line maintenance therapy in AAV and that azathioprine is a cheap and highly effective agent for maintenance therapy.

Conclusions

For the last 40–50 years, the management of AAV has been largely driven by observational studies and AAV is a relatively rare condition with a wide array of presentations which can make conducting large-scale randomized trials difficult. However, the last 10–15 years have seen a number of large, well-conducted RCTs that have informed and changed practice. As well as encompassing end points such as death and dialysis, tools to assess vasculitis activity such as BVAS have enabled disease activity to be more objectively assessed in clinical trials. Although

BVAS/WG may be seen as a subjective tool, it has been validated as a sensitive tool of disease activity with good inter- and intra-observer reliability [8]. Severe renal disease has been an exclusion criteria for many of the trials, yet this is precisely the cohort of patients that need to be targeted in future studies as prognosis for AAV patients with severe renal disease is poor. While it may be difficult to recruit such patients into RCTs, the MEPEX and RITUXIVAS studies demonstrate that this can be done. Given the chronic, relapsing nature of the disease, it is essential that RCTs have long-term follow-up data as short-term data may be misleading. This was seen with both the MEPEX and CYCLOPS data where the long-term outcomes were much less promising than that suggested by the initial studies. Furthermore, it needs to be recognized that changes in estimated glomerular filtration rate (rather than measured glomerular rate) may not be an appropriate surrogate end point to evaluate the nephroprotective effect of therapies in AAV [9].

For induction of remission, cyclophosphamide combined with corticosteroids has been the gold standard for the last two decades. Rituximab has emerged as an alternative to cyclophosphamide, but one has to bear in mind that patients with severe renal impairment and pulmonary hemorrhage were excluded from the RAVE trial. This was reflected in the latest KDIGO guidelines which recommend the use of cyclophosphamide-based regimen as an initial therapy for induction and rituximab-based regimen as an alternative [10]. Rituximab offers an effective alternative as induction therapy in patients where there is a concern about fertility or toxicity with cyclophosphamide. The use of plasma exchange as an adjuvant therapy in patients with AAV and severe renal impairment (serum creatinine >500 µmol/L) improves renal survival in the short term but has little impact on longer-term outcomes.

Azathioprine remains the agent of choice for maintenance therapy following cyclophosphamide and corticosteroids induction. Rituximab on the other hand, used as a single course for induction with corticosteroids, has shown good results in maintaining remission and was non-inferior to cyclophosphamide-azathioprine-based regimen. Furthermore, the data from RAVE suggests that it may be of particular benefit in chronic, relapsing disease.

Rituximab might be seen as a game changer in the treatment of AAV as it is the only licensed treatment, but questions around long-term safety and efficacy remain. Its efficacy in advanced kidney disease has not been demonstrated by RCT evidence and long-term chronic administration is complicated by hypogammaglobulinemia which is problematic. The Rituximab for ANCA-associated Vasculitis Long-Term Follow-Up Study (RAVELOS) may provide answers to some of these questions (ClinicalTrial.gov: NCT01586858). There are other ongoing trials to look into its role as a preemptive maintenance therapy and its role in relapsing disease. One of the other biologic agents of interest is abatacept. The ABROGATE trial is expected to start recruitment soon looking into its efficacy in treatment of relapsing non-severe GPA (ClinicalTrials.gov: NCT02108860). Toxicity of the current therapies remains a key clinical issue, which leaves the door open for research in new less toxic therapies.

References

1. Mukhtyar C, Guillevin L, Cid M, Dasgupta B, De Groot K, Gross W, Hauser T, Hellmich B, Jayne D, Kallenberg C, et al. EULAR recommendations for the management of primary small and medium vessel vasculitis. Ann Rheum Dis. 2009;68(3):310–7.
2. Jennette J, Falk R, Gasim A. Pathogenesis of antineutrophil cytoplasmic autoantibody vasculitis. Curr Opin Nephrol Hypertens. 2011;20(3):263–70.
3. Smith RM, Jones RB, Jayne DR. Progress in treatment of ANCA-associated vasculitis. Arthritis Res Ther. 2012;14(2):210.
4. Hoffman G, Kerr G, Leavitt R, Hallahan C, Lebovics R, Travis W, Rottem M, Fauci A. Wegener granulomatosis: an analysis of 158 patients. Ann Intern Med. 1992;116(6):488–98.
5. Harper L, Morgan M, Walsh M, Hoglund P, Westman K, Flossmann O, Tesar V, Vanhille P, De Groot K, Luqmani R, et al. Pulse versus daily oral cyclophosphamide for induction of remission in ANCA-associated vasculitis: long-term follow-up. Ann Rheum Dis. 2012;71(6):955–60.
6. Walsh M, Casian A, Flossmann O, Westman K, Höglund P, Pusey C, Jayne D. Long-term follow-up of patients with severe ANCA-associated vasculitis comparing plasma exchange to intravenous methylprednisolone treatment is unclear. Kidney Int. 2013;84(2):397–402.
7. Dooley M, Jayne D, Ginzler E, Isenberg D, Olsen N, Wofsy D, Eitner F, Appel G, Contreras G, Lisk L, et al. Mycophenolate versus azathioprine as maintenance therapy for lupus nephritis. N Engl J Med. 2011;365(20):1886–95.
8. Stone J, Hoffman G, Merkel P, Min Y, Uhlfelder M, Hellmann D, et al. A disease-specific activity index for Wegener's granulomatosis: modification of the Birmingham Vasculitis Activity Score. Arthritis Rheum. 2001;44(4):912–20.
9. Rosansky S, Glassock R. Is a decline in estimated GFR an appropriate surrogate end point for renoprotection drug trials. Kidney Int. 2014;85(4):723–7.
10. Radhakrishnan J, Cattran D. The KDIGO practice guideline on glomerulonephritis: reading between the (guide) lines—application to the individual patient. Kidney Int. 2012;82(8):840–56.

Yangmin Zeng and Adeera Levin

Introduction

Clinical trials in the area of acute kidney injury (AKI) over the last decade have focused on attenuating the incidence of AKI (contrast nephropathy), managing AKI (diuretics, dopamine), or improving the outcomes of established AKI and kidney failure (intensity or type of dialysis). As a community we have struggled with matching our understanding of the physiology of kidney failure with testing hypotheses within complex clinical conditions using robust clinical studies to determine the best care for patients with AKI. The current limitations of our knowledge are a function of the difficulty of executing large-scale clinical trials in this area given the complexity of the patient population. This chapter highlights key studies that examine the role of N-acetylcysteine, hydration, and type of contrast agent on the incidence, severity, and duration of contrast nephropathy; the role of diuretics and dopamine on duration and severity of AKI; the utility of different methods of fluid removal in acute decompensated heart failure (ultrafiltration vs. diuretics); and the impact of different dialysis prescriptions or methods on patient outcomes. All of the studies selected reflect important questions, relevant in clinical practice. Due to limited ability to truly diagnose AKI, we may not be able to intervene in a timely manner, and our therapies, once kidney failure is established, are surely predicated on the etiology and duration of the AKI insult. Nonetheless, the studies described herein reflect the best available data to guide therapy and suggest that IV hydration to approximately 1 l is of benefit in attenuation of the onset of AKI in a number of high-risk situations,

that bolus vs. continuous infusions of loop diuretics are not substantially different, that low-dose dopamine does not improve kidney outcomes, that intensity of CRRT may not impact long-term outcomes, and that PD in acute situations may be a viable renal replacement method. Some of the studies are small (<500 patients) and all have their limitations. They represent our best understanding at the current time. In the coming decade, we need more robust, inclusive, and large-scale studies which address other important questions such as best way to diagnosis early AKI, appropriate early interventions to avoid dialysis, and timing of dialytic intervention in AKI. Of additional note is the problem of defining hard outcomes in AKI. While need for dialysis or death are certainly hard outcomes, the importance of small changes in serum creatinine cannot be underestimated. In numerous clinical and administrative databases, any change in serum creatinine above 26 μmol/l is associated with increased risk of CKD, CVD, hospitalizations, and death. Thus, we have chosen in this series to "accept" a change in serum creatinine as reasonable "hard end point" while acknowledging that not all would agree. In order to acknowledge the problems with a change in biomarker being a primary end point, we have altered the scoring system for this parameter in the tables below. In the meantime, we would hope that the results of these trials could be incorporated into clinical practice.

Acute kidney injury, **Dialysis dose**, **N-acetylcysteine**, **Hydration**, **Dopamine**, **Lasix**, **Peritoneal dialysis**, **Randomized controlled trials**, **Dialysis**

Y. Zeng, MD
A. Levin, BSc (Honours), MD, FRCPC, FACP (✉)
Division of Nephrology, Department of Medicine,
St. Paul's Hospital, University of British Columbia
1081 Burrard St, Vancouver, BC V6Z 1Y6, Canada
e-mail: yangmin.zeng@gmail.com;
alevin@providencehealth.bc.ca

Contrast Induced Acute Kidney Injury: Acetylcysteine

Publication: Acetylcysteine for prevention of renal outcomes in patients undergoing coronary and peripheral vascular angiography: main results from the randomized Acetylcysteine for Contrast-induced nephropathy Trial (ACT).

Authors: The ACT Investigators

Reference: Acetylcysteine for prevention of renal outcomes in patients undergoing coronary and peripheral vascular angiography: main results from the randomized Acetylcysteine for Contrast-induced nephropathy Trial (ACT). Circulation. 2011;124(11):1250–9.

Abstract

Background: It remains uncertain whether acetylcysteine prevents contrast-induced acute kidney injury.

Methods and Results: We randomly assigned 2,308 patients undergoing an intravascular angiographic procedure with at least one risk factor for contrast-induced acute kidney injury (age >70 years, renal failure, diabetes mellitus, heart failure, or hypotension) to acetylcysteine 1,200 mg or placebo. The study drugs were administered orally twice daily for two doses before and two doses after the procedure. The allocation was concealed (central Web-based randomization). All analysis followed the intention-to-treat principle. The incidence of contrast-induced acute kidney injury (primary end point) was 12.7 % in the acetylcysteine group and 12.7 % in the control group (relative risk, 1.00; 95 % confidence interval, 0.81–1.25; $P=0.97$). A combined end point of mortality or need for dialysis at 30 days was also similar in both groups (2.2 and 2.3 %, respectively; hazard ratio, 0.97; 95 % confidence interval, 0.56–1.69; $P=0.92$). Consistent effects were observed in all subgroups analyzed, including those with renal impairment.

Conclusions: In this large randomized trial, we found that acetylcysteine does not reduce the risk of contrast-induced acute kidney injury or other clinically relevant outcomes in at-risk patients undergoing coronary and peripheral vascular angiography.

Critical Appraisal

Parameters	Yes	No	Comment
Validity			
Is the **Randomization** Procedure well described?	+1		1:1 to acetylcysteine or placebo generated by permuted blocks of variable size and stratified by site
Double **blinded**?	+2		Healthcare staff, data collectors, and outcome assessors were all blinded
Is the **sample size** calculation described/ adequate?	+3		Estimated event rate of 15 % based on a prior meta-analysis. To detect 30 % relative risk reduction with 90 % power strived to include 2,300 patients

Parameters	Yes	No	Comment
Does it have a hard primary **end point**?	+.5		25 % elevation of serum creatinine above baseline 48–96 h after angiography
Is the end point surrogate?		0	
Is the follow-up appropriate?	+1		Followed to 30 days for mortality and need for RRT
Was there a **Bias**?		+2	
Is the dropout >25 %?		+1	36 patients did not have primary end point follow-up; 29 patients did not return to collect serum creatinine
Is the analysis **ITT**?	+3		
Utility/usefulness			
Can the findings be generalized?	+1		Only 5 % had eGFR <30 so this may not be generalized to the highest risk population
Was the NNT <100?			N/a: negative study
Score	**97 %**		Well-designed and well-conducted study

Summary and Conclusions

Acetylcysteine is a vasodilator and antioxidant that has been extensively investigated for the prevention of contrast-induced acute kidney injury (CIAKI). This study builds on the data from previous studies that demonstrated benefits of the agent in CIAKI. In 2000, Tepel et al. randomized 83 patients undergoing contrast-enhanced CT scanning to either oral acetylcysteine 600 mg twice daily on the day before and the day of the CT scan or placebo. They found that acetylcysteine in combination with adequate hydration reduced the incidence of CIAKI from 21 to 2 %, with a relative risk reduction of 90.5 % [1]. Since this seminal paper, more than 40 RCTs have compared acetylcysteine to placebo on the impact of patient mortality, need for RRT, or prevention of CIAKI. Unfortunately, these clinical trials have resulted in conflicting results with some finding substantial benefit, while others reporting no effect [2, 3]. Many of these trials were small and underpowered, so meta-analyses were performed in an attempt to improve the estimate of treatment effect [4]. Seven out of 11 meta-analyses found a net benefit of acetylcysteine for prevention of CIAKI, with some reporting up to 50 % relative risk reduction. However, there was significant clinical heterogeneity among the pooled RCTs. Meta-analyses that reported benefits of acetylcysteine generally did not account for heterogeneity between included trials [5]. As a result, treatment recommendations were difficult to make. This called for larger, well-powered, multicenter studies in order to clarify the muddy literature and determine the true effect of acetylcysteine in contrast nephropathy.

The ACT is the largest multicenter, double-blinded RCT testing the effects of acetylcysteine for the prevention of CIAKI to date. The authors decided on oral acetylcysteine 1,200 mg twice daily because of previous trials that showed benefit at higher doses [6]. There was no difference in the development of CIAKI, defined as a ≥25% increase above baseline in serum creatinine within 48–96 h after angiography. Secondary end points, including death and the need for dialysis at 30 days, were also similar.

This trial has noteworthy strengths including a large sample size, adequately powered; 98 % of patients with complete follow-up; and a 95 % compliance with study drugs. In addition, the trial represented a population at risk for CIAKI with 60 % with history of diabetes, 85 % with hypertension, and 10 % with known heart failure. Thus, the target population at high risk of CIAKI is included in this study.

Nonetheless, there are some drawbacks that limit the generalizability of this trial. Although the trial included 823 patients who had CKD, a majority of patients had mild CKD with eGFR 30–60. In fact, only 5 % of the patients had an eGFR <30. Therefore, ACT was underpowered to exclude a benefit of acetylcysteine for patients at highest risk for AKI [7]. Furthermore, albuminuria (urine albumin to creatinine ration UACR) was not factored in, despite it being a known risk factor. In addition, the baseline creatinine was obtained several months prior to enrolment, so that baseline renal function as reported may not be accurate in a temporal sense.

At present, there is no evidence that either oral or intravenous acetylcysteine can alter mortality or need for RRT after contrast-media administration to patients at risk for CIAKI [7]. Despite the lack of convincing evidence for benefit, the 2012 KDIGO guidelines suggest administration of acetylcysteine to patients at high risk as the agent is potentially beneficial, well-tolerated, and inexpensive [7]. This study suggests that despite these recommendations, it is not likely that the agent is of benefit. Given the quality and the totality of accumulating evidence, the use of *N*-acetylcysteine should not be recommended in guidelines, despite the acknowledgment that the medication is unlikely to be of harm.

Contrast Induced Acute Kidney Injury: Type of Contrast Media

Publication: Nephrotoxicity of ionic and nonionic contrast media in 1196 patients: A randomized trial

Author: Rudnick M et al.

Reference: Rudnick MR, Goldfarb S, Wexler L, Ludbrook PA, Murphy MJ, Halpern EF, Hill JA, Winniford M, Cohen MB, VanFossen DB. Nephrotoxicity of ionic and nonionic contrast media in 1196 patients: a randomized trial. The Iohexol Cooperative Study. Kidney Int. 1995;47(1):254–61.

Abstract

The incidence of nephrotoxicity occurring with the nonionic contrast agent, iohexol, and the ionic contrast agent, meglumine/sodium diatrizoate, was compared in 1,196 patients undergoing cardiac angiography in a prospective, randomized, double-blind multicenter trial. Patients were stratified into four groups: renal insufficiency (RI), diabetes mellitus (DM) both absent ($N=364$); RI absent, DM present ($N=318$); RI present, DM absent ($N=298$); and RI and DM both present ($N=216$). Serum creatinine levels were measured at −18–24, 0, and 24, 48, and 72 h following contrast administration. Prophylactic hydration was administered pre- and post-angiography. Acute nephrotoxicity (increase in serum creatinine of ≥1 mg/dl 48–72 h post-contrast) was observed in 42 (7 %) patients receiving diatrizoate compared to 19 (3 %) patients receiving iohexol, $P<0.002$. Differences in nephrotoxicity between the two contrast groups were confined to patients with RI alone or combined with DM. In a multivariate analysis, baseline serum creatinine, male gender, DM, volume of contrast agent, and RI were independently related to the risk of nephrotoxicity. Patients with RI receiving diatrizoate were 3.3 times as likely to develop acute nephrotoxicity compared to those receiving iohexol. Clinically severe adverse renal events were uncommon ($N=15$) and did not differ in incidence between contrast groups (iohexol $N=6$; diatrizoate $N=9$). In conclusion, in patients undergoing cardiac angiography, only those with preexisting RI alone or combined with DM are at higher risk for acute contrast nephrotoxicity

Critical Appraisal

Parameters	Yes	No	Comment
Validity			
Is the **Randomization** Procedure well described?		−1	No description given of randomization or allocation concealment. However, groups were well balanced in characteristics
Double **blinded**?	+2		Article claims it to be but not described
Is the **sample size** calculation described/adequate?	+3		Overall, 90 % power to detect difference of 10 and 5 %. Sample size 290 per each 4 groups provides 80 % for incidence of 15 and 7.5 %
Does it have a hard primary **end point**?	+.5		Increase in creatinine of 1 mg/dl or more within 48–72 h
Is the end point surrogate?		0	

Parameters	Yes	No	Comment
Is the follow-up appropriate?		−1	Follow up was from 48 to 72 h. 99 % had renal data at 48 h, but only 27 % had renal data at 72 h. No other clinical outcome data were recorded. This may have missed any CIAKI occurring *after* 48 h
Was there a **Bias**?		+2	Well balanced characteristics
Is the dropout <25 %?		+1	Paper did not specify how many were lost to follow-up explicitly, but out of 1,196 enrolled, 1,183 had outcome data in final analysis
Is the analysis **ITT**?		−3	Not stated
Utility/usefulness			
Can the findings be generalized?	+1		
Was the NNT <100?	+1		NNT = 26 overall; NNT = 6 in those with CKD and DM2
Score	**28 %**		Study with serious limitations

Summary and Conclusions

The osmolality of a contrast medium (CM) has been implicated in the pathophysiology of CIAKI. Hyperosmolar CM can cause direct injury of renal tubular cells if tubular fluid osmolality is more than its surrounding medullary osmolality. High osmolality may increase the intrinsic cytotoxicity of CM [8]. In addition, increased osmotic work load increases renal oxygen consumption by enhanced tubular sodium reabsorption, contributing to medullary hypoxia [9]. Finally, higher osmolality contributes to medullary hypoperfusion by changing the shape and rigidity of erythrocytes, making its passage through small renal vessels more difficult.

Contrast media are tri-iodinated benzene derivatives that use iodine for their radiopacity. Since a minimum concentration of iodine (250–400 mg I/mL) is required to achieve adequate opacification, the ratio of iodine atoms to dissolved particles and the iconicity of any contrast medium determine its osmolality [10]. High osmolality CM are ionic monomers with very high osmolalities ranging from 1,500 to 2,000 mOsm/kg. Second-generation low osmolar CM were developed using ionic dimers or nonionic monomers. Low osmolar CM achieved an osmolality of 500–850 mosmol/kg, which is still higher than that of plasma.

The best data comparing ionic, high osmolality contrast to nonionic low osmolality contrast iohexol in CI-AKI comes from Rudnick et al. Patients undergoing non-emergent diagnostic cardiac angiography stratified into four groups based on whether they had diabetes or CKD (defined as Scr >1.5 mg/dl for more than 6 weeks): Group 1: Non-diabetic and no CKD; Group 2 Diabetic and no CKD; Group 3: Nondiabetic and CKD; Group 4 Diabetic and CKD. Each of the four groups randomly received either high or low osmolar CM. The authors found that the nonionic, low osmolar CM was associated with significantly less nephrotoxicity than ionic, high osmolar CM in high-risk patients (CKD and diabetes) undergoing elective cardiac angiography.

The results of this landmark study revealed several important facts that have now become widely accepted in clinical practice. The realization that high osmolar contrast agents are associated with an increased risk of CIAKI has led to the use of low or iso-osmolar CM in the Western world [11]. However, studies comparing the nephrotoxicity of low osmolar versus iso-osmolar CM have been conflicting and unresolved.

Secondly, this study identified the fact that baseline renal impairment is the principal risk factor for CIAKI. This potentially heightens our awareness of the need to identify patients with decreased kidney function prior to the administration of contrast. This premise is key to many of the current guideline recommendations from national and international radiology groups. The identification of high-risk groups is essential in order to target preventive care. Diabetes is also a risk multiplier for CIAKI in a patient with CKD. Finally, the study found that higher volumes of contrast increased the risk of CIAKI. Subsequent studies also confirmed this finding.

Thus, KDIGO recommendations are that it is important to minimize contrast exposure in high-risk patients. Despite this, there is an important caveat: studies have suggested that concern over contrast-induced AKI leads to underutilization of imaging techniques, particularly coronary angiography, in high-risk patients with CKD [12] and that this ultimately may adversely impact patient care. The final decision to undergo diagnostic or therapeutic interventions with contrast exposure should be individualized, after considering risks and benefits and recognizing that the CIAKI can be mitigated with a number of strategies. The totality of evidence would suggest that performing contrast studies in CKD patients with appropriate proactive interventions would be prudent, where the information would be used to guide care.

Contrast Induced Acute Kidney Injury: Effects of Intravenous Hydration

Publication: Effects of hydration in contrast-induced acute kidney injury after primary angioplasty: a randomized, controlled trial.

Author: Maioli M, Toso A, Leoncini M, Gallopin M, Tedeschi D, Micheletti C, Bellandi F

Reference: Maioli M, Toso A, Leoncini M, Micheletti C, Bellandi F. Effects of hydration in contrast-induced acute kidney injury after primary angioplasty: a randomized, controlled trial. Circ Cardiovasc Interv. 2011;4(5):456–62.

Abstract

Background: Intravascular volume expansion represents a beneficial measure against contrast-induced acute kidney injury (CI-AKI) in patients undergoing elective angiographic procedures. However, the efficacy of this preventive strategy has not yet been established for patients with ST-elevation myocardial infarction (STEMI), who are at higher risk of this complication after primary percutaneous coronary intervention (PCI). In this randomized study we investigated the possible beneficial role of periprocedural intravenous volume expansion and we compared the efficacy of two different hydration strategies in patients with STEMI undergoing primary PCI. Methods and Results: We randomly assigned 450 STEMI patients to receive (1) preprocedure and postprocedure hydration of sodium bicarbonate (early hydration group), (2) postprocedure hydration of isotonic saline (late hydration group), or (3) no hydration (control group). The primary end point was the development of CI-AKI, defined as an increase in serum creatinine of ≥ 25 % or 0.5 mg/dL over the baseline value within 3 days after administration of the contrast medium. Moreover, we evaluated a possible relationship between the occurrence of CI-AKI and total hydration volume administered. There were no significant differences in baseline clinical, biochemical, and procedural characteristics in the three groups. Overall, CI-AKI occurred in 93 patients (20.6 %): the incidence was significantly lower in the early hydration group (12 %) with respect to both the late hydration group (22.7 %) and the control group (27.3 %) (P for trend=0.001). In hydrated patients (early and late hydration groups), lower infused volumes were associated with a significant increase in CI-AKI incidence, and the optimal cutoff point of hydration volume that best discriminates patients at higher risk was ≤ 960 mL.

Conclusions: Adequate intravenous volume expansion may prevent CI-AKI in patients undergoing primary PCI. A regimen of preprocedure and postprocedure hydration therapy with sodium bicarbonate appears to be more efficacious than postprocedure hydration only with isotonic saline.

Critical Appraisal

Parameters	Yes	No	Comment
Validity			
Is the **Randomization** Procedure well described?	+1		
Double **blinded**?		−2	
Is the **sample size** calculation described/ adequate?	+3		Powered to detect reduction of the primary end point of CIAKI from 25 % in the control group to 12.5 % in the hydration groups. The inclusion of 130 patients in each group allowed for a statistical power of 80 %
Does it have a hard primary **end point**?	+.5		Primary end point of the study was the development of CI-AKI, defined as an increase in serum creatinine of >25 % or 0.5 mg/dL over the baseline value within 3 days after administration of contrast medium
Is the end point surrogate?		0	CIAKI incidence was only outcome. No mortality/ morbidity or long-term outcome
Is the follow-up appropriate?	+1		
Was there a **Bias**?		+2	Despite using sodium bicarbonate for early hydration group and NS for late hydration group
Is the dropout >25 %?		+1	
Is the analysis **ITT**?		−3	Not explicitly stated
Utility/usefulness			
Can the findings be generalized?	+1		Generalizable to PCI population, but single-center study
Was the NNT <100?	+1		NNT=7
Score	**40 %**		Study with limitations

Summary and Conclusions

The protective effect of volume expansion in patients at risk for CIAKI come from the cumulative evidence of animal studies, observational analyses, and randomized clinical trials [13]. However, the exact mechanism by which volume expansion protects against CIAKI is speculative and remains unknown. Volume expansion may ameliorate the vasoconstrictive and cytotoxic effects of contrast through dilution. Maioli et al. conducted a three-arm open-label, single-center RCT to investigate the effect of intravenous hydration in patients at risk for CIAKI.

Patients presenting with STEMI undergoing urgent primary PCI, a particularly high-risk group, were randomly assigned in a 1:1:1 ratio to early hydration, late hydration, or no hydration. The early hydration group received a bolus of

3 cc/kg of sodium bicarbonate for a total of 1 h before PCI, followed by 1 cc/kg infusion for 12 h after PCI. The late hydration group received 0.9 % normal saline at 1 cc/kg for 12 after PCI. The decision to use sodium bicarbonate as a rapid bolus and normal saline as a slow infusion was based on the study done by Merten et al. Hydration rate was reduced to 0.5 mL/kg/h in patients with ejection fraction <40 % or NYHA class III–IV.

The early hydration had significantly less CIAKI compared to both late hydration and no hydration groups (12 % vs. 22 % and 27 %, respectively). The total volume of fluid administered had the greatest impact on the incidence of CIAKI. For instance, when patients were divided into tertiles of total volume of fluids received, the authors observed that those who received more volume had a lower incidence of CIAKI. Importantly, CIAKI rates were *similar* between early and late hydration groups when separated into tertiles of volume administered, suggesting the timing of fluid administration may be of less importance. A hydration volume of <960 cc was identified as the optimal cutoff point to predict risk for CIAKI incidence. Major adverse outcomes including mortality, need for hemofiltration, cardiogenic shock, and repeat vascularization did not differ between the three groups. Furthermore, patients with CIAKI had significantly higher mortality, cardiogenic shock, and longer hospitalization.

The significant benefit derived from volume expansion may have been partially due to the rehydration of those patients whose intravascular volume was depleted due to nausea, diaphoresis, or decreased oral intake. Volume resuscitation may have also benefitted those who were in preload-dependent cardiogenic shock.

This trial, focused on a high-risk patient group, has elegantly demonstrated that periprocedural volume expansion appears to mitigate the risk for CIAKI. Another randomized controlled trial of 1,620 patients undergoing elective and emergent cardiac angiography also found that volume expansion with NS was more beneficial than half NS [14]. Furthermore, the hydration protocol used in this trial did not result in more adverse events such as heart failure. The optimal volume administered probably needs to be individualized, but the results of this study estimate that 1 L of isotonic crystalloid is reasonable and safe in hydration protocols in high-risk patients undergoing contrast administration.

Contrast Induced Acute Kidney Injury: Comparison of Sodium Bicarbonate Versus Normal Saline in Prevention of Contrast Nephropathy

Publication: Sodium bicarbonate vs sodium chloride for the prevention of contrast medium-induced nephropathy in patients undergoing coronary angiography: a randomized trial

Authors: Brar SS, Shen AY, Jorgensen MB, Kotlewski A, Aharonian VJ, Desai N, Ree M, Shah AI, Burchette RJ

Reference: : Brar SS, Shen AY, Jorgensen MB, Kotlewski A, Aharonian VJ, Desai N, Ree M, Shah AI, Burchette RJ (2008) Sodium bicarbonate vs sodium chloride for the prevention of contrast medium-induced nephropathy in patients undergoing coronary angiography: a randomized trial. JAMA 2008;300(9):1038–46.

Abstract

Context: Sodium bicarbonate has been suggested as a possible strategy for prevention of contrast medium-induced nephropathy, a common cause of renal failure associated with prolonged hospitalization, increased health care costs, and substantial morbidity and mortality.

Objectives: To determine if sodium bicarbonate is superior to sodium chloride for preventing contrast medium-induced nephropathy in patients with moderate to severe chronic kidney dysfunction who are undergoing coronary angiography.

Design, Setting, and Patients: Randomized, controlled, single-blind study conducted between January 2, 2006, and January 31, 2007, and enrolling 353 patients with stable renal disease who were undergoing coronary angiography at a single US center. Included patients were 18 years or older and had an estimated glomerular filtration rate of 60 mL/min per 1.73 m(2) or less and 1 or more of diabetes mellitus, history of congestive heart failure, hypertension, or age older than 75 years.

Interventions: Patients were randomized to receive either sodium chloride (n=178) or sodium bicarbonate (n=175) administered at the same rate (3 mL/kg for 1 hour before coronary angiography, decreased to 1.5 mL/kg per hour during the procedure and for 4 hours after the completion of the procedure).

Main outcome measure: The primary end point was a 25 % or greater decrease in the estimated glomerular filtration rate on days 1 through 4 after contrast exposure.

Results: Median patient age was 71 (interquartile range, 65–76) years, and 45 % had diabetes mellitus. The groups were well matched for baseline characteristics. The primary end point was met in 13.3 % of the sodium bicarbonate group and 14.6 % of the sodium chloride group (relative risk, 0.94; 95 % confidence interval, 0.55–1.60; $P = .82$). In patients randomized to receive sodium bicarbonate vs. sodium chloride, the rates of death, dialysis, myocardial infarction, and cerebrovascular events did not differ significantly at 30 days (1.7 % vs. 1.7 %, 0.6 % vs. 1.1 %, 0.6 % vs. 0 %, and 0 % vs. 2.2 %, respectively) or at 30 days to 6 months (0.6 % vs. 2.3 %, 0.6 % vs. 1.1 %, 0.6 % vs. 2.3 %, and 0.6 % vs. 1.7 %, respectively) ($P > .10$ for all).

Conclusions: The results of this study do not suggest that hydration with sodium bicarbonate is superior to hydration with sodium chloride for the prevention of contrast medium-induced nephropathy in patients with moderate to severe chronic kidney disease who are undergoing coronary angiography.

Critical Appraisal

Parameters	Yes	No	Comment
Validity			
Is the **Randomization** Procedure well described?	+1		Yes
Double **blinded**?		−2	Patient not blinded. Physician and lab personnel blinded
Is the **sample size** calculation described/ adequate?	+3		
Does it have a hard primary **end point**?	+1		Outcome of 25 % reduction in eGFR, 25 % increase in serum creatinine, 30 day mortality and need for RRT
Is the end point surrogate?		0	
Is the follow-up appropriate?	+1		Clinical outcomes followed for up to 6 months post study
Was there a **Bias**?		+2	
Is the dropout <25 %?		+1	No loss to follow up. But 12 % of patients had no baseline eGFR and excluded
Is the analysis **ITT**?	+3		Yes
Utility/usefulness			
Can the findings be generalized?	+1		Patients for elective PCI, single-center study
Was the NNT <100?			N/a: negative study
Score	**73 %**		Well-designed and well-conducted study

Summary and Conclusions

The alkalizing property of sodium bicarbonate solutions has been thought to give protection against free radicals. There has been considerable interest regarding the use of sodium bicarbonate in the prevention of CIAKI.

Brar et al. conducted the best randomized controlled trial to date addressing this question. The trial was a single-center, single-blind study that randomized 353 patients undergoing elective coronary angiography to either saline or sodium bicarbonate before and after iso-osmolar contrast medium administration. Importantly, the infusion protocol was identical for both fluid types.

The overall rate of CIAKI, defined by a >25 % reduction of eGFR or >25 % increase of serum creatinine, was similar in both groups. The overall mortality at 6 months was 3.1 % among all randomized patients vs. 9.8 % among the patients developing contrast-induced nephropathy. At 6 months follow-up, the mortality rate was similar between sodium chloride and sodium bicarbonate (3.9 % and 2.3). Only six patients needed dialysis at 6 months with similar rates

between the two groups. Notably, all four patients who needed dialysis due to CIAKI died at 6 months, illustrating that the need for dialysis after CIAKI portends a poor prognosis after PCI.

A major strength of this study is that it reported clinical adverse events at 30 days and 6 months after contrast exposure among all randomized patients. Most previous trials have had limited follow-up post contrast administration. The trial was adequately powered and met its enrolment goals.

The population represented in this trial was at moderate risk for CIAKI. The trial excluded very high-risk patient populations, such as those with cardiogenic shock and acute myocardial infarction. Also, only ~6 % of patients had severe renal impairment eGFR <30 at baseline. Other limitations included the fact the physicians performing the procedure were not blinded and its single-center design.

The cumulative evidence from several meta-analyses and randomized controlled trials examining the benefit of sodium bicarbonate in CIKAI yields conflicting results. A systematic review recently concluded a lack of evidence for sodium bicarbonate. It commented that the earlier, smaller trials tended to show more benefit, whereas more recent, larger trials showed neutral effect [15, 16]. Since no trial has demonstrated that sodium bicarbonate is inferior to normal saline, the most recent KDIGO recommendations are that either normal saline or sodium bicarbonate can be used in high-risk patients [17]. However, since isotonic bicarbonate solutions are not as readily available, there is a potential for mixing errors with using sodium bicarbonate.

Thus, pragmatically, any isotonic hydration strategy may be of benefit. Difficulties with access and mixing issues are not seen with the use of premixed normal saline. In addition, depending on the facility, preparation of isotonic sodium bicarbonate solutions takes time and resources. Given the totality of evidence, it may be that isotonic saline solution may be preferable in emergent situations prior to contrast administration. Nonetheless, any hydration protocol is better than no hydration protocol in vulnerable populations.

Prevention of Acute Kidney Injury: Role of Loop Diuretics

Publication: High-dose furosemide for established ARF: a prospective, randomized, double-blind, placebo-controlled, multicenter trial

Authors: Cantarovich F, Rangoonwala B (High-Dose Furosemide in Acute Renal Failure Study Group)

Reference: Cantarovich F, Rangoonwala B, Lorenz H, Verho M, Esnault VLM, High-Dose Furosemide in Acute Renal Failure Study G. High-dose furosemide for established ARF: a prospective, randomized, double-blind, placebo-controlled, multicenter trial. Am J Kidney Dis. 2004;44(3): 402–9.

Abstract

Background: The effect of furosemide on the survival and renal recovery of patients presenting with acute renal failure (ARF) is still debated.

Methods: Three hundred thirty-eight patients with ARF requiring dialysis therapy were randomly assigned to the administration of either furosemide (25 mg/kg/day intravenously or 35 mg/kg/day orally) or matched placebo, with stratification according to severity at presentation. The primary end point was survival. The secondary end point was number of dialysis sessions. Tertiary end points included time on dialysis therapy, time to achieve a serum creatinine level less than 2.26 mg/dL (<200 μmol/l), and time to reach a 2 L/day diuresis.

Results: There were no differences in survival and renal recovery rates between the two groups. Time to achieve a 2-L/day diuresis was shorter with furosemide (5.7 ± 5.8 days) than placebo (7.8 ± 6.8 days; $P = 0.004$). Overall, 148 patients achieved a urine output of at least 2 L/day during the study period (94 of 166 patients; 57 %) with furosemide versus 54 of 164 patients (33 %) with placebo ($P < 0.001$). However, there were no significant differences in number of dialysis sessions and time on dialysis therapy between the furosemide and placebo groups, even in the subgroup of patients reaching a 2-L/day diuresis.

Conclusion: High-dose furosemide helps maintain urinary output, but does not have an impact on the survival and renal recovery rate of patients with established ARF.

Critical Appraisal

Parameters	Yes	No	Comment
Validity			
Is the **Randomization** Procedure well described?		−1	Assigned by "random plan" and stratified based on severity of illness. Allocation concealment not fully described
Double **blinded**?	+2		A pharmaceutical company provided blinded medications
Is the **sample size** calculation described/adequate?	+3		80 % power, 45 % of event rate, 15 % difference
Does it have a hard primary **end point**?	+1		The primary end point was survival at the end of the 1-month for patients not showing a recovery in renal function or 7 days after RRT discontinuation for patients showing a recovery in renal function
Is the end point surrogate?		0	

Parameters	Yes	No	Comment
Is the follow-up appropriate?	+1		
Was there a **Bias**?		−2	Imbalanced baseline characteristics: Lasix group had more diabetics, more severe renal failure, and more septic shock patients
Is the dropout <25 %?		+1	None lost to follow-up
Is the analysis **ITT**?	+3		
Utility/usefulness			
Can the findings be generalized?		−1	AKI due to mostly shock and sepsis. Few diabetics enrolled
Was the NNT <100?			N/a: negative study
Score	**33 %**		Study with serious limitations

Summary and Conclusions

Loop diuretics have been postulated to protect against AKI via several mechanisms. Loop diuretics have been shown in animal models to reduce metabolic demands of injured tubular cells, prevent tubular obstruction by flushing tubular debris, improve renal blood flow, and even attenuate apoptosis in renal tubular cells [18–20]. Also, oliguria is a known poor prognostic indicator in patients with AKI and further increases the risk of death compared to nonoliguric AKI [21, 22]. Oliguric AKI makes fluid management difficult and there is mounting evidence that fluid overload in AKI is independently associated with increased mortality [23]. Therefore, many clinicians wondered whether diuretics converting an oliguric AKI to a nonoliguric one impacts clinical outcomes [24–27].

Catarovich et al. conducted the largest prospective, double-blinded, placebo-controlled trial examining whether furosemide improves the survival rate in patients with established AKI to date. There was no difference in survival or renal recovery at 1 month despite the time to reach 2 L per day of diuresis was shorter in the furosemide arm.

Some key elements of the trial design need to be highlighted. First, this is a study of patients with established ATN since the authors carefully excluded patients with dehydration and prerenal failure using urinary-plasma osmolarity ratio, urinary sodium, and volume filling measurements. Secondly, the trial excluded any patients showing renal recovery, so that all the patients included in the final analysis eventually needed renal replacement therapy. Finally, a high dose of 25 mg/kg furosemide IV to a maximum of 2 g/day was used in the study to ensure effective delivery of the drug to its site of action in the tubular lumen. Interestingly, although this dose was in the upper range when compared prior controlled trials, there were no increased ototoxicity in the furosemide arm.

The results of this trial need to be considered within its limitations. Only a minority of patients, approximately 14 % had diabetes. Baseline renal functions of the patients were not available. Other comorbidities were not mentioned nor controlled for. More importantly, the furosemide and placebo groups were not balanced at randomization: more patients with diabetes and septic shock were in the furosemide arm. Renal impairment was also worse in the furosemide group at randomization, despite being similar before the first dialysis session. These factors may have masked a possible beneficial effect of furosemide.

Despite these limitations, this study in conjunction with other studies reveals that there is no convincing evidence to support the use of loop diuretics in order to attenuate the severity of AKI or improve outcomes. A systematic review and meta-analysis by Ho and Power included six studies that used furosemide to treat AKI, with doses ranging from 600 to 3,400 mg/day [27]. No significant reduction was found for in-hospital mortality or for RRT requirement. Thus, loop diuretics in early or established AKI may help with fluid management, but the strategy does not have proven benefit to attenuate the course of AKI or patient outcomes.

Prevention of Acute Kidney Injury: Synthetic Colloids

Publication: Hydroxyethyl starch or saline for fluid resuscitation in intensive care (CHEST)

Authors: Myburgh et al.

Reference: Myburgh JA, Finfer S, Bellomo R, Billot L, Cass A, Gattas D, Glass P, Lipman J, Liu B, McArthur C, McGuinness S, Rajbhandari D, Taylor CB, Webb SA. Hydroxyethyl starch or saline for fluid resuscitation in intensive care. N Engl J Med. 2012;367(20):1901–11.

Abstract

Background: The safety and efficacy of hydroxyethyl starch (HES) for fluid resuscitation have not been fully evaluated, and adverse effects of HES on survival and renal function have been reported.

Methods: We randomly assigned 7,000 patients who had been admitted to an intensive care unit (ICU) in a 1:1 ratio to receive either 6 % HES with a molecular weight of 130 kD and a molar substitution ratio of 0.4 (130/0.4, Voluven) in 0.9 % sodium chloride or 0.9 % sodium chloride (saline) for all fluid resuscitation until ICU discharge, death, or 90 days after randomization. The primary outcome was death within 90 days. Secondary outcomes included acute kidney injury and failure and treatment with renal replacement therapy.

Results: A total of 597 of 3,315 patients (18.0 %) in the HES group and 566 of 3,336 (17.0 %) in the saline group died (relative risk in the HES group, 1.06; 95 % confidence interval [CI], 0.96–1.18; $P=0.26$). There was no significant difference in mortality in six predefined subgroups. Renal replacement therapy was used in 235 of 3,352 patients (7.0 %) in the HES group and 196 of 3,375 (5.8 %) in the saline group (relative risk, 1.21; 95 % CI, 1.00–1.45; $P=0.04$). In the HES and saline groups, renal injury occurred in 34.6 and 38.0 % of patients, respectively ($P=0.005$), and renal failure occurred in 10.4 and 9.2 % of patients, respectively ($P=0.12$). HES was associated with significantly more adverse events (5.3 % vs. 2.8 %, $P<0.001$).

Conclusions: In patients in the ICU, there was no significant difference in 90-day mortality between patients resuscitated with 6 % HES (130/0.4) or saline. However, more patients who received resuscitation with HES were treated with renal replacement therapy.

Critical Appraisal

Parameters	Yes	No	Comment
Validity			
Is the **Randomization** Procedure well described?	+1		
Double **blinded**?	+2		
Is the **sample size** calculation described/adequate?	+3		Power of 90 % to detect an absolute difference of 3.5 percentage points in 90-day mortality on the basis of an estimated baseline mortality of 26 %
Does it have a hard primary **end point**?	+1		Primary: 90 days mortality. Secondary: incidence of AKI by RIFLE and use of RRT
Is the end point surrogate?		0	
Is the follow-up appropriate?	+1		
Was there a **Bias**?		+2	
Is the dropout <25 %?		+1	Approximately 2.5 % were lost to follow-up
Is the analysis **ITT**?	+3		
Utility/usefulness			
Can the findings be generalized?		−1	Almost half of all screened patient excluded in trial, limiting its generalizability
Was the NNT <100?			N/a: negative study
Score	**87 %**		Well-designed and well-conducted study

Summary and Conclusions

Colloids are used in for patients with hypovolemia secondary to sepsis because they are thought to remain in the intravascular space longer and require less amount of fluid for resuscitation compared with crystalloids. Hydroxyethyl starches (HES) are synthetic colloids that vary in concentration, molecular weight, and hydroxyethyl moieties. The concentration of colloid in solution determines its osmotic pressure effect. A 10 % HES is hyper-oncotic to plasma and is a better blood volume expander than 6 % iso-oncotic HES [28]. Recently, concerns about hyper-oncotic HES emerged after RCTs and meta-analyses reported increasing rates of AKI associated with its use [29]. HES may cause AKI by increased uptake of the starch into the proximal renal epithelial cells inducing "osmotic nephrosis-like lesions," tubular obstruction caused by the production of hyperviscous urine, and renal interstitial inflammation [30]. In addition, high molecular substitution starch may impair coagulation by decreasing factor VIII and vWF. These concerns have led to a widespread usage of iso-oncotic starches with lower molecular and substitution ratios for fluid resuscitation over the last decade in critically ill patients.

However, the large multicenter, double-blinded randomized controlled trial by Myburg et al. demonstrated that iso-oncotic 6 % HES is *still* associated with an increased risk of AKI compared to crystalloid. The study randomized 7,000 patients admitted to the ICU to receive either 6 % HES (130/0.4) in 0.9 % saline (Voluven) or normal saline for 90 days. The HES group and normal saline group had similar mortality at 90 days (18 % vs. 17 %). Significantly more renal replacement therapy was required in the HES compared to the saline group (7 % vs. 5.8 %), with a number needed to harm of 83. Subgroup analysis showed a trend towards greater mortality in the HES group. Furthermore, HES had higher rates of pruritus and rash. Interestingly the study did not find a large volume sparing effect of HES, in agreement with prior blinded studies.

This trial was well designed and adequately powered. Bias was minimized by concealing allocation and blinding all trial procedures. Study outcomes were meaningful and follow-up of 90 days was reasonable for this population. Limitation of this study includes its extensive exclusion criteria such as patients considered unlikely to survive, intracranial hemorrhage, transfers from another ICU, and postcardiac surgery. In fact, out of 19,475 patients screened, 10,612 were excluded for ineligibility. These exclusions may limit the generalizability of the results.

This study adds to the growing body of literature that synthetic starches used for resuscitation increase the risk of AKI in critically ill patients. Perner et al. also conducted a well-designed study that found that the use of 6 % HES (130/0.42) needed more renal replacement therapy compared to Lactated Ringer's in patients with septic shock (NNH=17) as well as increased mortality at 90 days in the HES group (NNH=13). The discrepancy in the mortality may be due to the fact CHEST enrolled a less sick population compared to Perner et al.

Overall, given the evidence of harm and lack of clinical benefit, HES should not be used for fluid resuscitation for critically ill patients with severe sepsis.

Prevention of Acute Kidney Injury: Dopamine

Publication: Low-dose dopamine in patients with early renal dysfunction: a placebo-controlled randomised trial

Authors: Bellomo et al.

Reference: Bellomo R, Chapman M, Finfer S, Hickling K, Myburgh J. Low-dose dopamine in patients with early renal dysfunction: a placebo-controlled randomised trial. Australian and New Zealand Intensive Care Society (ANZICS) Clinical Trials Group. Lancet. 2000;356(9248):2139–43.

Abstract

Background: Low-dose dopamine is commonly administered to critically ill patients in the belief that it reduces the risk of renal failure by increasing renal blood flow. However, these effects have not been established in a large randomized controlled trial, and use of dopamine remains controversial. We have done a multicenter, randomized, double-blind, placebo-controlled study of low-dose dopamine in patients with at least two criteria for the systemic inflammatory response syndrome and clinical evidence of early renal dysfunction (oliguria or increase in serum creatinine concentration).

Methods: 328 patients admitted to 23 participating intensive care units (ICUs) were randomly assigned a continuous intravenous infusion of low-dose dopamine (2 microg kg(-1) min(-1)) or placebo administered through a central venous catheter while in the ICU. The primary end point was the peak serum creatinine concentration during the infusion. Analyses excluded four patients with major protocol violations.

Findings: The groups assigned dopamine ($n=161$) and placebo ($n=163$) were similar in terms of baseline characteristics, renal function, and duration of trial infusion. There was no difference between the dopamine and placebo groups in peak serum creatinine concentration during treatment (245 [SD 144] vs. 249 [147] µmol/l; $p=0.93$), in the increase from baseline to highest value during treatment (62 [107] vs. 66 [108] µmol/l; $p=0.82$), or in the numbers of patients whose serum creatinine concentration exceeded 300 µmol/l (56 vs. 56; $p=0.92$) or who required renal replacement therapy (35 vs. 40; $p=0.55$). Durations of ICU stay (13 [14] vs. 14 [15] days; $p=0.67$) and of hospital stay (29 [27] vs. 33 [39] days; $p=0.29$) were also similar. There were 69 deaths in the dopamine group and 66 in the placebo group.

Interpretation: Administration of low-dose dopamine by continuous intravenous infusion to critically ill patients at risk of renal failure does not confer clinically significant protection from renal dysfunction.

Critical Appraisal

Parameters	Yes	No	Comment
Validity			
Is the **Randomization** Procedure well described?	+1		Coded medication packs
Double **blinded**?	+2		Caregivers, outcomes assessors, data analysts
Is the **sample size** calculation described/adequate?	+3		From the final SD for the control and intervention groups, this study had 90 % power to detect a difference of more than 25 % in peak serum creatinine between the groups
Does it have a hard primary **end point**?		−1	Peak serum creatinine not an appropriate primary end point in this study
Is the end point surrogate?		0	Secondary end point reported survival until hospital or ICU discharge and need for RRT
Is the follow-up appropriate?	+1		
Was there a **Bias**?		+2	
Is the dropout <25 %?		+1	
Is the analysis **ITT**?	+3		Not stated, but they included patients with minor protocol violations. The inclusion/exclusion of these patients did not affect final results
Utility/usefulness			
Can the findings be generalized?	+1		
Was the NNT <100?			N/a: negative study
Score	87 %		Well-designed and well-conducted study

Summary and Conclusions

Dopamine infused at low doses (0.5–3 mcg/kg/min) dilates interlobular arteries as well as afferent and efferent arterioles [31]. In animals and healthy volunteers, low-dose dopamine increases renal blood flow and glomerular filtration rate [32]. At higher concentrations above 5 mcg/kg/min, dopamine activates alpha receptors and causes renal vasoconstriction [31]. Dopamine also promotes natriuresis by inhibiting proximal tubule sodium reabsorption [33]. These appealing properties lead to the embracement use of low-dose dopamine to preserve renal function in patients at risk for AKI. However, multiple recent studies including well-designed RCTs and systematic reviews have shown such therapy is ineffective and may cause harm.

The ANZICS Trial is the second largest study to date examining this topic. This multicenter, double-blinded study randomized critically ill patients with early AKI to low-dose dopamine infusion or placebo. The study reflected a sick population with over >40 % mortality and 25 % of the patients requiring RRT. This study unequivocally showed that low-dose dopamine has no effect on serum creatinine, requirements for renal replacement therapy, or duration of stay in the intensive care unit. The mortality rate was similar in the dopamine and placebo groups. In contrast to previous studies, ANZICS did not find more adverse events in the dopamine group.

A comprehensive systematic review and meta-analysis by Friedrich et al. also concluded that low-dose dopamine had no effect on mortality or renal replacement therapy [34]. Post hoc analysis excluding the large ANZICS study did not change the results. Although the meta-analysis did not find evidence for harm, there is ample literature suggesting dopamine can trigger arrhythmias and myocardial ischemia, decrease intestinal blood flow, cause hypopituitarism, and suppress T-cell function [35]. As a result KDIGO recommends abandoning the use of low-dose dopamine for the prevention and therapy of AKI. All of the evidence supports the nonuse of low-dose dopamine in AKI.

Renal Replacement Therapy in Acute Kidney Injury: Intermittent Versus Continuous Hemodialysis

Publication: Intermittent versus continuous renal replacement therapy for acute kidney injury patients admitted to the intensive care unit: results of a randomized clinical trial

Authors: Robert L. Lins, Monique M. Elseviers, Patricia Van der Niepen, Eric Hoste, Manu L. Malbrain, Pierre Damas and Jacques Devriendt for the SHARF investigators

Reference: Lins RL, Elseviers MM, Van der Niepen P, Hoste E, Malbrain ML, Damas P, Devriendt J. Intermittent versus continuous renal replacement therapy for acute kidney injury patients admitted to the intensive care unit: results of a randomized clinical trial. Nephrol Dial Transplant. 2009;24(2):512–8. doi:10.1093/ndt/gfn560.

Abstract

Background: There is uncertainty on the effect of different dialysis modalities for the treatment of patients with acute kidney injury (AKI) admitted to the intensive care unit (ICU). This controlled clinical trial performed in the framework of the multicenter SHARF 4 study (Stuivenberg Hospital Acute Renal Failure) aimed to investigate the outcome in patients with AKI, stratified according to severity of disease and randomized to different treatment options.

Methods: This was a multicenter prospective randomized controlled trial with stratification according to severity of disease expressed by the SHARF score. ICU patients were eligible for inclusion when serum creatinine was >2 mg/dL, and RRT was initiated. The selected patients were randomized to intermittent (IRRT) or continuous renal replacement therapy (CRRT).

Results: A total of 316 AKI patients were randomly assigned to IRRT ($n = 144$) or CRRT ($n = 172$). The mean age was 66 (range 18–96); 59 % were male. Intention-to-treat analysis revealed a mortality of 62.5 % in IRRT compared to 58.1 % in CRRT ($P = 0.430$). No difference between IRRT and CRRT could be observed in the duration of ICU stay or hospital stay. In survivors, renal recovery at hospital discharge was comparable between both groups. Multivariate analysis, including the SHARF score and APACHE II and SOFA scores for correction of disease severity, showed no difference in mortality between both treatment modalities. This result was confirmed in prespecified subgroup analysis (elderly, patients with sepsis, heart failure, ventilation) and after exclusion of possible confounders (early mortality, delayed ICU admission).

Conclusions: Modality of RRT, either CRRT or IRRT, had no impact on the outcome in ICU patients with AKI. Both modalities need to be considered as complementary in the treatment of AKI.

Critical Appraisal

Parameters	Yes	No	Comment
Validity			
Is the **Randomization** Procedure well described?	+1		Stratified block randomization by severity of illness using a computer system
Double **blinded**?		−2	
Is the **sample size** calculation described/ adequate?		−3	80 % power to detect a 10 % difference between two arms, assuming overall mortality of 50 %. 407 patients needed in each treatment group. Recruitment ended early due to change in policies and limited centers eligible
Does it have a hard primary **end point**?	+1		Mortality, duration of ICU, and hospital stay
Is the end point surrogate?		0	
Is the follow-up appropriate?	+1		Outcomes evaluated at 10 and 30 days

Parameters	Yes	No	Comment
Was there a **Bias**?		+2	
Is the dropout <25 %?		+1	None lost to follow-up
Is the analysis **ITT?**	+3		
Utility/usefulness			
Can the findings be generalized?	+1		Multicenter, but excluded patients with CKD (sCr >1.5) at baseline. 50 % of eligible population was excluded for nonmedical reasons
Was the NNT <100?			N/A: negative study
Score	**33 %**		Study with serious limitations as it was severely underpowered due to poor recruitment

Summary and Conclusions

In intensive care units, nearly a quarter of patients are diagnosed with AKI and a significant proportion will require renal replacement therapy (RRT). Compared to intermittent hemodialysis (IHD), continuous renal replacement therapy (CRRT) theoretically offers the advantage of improved tolerability in patients with hemodynamic instability and its ability to remove pro-inflammatory cytokines [36]. The ideal modality for RRT in critically ill patients has been debated over the last two decades. The results from retrospective and observational trials have been conflicting with varying conclusions ranging from improved survival [37] to increased mortality [38] to no difference in outcome [39] associated with CRRT. Comparing outcomes between IHD and CRRT in retrospective cohorts is subject to selection bias since patients treated with CRRT are more likely to have greater severity of illness and more hemodynamically unstable. Subsequent high quality RCTs and prospective cohort studies showed no evidence for better survival or better clinical outcome in patients treated with CRRT.

Lins et al. conducted a multicenter trial that randomized 316 patients from nine Belgian centers to receive either CRRT or daily IHD. Within each center, patients were stratified to severity of illness using the SHARF score, a validated scoring system previously developed by the authors. For comparison purposes, the SOFA and APACHE scores were reported and well matched at baseline. Daily IHD were treated for four sessions averaging four hours per session. The CRRT group was treated for a median of 4 days at an average dose of 21 cc/kg. Eleven patients crossed over from IHD to CRRT for mainly hemodynamic instability, while 12 patients crossed over from CRRT to IHD for coagulation problems. The authors observed no difference in overall mortality in daily IHD versus CRRT at 10 and 30 days after diagnosis of AKI. The overall mortality in the population studied was high at approximately 60 %. In addition, there was no mortality difference within each of the SHARF classes. Finally, no difference was observed in the duration of ICU stay, hospital stay, or eGFR between the two treatment groups.

A major limitation of this study was that it failed to meet its initial recruitment goal by approximately 500 patients. The major barrier to recruitment was that there were limited sites that provided both CRRT and IHD. Therefore, this study is underpowered to detect a difference in its primary outcome. Furthermore, out of the eligible population, only half were randomized and included in the trial. This may have introduced selection bias into the study. However, the authors also analyzed the excluded, nonrandomized patients and did not detect any differences in outcome.

Three systematic reviews and meta-analyses of modality for renal support in AKI have been published in the last 5 years, and none have found differences in mortality or renal recovery [40]. The latest KDIGO guidelines also recommend that both intermittent and continuous renal replacement therapies be used as complementary therapies. CRRT may be used preferentially for patients with hemodynamic instability and those with acute brain injury, increased intracranial pressure, or generalized brain edema as there is some evidence that IHD is associated with greater decreases in cerebral perfusion compared to CRRT [41].

Results: Of the 1,508 enrolled patients, 747 were randomly assigned to higher-intensity therapy, and 761 to lower-intensity therapy with continuous venovenous hemodiafiltration. Data on primary outcomes were available for 1,464 patients (97.1 %): 721 in the higher-intensity group and 743 in the lower-intensity group. The two study groups had similar baseline characteristics and received the study treatment for an average of 6.3 and 5.9 days, respectively ($P=0.35$). At 90 days after randomization, 322 deaths had occurred in the higher-intensity group and 332 deaths in the lower-intensity group, for a mortality of 44.7 % in each group (odds ratio, 1.00; 95 % confidence interval [CI], 0.81–1.23; $P=0.99$). At 90 days, 6.8 % of survivors in the higher-intensity group (27 of 399), as compared with 4.4 % of survivors in the lower-intensity group (18 of 411), were still receiving renal replacement therapy (odds ratio, 1.59; 95 % CI, 0.86–2.92; $P=0.14$). Hypophosphatemia was more common in the higher-intensity group than in the lower-intensity group (65 % vs. 54 %, $P<0.001$).

Conclusions: In critically ill patients with acute kidney injury, treatment with higher-intensity continuous renal replacement therapy did not reduce mortality at 90 days.

Renal Replacement Therapy in Acute Kidney Injury: Intensity of Continuous Renal Replacement Therapy

Publication: Intensity of renal support in critically ill patients with acute kidney injury

Authors: Bellomo R et al. (RENAL Replacement Therapy Study Investigators)

Reference: Bellomo R, Cass A, Cole L, Finfer S, Gallagher M, Lo S, McArthur C, McGuinness S, Myburgh J, Norton R, Scheinkestel C, Su S. Intensity of continuous renal-replacement therapy in critically ill patients. N Engl J Med. 2009;361(17):1627–38.

Abstract

Background: The optimal intensity of continuous renal replacement therapy remains unclear. We conducted a multicenter, randomized trial to compare the effect of this therapy, delivered at two different levels of intensity, on a 90-day mortality among critically ill patients with acute kidney injury.

Methods: We randomly assigned critically ill adults with acute kidney injury to continuous renal replacement therapy in the form of postdilution continuous venovenous hemodiafiltration with an effluent flow of either 40 ml per kilogram of body weight per hour (higher intensity) or 25 ml per kilogram per hour (lower intensity). The primary outcome measure was death within 90 days after randomization.

Critical Appraisal

Parameters	Yes	No	Comment
Validity			
Is the **Randomization** Procedure well described?	+1		
Double **blinded**?		−2	
Is the **sample size** calculation described/adequate?	+3		Target of 1,500 for 90 % power to detect 8.5 % in a 90-day mortality
Does it have a hard primary **end point**?	+1		90-day mortality all-cause
Is the end point surrogate?		0	
Is the follow-up appropriate?	+1		
Was there a **Bias**?		+2	
Is the dropout <25 %?		+1	Only 1 was lost to follow-up. 4 withdrew consent and 39 refused delayed consent
Is the analysis **ITT**?	+3		
Utility/usefulness			
Can the findings be generalized?	+1		
Was the NNT <100?			N/A: negative study
Score	73 %		Well-conducted and well-designed study

Summary and Conclusions

Providing more intensive renal replacement therapy in critically ill patients has been previously thought to improve patient outcomes. This is based on the premise that during continuous therapy, there is equilibration of low molecular weight solutes between blood, dialysate, and the ultrafiltrate, so that more intensive therapy would lead to more stable and normalized parameters. Notably, this assumption is confounded by factors such as amount of replacement fluids infused prefilter and clotting within the membrane. With this in mind, the dose of continuous renal replacement therapy (CRRT) is typically based on effluent flow rates, which is the sum of the ultrafiltrate and dialysate, normalized to body weight. The seminal study by Ronco et al. reported increased survival in patients receiving higher effluent flow rates (35 or 45 cc/kg/h) compared to lower effluent flow rates (20 cc/kg/h) [42]. However, subsequent small studies yielded conflicting results, which led to the lack of consensus regarding the optimal dosing of CRRT [43].

The RENAL Trial provided definitive evidence that higher intensity therapy did not reduce mortality or increase the rate of renal recovery compared with lower intensity therapy. The trial's large number of patients, multicenter design, and rigorous methodology allow the results to be widely applicable to clinical practice. In this landmark study, 1,508 patients in 35 ICUs in Australia and New Zealand were randomly assigned to two doses (25 or 40 mL/kg/h) of CVVHDF. There was no difference in the net ultrafiltration or fluid balance between the two groups. Also, both groups achieved similar target doses of 84 %. Survival at 90 days was abysmal at 45 % in both treatment arms, which was similar to previous studies of this population.

Although the current evidence does not support that more RRT is better, data suggest that there must be a minimum adequate dose below which mortality will increase. This precise threshold is unknown. KDIGO Guidelines recommend delivering 20–25 cc/kg/h for CRRT and a Kt/Vurea of 3.9 per week (the equivalent of 1.2–1.4 three times per week) when using conventional or SLED [44]. Importantly, the actual delivered dose of RRT in the acute setting often falls short of prescribed dose due to frequent interruptions due to filter clotting, surgery, or diagnostic investigations. Thus, the delivered dose of therapy should be closely monitored and individualized to ensure that the targeted dose is actually achieved.

The interpretation of these studies is not that dose does not matter, but rather that delivered dose of dialysis in critically ill patient needs to be monitored and reviewed to ensure volume and solute removal meet clinical needs. Treatment of kidney failure requiring dialysis in severely ill patients (ill from diverse causes) is not likely and should not be expected to alter outcomes. After all, the kidney failure is really a reflection of the severity of the overarching condition.

Renal Replacement Therapy in Acute Kidney Injury: Intensity of Continuous Renal Replacement Therapy

Publication: Intensity of renal support in critically ill patients with acute kidney injury. The New England Journal of Medicine

Authors: Palevsky et al

Reference: Palevsky PM, Zhang JH, O'Connor TZ, Chertow GM, Crowley ST, Choudhury D, Finkel K, Kellum JA, Paganini E, Schein RM, Smith MW, Swanson KM, Thompson BT, Vijayan A, Watnick S, Star RA, Peduzzi P. Intensity of renal support in critically ill patients with acute kidney injury. N Engl J Med. 2008;359(1):7–20.

Abstract

Background: The optimal intensity of renal replacement therapy in critically ill patients with acute kidney injury is controversial.

Methods: We randomly assigned critically ill patients with acute kidney injury and failure of at least one nonrenal organ or sepsis to receive intensive or less-intensive renal replacement therapy. The primary end point was death from any cause by day 60. In both study groups, hemodynamically stable patients underwent intermittent hemodialysis, and hemodynamically unstable patients underwent continuous venovenous hemodiafiltration or sustained low-efficiency dialysis. Patients receiving the intensive treatment strategy underwent intermittent hemodialysis and sustained low-efficiency dialysis six times per week and continuous venovenous hemodiafiltration at 35 ml per kilogram of body weight per hour; for patients receiving the less-intensive treatment strategy, the corresponding treatments were provided thrice weekly and at 20 ml per kilogram per hour.

Results: Baseline characteristics of the 1,124 patients in the two groups were similar. The rate of death from any cause by day 60 was 53.6 % with intensive therapy and 51.5 % with less-intensive therapy (odds ratio, 1.09; 95 % confidence interval, 0.86–1.40; $P = 0.47$). There was no significant difference between the two groups in the duration of renal replacement therapy or the rate of recovery of kidney function or nonrenal organ failure. Hypotension during intermittent dialysis occurred in more patients randomly assigned to receive intensive therapy, although the frequency of hemodialysis sessions complicated by hypotension was similar in the two groups.

Conclusions: Intensive renal support in critically ill patients with acute kidney injury did not decrease mortality, improve recovery of kidney function, or reduce the rate of nonrenal organ failure as compared with less-intensive therapy involving a defined dose of intermittent hemodialysis three times per week and continuous renal replacement therapy at 20 mL/kg/h.

Critical Appraisal

Parameters	Yes	No	Comment
Validity			
Is the **Randomization** Procedure well described?	+1		Randomization was stratified according to and within site on the basis of the SOFA cardiovascular score and by the presence or absence of oliguria
Double **blinded**?		−2	
Is the **sample size** calculation described/adequate?	+3		1,164 patients would need to be enrolled to detect a decrease in the 60 day rate of death from any cause from 55 % (with less-intensive therapy) to 45 % (with intensive therapy) with a statistical power of 90 %
Does it have a hard primary **end point**?	+1		60 days mortality all cause
Is the end point surrogate?		0	
Is the follow-up appropriate?	+1		
Was there a **Bias**?		+2	
Is the dropout <25 %?		+1	29 patients withdrawn from study post randomization. Total of 5 patients lost to follow-up
Is the analysis **ITT**?	+3		
Utility/usefulness			
Can the findings be generalized?	+1		Excluded patients with CKD and therefore cannot generalize results to CKD population
Was the NNT <100?			N/A: negative study
Score	**73 %**		Well-conducted and well-designed study

Summary and Conclusions

The Acute Renal Failure Trial Network (ATN) study randomized 1,124 critically ill patients with AKI to a more intensive (CVVHDF at 35 mL/kg/h or intermittent hemodi-alysis or sustained low-efficiency dialysis (SLED) on a 6-day-per-week schedule) or less-intensive (CVVHDF at 20 mL/kg/h or intermittent hemodialysis or SLED on a 3-day-per-week schedule) strategy [45]. The trial enrolled predominantly males (70 %) and more than half had AKI in the setting of sepsis. Notably, the trial excluded patients with CKD 4–5 at baseline. Patients were allowed to have undergone less than two sessions of IHD/SLED or less than 24 h of CRRT prior to randomization. In contrast, the RENAL study excluded patients with prior RRT.

Importantly, the study allocated patients to CRRT or IHD based on patients' Sequential Organ Failure Assessment (SOFA) score: IHD if SOFA <2 and CRRT if SOFA was 3–4. In centers where CRRT was not available, a very small number of patients received SLED in the study [46]. Patients switched from CRRT to IHD if their SOFA score was 0 or 1 for more than 24 h. Rates of switching across modalities were similar in the high and low intensity groups. Overall, a majority of patients (84 %) received IHD at some stage during their ICU stay at 60 days. Due to the controversies of including three dialysis modalities, the ATN trial might be better described as a test of the effects of maximizing RRT intensity rather than a direct test of a dose–response relationship for CRRT.

The authors demonstrated there was no difference in a 60-day all-cause mortality between the intensive and the less-intensive arm. There was also no significant difference in the rate of recovery of kidney function, duration of renal replacement therapy, or evolution of nonrenal organ failure. In the critically ill population studied, the outcomes are not improved by providing intermittent hemodialysis to hemodynamically stable patients more frequently than three times per week, with a target achieved Kt/Vurea value of 1.2–1.4 per treatment, or providing continuous renal replacement therapy to hemodynamically unstable patients at an effluent flow rate of more than 20 ml per kilogram per hour. Hypotension occurred at a similar rate during intermittent-hemodialysis sessions in the two groups, but in a greater percentage of patients in the intensive-therapy group due to greater dialysis exposure. In summary, along with the results of RENAL and two recent systematic reviews, there is no evidence that more intensive RRT leads to improved outcomes in AKI [47, 48].

Cardiorenal Syndrome: Diuretic Prescription in Decompensated Heart Failure

Publication: Diuretic Strategies in Patients with Acute Decompensated Heart Failure (DOSE)

Authors: Felker et al.

Reference: Felker GM, Lee KL, Bull DA, Redfield MM, Stevenson LW, Goldsmith SR, LeWinter MM, Deswal A, Rouleau JL, Ofili EO, Anstrom KJ, Hernandez AF, McNulty SE, Velazquez EJ, Kfoury AG, Chen HH, Givertz MM,

Semigran MJ, Bart BA, Mascette AM, Braunwald E, O'Connor CM. Diuretic strategies in patients with acute decompensated heart failure. N Engl J Med. 2011;364(9):797–805.

Abstract

Loop diuretics are an essential component of therapy for patients with acute decompensated heart failure, but there are few prospective data to guide their use.

Methods: In a prospective, double-blind, randomized trial, we assigned 308 patients with acute decompensated heart failure to receive furosemide administered intravenously by means of either a bolus every 12 h or continuous infusion and at either a low dose (equivalent to the patient's previous oral dose) or a high dose (2.5 times the previous oral dose). The protocol allowed specified dose adjustments after 48 h. The coprimary end points were patients' global assessment of symptoms, quantified as the area under the curve (AUC) of the score on a visual analogue scale over the course of 72 h, and the change in the serum creatinine level from baseline to 72 h.

Results: In the comparison of bolus with continuous infusion, there was no significant difference in patients' global assessment of symptoms (mean AUC, $4{,}236 \pm 1{,}440$ and $4{,}373 \pm 1{,}404$, respectively; $P=0.47$) or in the mean change in the creatinine level (0.05 ± 0.3 mg/dl [4.4 ± 26.5 μmol/l] and 0.07 ± 0.3 mg/dl [6.2 ± 26.5 μmol/l], respectively; $P=0.45$). In the comparison of the high-dose strategy with the low-dose strategy, there was a nonsignificant trend towards greater improvement in patients' global assessment of symptoms in the high-dose group (mean AUC, $4{,}430 \pm 1{,}401$ vs. $4{,}171 \pm 1{,}436$; $P=0.06$). There was no significant difference between these groups in the mean change in the creatinine level (0.08 ± 0.3 mg/dl [7.1 ± 26.5 μmol/l] with the high-dose strategy and 0.04 ± 0.3 mg/dl [3.5 ± 26.5 μmol/l] with the low-dose strategy, $P=0.21$). The high-dose strategy was associated with greater diuresis and more favorable outcomes in some secondary measures but also with transient worsening of renal function.

Conclusions: Among patients with acute decompensated heart failure, there were no significant differences in patients' global assessment of symptoms or in the change in renal function when diuretic therapy was administered by bolus as compared with continuous infusion or at a high dose as compared with a low dose.

Critical Appraisal

Parameters	Yes	No	Comment
Validity			
Is the **Randomization** Procedure well described?	+1		

Parameters	Yes	No	Comment
Double **blinded**?	+2		
Is the **sample size** calculation described/adequate?	+3		We estimated that with a sample of 300 patients, the study would have 88 % power to detect a 600-point difference between groups in the AUC of the patients' global assessment score and 88 % power to detect a difference of 0.2 mg/dl (17.7 μmol/l) in the change in the creatinine level between groups
Does it have a hard primary **end point**?		−1	Visual analogue scale for symptoms Change in serum creatinine not appropriate end point for study
Is the end point surrogate?	−2		
Is the follow-up appropriate?	+1		Primary outcome evaluated at 72 h and serum creatinine measured at 60 days of follow-up
Was there a **Bias**?		+2	
Is the dropout <25 %?		+1	
Is the analysis **ITT**?	+3		
Utility/usefulness			
Can the findings be generalized?	+1		
Was the NNT <100?			N/A: negative study
Score	73 %		Well-designed and well-conducted study

Summary and Conclusions

Loop diuretics have been the mainstay of therapy in treating acute decompensated heart failure (ADHF). However, the dosing and mode of loop diuretic administration vary greatly among clinicians. Loop diuretics are effective at decreasing congestion, reducing afterload, and alleviating heart failure symptoms. Yet multiple observational studies suggested that loop diuretics, especially when used at higher doses, were associated with increased risk of heart failure progression, renal failure, and mortality [49]. These observations are confounded by the fact that patients receiving higher doses of diuretics tend to have greater disease severity or comorbidity, making it difficult to establish whether the relationship between diuretic dose and outcomes is causal. Potential mechanisms for worse outcomes with loop diuretics include decreasing effective circulation blood volume and activating the renin-angiotensin-aldosterone and sympathetic systems. Upregulation of these neurohormonal axes can worsen renal function and lead to the progression of heart failure [50]. In addition, diuretics use results in a variety of electrolyte abnormalities that may trigger potentially dangerous arrhythmias in decompensated heart failure. Continuous IV infusion of loop diuretics has several theoretical benefits compared to IV bolus dosing. Continuous infusions result in lower peak concentrations and may reduce renal failure, electrolyte disturbances, and ototoxicity. Bolus dosing has peaks and troughs and potential with periods of subtherapeutic levels, which may result in rebound sodium reabsorption and diuretic resistance.

The Diuretic Optimization Strategies Evaluation (DOSE) was the largest randomized, double-blind study designed to answer to the question: what is the best way to deliver IV loop diuretics to hospitalized patients with acute decompensated heart failure? Three hundred and eight patients with ADHF were randomized into one of four treatment arms in a 2 by 2 factorial design: low-dose diuretics delivered in twice daily IV boluses, low-dose diuretics delivered by continuous infusion, high-dose diuretics delivered in twice daily IV boluses, and high-dose diuretics delivered by continuous infusion. This pivotal study allowed for the comparison of continuous infusion versus IV boluses and of high- versus low-dose strategies.

Patients had to have a history of chronic heart failure and have received an oral loop diuretic for at least 1 month prior. The low-dose strategy was defined as a total IV furosemide dose equal to the patient's total daily oral loop diuretic dose in furosemide equivalents. The high-dose group was defined as a total daily IV furosemide dose 2.5 times the patient's daily oral dose. After 48 h of study protocol, the treating physician was allowed to adjust the diuretic strategy depending on clinical response, by either increasing the IV dose by 50 %, switching IV therapy to open-label oral dosing, or continuing protocol therapy for another 24 h. After 72 h, all patients were switched to open-labeled furosemide therapy at the treating clinician's discretion. All other therapeutic interventions were allowed, including fluid restriction, sodium restriction, and standardized medical therapy. The coprimary end point of the study was (1) symptom improvement using a visual analogue scale and (2) change in serum creatinine from baseline at 72 h. Patients were followed for 60 days after discharge.

The DOSE Trial found no significant differences in the primary and secondary clinical end points between continuous infusion and bolus dosing. There was a nonsignificant trend towards improvement of symptoms in the high-dose group ($p = 0.06$) and no difference in serum creatinine. The high-dose group were more likely to switch to oral diuretics at 48 h, whereas the low-dose group required an increase in diuretic dose at 48 h. The high-dose group resulted in greater weight loss, fluid loss, and relief of dyspnea. Worsening renal function, defined as a rise of serum creatinine of more than 0.3 mg/dL at 72 h, occurred more in the high-dose arm versus the low-dose arm (23 % vs. 14 %, $p = 0.004$). However, serum creatinine was similar at 60 days post discharge. There was also no difference in the composite outcome of death, emergency department visits, or hospitalizations between the bolus versus infusion and high- versus low-dose groups.

The results of DOSE taught us two important lessons. First, administering loop diuretics by continuous infusion or twice-a-day IV bolus has equal efficacy and safety. This result refutes the clinical dogma that continuous infusion of diuretics is better than bolus dosing in the patient population studied. Also, the theories of greater toxicity with bolus dosing caused by higher peak serum concentrations were not supported in this trial. This has important clinical implications because compared to a continuous infusion, IV bolus dosing does not require infusion pumps and frees the patient from being attached to an IV pole. Secondly, high-dose therapy achieved greater relief of dyspnea and diuresis without worsening renal function compared to low-dose therapy. That is, there was no evidence that "gentle diuresis" results in greater renal preservation than a higher-dose therapy.

Several limitations of the trial need to be highlighted. The study enrolled patients with a history of diuretic use between 80 and 240 mg of furosemide or equivalent per day. This excludes patients on lower chronic doses or those who are diuretic naïve. It is unknown whether these patients would respond differently to the regimens used in DOSE. Importantly, the trial was not powered to detect differences in clinical outcomes at 60 days. Previous studies found that worsening renal function in the setting of diuresis was a poor predictor of outcomes. However, DOSE and other recent studies have called this into question, suggesting that transient AKI during ADHF does not affect post-discharge outcomes [51]. Since the lack of adequate symptom relief with diuretics has been associated with longer hospital stays and increased mortality [52], perhaps transient AKI may be a reasonable trade-off for more expedient decongestion.

In summary, the results of DOSE suggest that higher doses of diuretic may be safely used to achieve greater diuresis, weight loss, and relief of dyspnea in patients with ADHF. Despite the fact that the high-dose group had higher rates of AKI at 72 h, these effects were not associated with any long-term consequences. Also, in agreement with a recent systematic review and meta-analysis by Wu et al. [53], DOSE demonstrated that continuous diuretic infusion did not offer significant benefits over IV bolus dosing across a variety of clinical end points.

In clinical practice, would this translate to a movement away from diuretic infusions and increased appreciation of diuretic resistance in critical care settings? This will need to be studied.

Cardiorenal Syndrome: Role of Ultrafiltration in Decompensated Heart Failure

Publication: Ultrafiltration in decompensated heart failure with cardiorenal syndrome

Author: Bart et al.

Reference: Bart BA, Goldsmith SR, Lee KL, Givertz MM, O'Connor CM, Bull DA, Redfield MM, Deswal A, Rouleau JL, LeWinter MM, Ofili EO, Stevenson LW, Semigran MJ, Felker GM, Chen HH, Hernandez AF, Anstrom KJ, McNulty SE, Velazquez EJ, Ibarra JC, Mascette AM, Braunwald E. Ultrafiltration in decompensated heart failure with cardiorenal syndrome. N Engl J Med. 2012;367(24):2296–304.

Abstract

Background: Ultrafiltration is an alternative strategy to diuretic therapy for the treatment of patients with acute decompensated heart failure. Little is known about the efficacy and safety of ultrafiltration in patients with acute decompensated heart failure complicated by persistent congestion and worsened renal function.

Methods: We randomly assigned a total of 188 patients with acute decompensated heart failure, worsened renal function, and persistent congestion to a strategy of stepped pharmacologic therapy (94 patients) or ultrafiltration (94 patients). The primary end point was the bivariate change from baseline in the serum creatinine level and body weight, as assessed 96 h after random assignment. Patients were followed for 60 days.

Results: Ultrafiltration was inferior to pharmacologic therapy with respect to the bivariate end point of the change in the serum creatinine level and body weight 96 h after enrollment ($P = 0.003$), owing primarily to an increase in the creatinine level in the ultrafiltration group. At 96 h, the mean change in the creatinine level was -0.04 ± 0.53 mg/dl (-3.5 ± 46.9 µmol/l) in the pharmacologic-therapy group, as compared with $+0.23 \pm 0.70$ mg/dl (20.3 ± 61.9 µmol/l) in the ultrafiltration group ($P = 0.003$). There was no significant difference in weight loss 96 h after enrollment between patients in the pharmacologic-therapy group and those in the ultrafiltration group (a loss of 5.5 ± 5.1 kg [12.1 ± 11.3 lb] and 5.7 ± 3.9 kg [12.6 ± 8.5 lb], respectively; $P = 0.58$). A higher percentage of patients in the ultrafiltration group than in the pharmacologic-therapy group had a serious adverse event (72 % vs. 57 %, $P = 0.03$).

Conclusions: In a randomized trial involving patients hospitalized for acute decompensated heart failure, worsened renal function, and persistent congestion, the use of a stepped pharmacologic-therapy algorithm was superior to a strategy of ultrafiltration for the preservation of renal function at 96 h, with a similar amount of weight loss with the two approaches. Ultrafiltration was associated with a higher rate of adverse events.

Critical Appraisal

Parameters	Yes	No	Comment
Validity			
Is the **Randomization** Procedure well described?	+1		
Double **blinded**?		−2	
Is the **sample size** calculation described/ adequate?	+3		Based on results from previous trial UNLOAD
Does it have a hard primary **end point**?		−1	Composite bivariable of change in weight and change in serum Cr at 96 h. Creatinine was not an ideal biomarker of renal function as creatinine clearance may be different with diuresis versus ultrafiltration. Hemoconcentration will also affect sCr levels
Is the end point surrogate?	−2		
Is the follow-up appropriate?	+1		Trial stopped short of 200 goal of patient enrolment due to lack of benefit and potential harm with UF group
Was there a **Bias**?	−2		Crossover occurred 18 % in pharmacology group and 23 % in UF group. UF group were not allowed to use vasodilators or inotropes, whereas the pharmacotherapy group was
Is the dropout <25 %?		+1	
Is the analysis **ITT**?	+3		
Utility/usefulness			
Can the findings be generalized?		−1	Exclusion of very sick patients (needing inotropes, vasodilators) and those with recent ACS. Not diuretic resistant patient
Was the NNT <100?			N/A: negative study
Score	7 %		Study with serious limitations, results inconclusive

Summary and Conclusions

Ultrafiltration (UF) allows for the extracorporeal removal of plasma water from whole blood by applying a transmembrane pressure gradient across a semipermeable membrane.

The recent development of UF devices using central or peripheral IV accesses has generated great interest as a potential alternative to loop diuretics in the treatment of ADHF. Modern UF devices are mobile and allow for the removal of fluid at the bedside without specialized personnel [54]. Full anticoagulation therapy with continuous infusion of heparin is recommended to preserve filter function.

The theoretical benefits of UF over diuretics are that UF may potentially avoid neurohormonal activation, renal impairment, electrolyte abnormalities, and diuretic resistance [55]. Unlike diuretics, the rate and volume of fluid removal can be controlled by UF. Also, the ultrafiltrate is isotonic, while diuretics produce hypotonic urine. Therefore, UF may remove more sodium per equivalent volume loss and avoid the electrolyte disturbances seen in diuresis [55].

CARRESS was a multicenter, prospective, randomized, non-blinded trial that enrolled 188 ADHF patients with cardiorenal syndrome. However, patients with acute coronary syndrome, severe renal dysfunction (>3.5 mg/dl SCr), and shock needing vasodilators or inotropes were excluded. Eligible patients were randomized to either UF versus a stepped pharmacological therapy. UF was performed using the Aquadex System 100 at a fluid removal rate of 200 ml/h. Loop diuretics were discontinued in patients randomized to the UF arm. Pharmacological therapy consisted of loop diuretics, thiazide diuretics, inotropes, and vasodilators titrated to maintain a urine output of 3–5 L/day. The coprimary end points were changed in serum creatinine from baseline and weight at 96 h post randomization. Patients were followed for 60 days after discharge.

CARRESS found that there was no significant difference in weight loss between UF and pharmacotherapy. However, the UF group had a significant increase in creatinine compared to the pharmacotherapy group (0.23 mg/dl ± 0.70 mg/dL vs. −0.04 mg/dl ± 0.53 mg/dL $p = 0.003$). At 60 days, the UF group had a slightly higher creatinine. There were no differences in secondary outcomes such as subjective well-being and dyspnea. Importantly, at 60-day follow-up, the UF group had more adverse events compared to pharmacotherapy (72 % vs. 57 % $P = 0.03$). Specifically, the UF group experienced more incomplete decongestion, renal failure, bleeding, and catheter-associated complications. Despite this, there was no significance difference in 60-day mortality or heart failure readmissions, although the trial was not powered to detect this. The overall outcome in this cohort was poor in both groups, with more than a third either dying or readmitted for heart failure within 60 days. As a result of these findings, the authors concluded that pharmacotherapy was superior to UF because it produced similar weight loss, preserved renal function, and had less adverse events.

After the publication of this trial, letters written to the *NEJM* that pointed out several weaknesses [56]. Creatinine was not an ideal biomarker of renal function in the trial because creatinine clearance may be different via glomerular filtration versus ultrafiltration. In UF, plasma creatinine freely passes through the membrane, so the concentration of creatinine in the ultrafiltrate is equal to that of plasma. Diuresis may be better at creatinine clearance per volume removed than ultrafiltration due to increased tubular flow. Since the UF group received no diuretics, they had lower urine output compared to the pharmacotherapy group. Consequently, the pharmacotherapy group would have been expected to have a lower serum creatinine when compared to the UF group at 96 h [56]. Secondly, the UF group were not allowed to receive any IV vasodilators or inotropes unless deemed necessary as rescue therapy. This adjunctive therapy may have helped improve or preserve renal perfusion in the pharmacotherapy group. Finally, the optimal rate and duration of ultrafiltration are not known, and a different intensity protocol could have resulted in improved outcomes.

Currently guidelines from ACC/AHA state that UF is reasonable for ADHF in select patients deemed refractory to medical therapy. The Canadian Cardiovascular Society also highlights that UF is potentially associated with risks including hypotension, catheter-related complications, and bleeding due to systemic anticoagulation. Taken together, the totality of the data would suggest that UF may be useful in the selected patients cared for by experienced teams. Future research is needed to identify better biomarkers that reliably reflect renal function and also incorporate intravascular volume monitoring to guide volume removal therapy. The question as to whether rapid removal of fluid with extraordinary means is better than conventional volume removal with medication remains unanswered.

Renal Replacement Therapy in Acute Kidney Injury: Acute Peritoneal Dialysis

Publication: High volume peritoneal dialysis vs daily hemodialysis: a randomized, controlled trial in patients with acute kidney injury

Authors: Gabriel et al.

Reference: Gabriel DP, Caramori JT, Martim LC, Barretti P, Balbi AL. High volume peritoneal dialysis vs daily hemodialysis: a randomized, controlled trial in patients with acute kidney injury. Kidney Int Suppl. 2008.

Abstract

There is no consensus in the literature on the best renal replacement therapy (RRT) in acute kidney injury (AKI), with both hemodialysis (HD) and peritoneal dialysis (PD) being used as AKI therapy. However, there are concerns about the inadequacy of PD as well as about the intermittency of HD complicated by hemodynamic instability. Recently, continuous replacement renal therapy (CRRT) has become the most commonly used dialysis method for AKI around the world. A prospective randomized controlled trial was performed to compare the effect of high volume peritoneal dialysis (HVPD) with daily hemodialysis (DHD) on AKI patient survival. A total of 120 patients with acute tubular necrosis (ATN) were assigned to HVPD or DHD in a tertiary-care university hospital. The primary end points were hospital survival rate and renal function recovery, with metabolic control as the secondary end point. Sixty patients were treated with HVPD and 60 with DHD. The HVPD and DHD groups were similar for age (64.2 ± 19.8 and 62.5 ± 21.2 years); gender (male: 72 and 66 %); sepsis (42 and 47 %); hemodynamic instability (61 and 63 %); severity of AKI (Acute Tubular Necrosis-Index Specific Score (ATN-ISS): 0.68 ± 0.2 and 0.66 ± 0.2); Acute Physiology, Age, and Chronic Health Evaluation Score (APACHE II) (26.9 ± 8.9 and 24.1 ± 8.2); pre-dialysis BUN (116.4 ± 33.6 and 112.6 ± 36.8 mg/100 ml); and creatinine (5.8 ± 1.9 and 5.9 ± 1.4 mg/100 ml). Weekly delivered Kt/V was 3.6 ± 0.6 in HVPD and 4.7 ± 0.6 in DHD ($P < 0.01$). Metabolic control, mortality rate (58 and 53 %), and renal function recovery (28 and 26 %) were similar in both groups, whereas HVPD was associated with a significantly shorter time to the recovery of renal function. In conclusion, HVPD and DHD can be considered as alternative forms of RRT in AKI.

Critical Appraisal

Parameters	Yes	No	Comment
Validity			
Is the **Randomization** Procedure well described?		−1	Sealed envelope, but manner of randomization not described
Double **blinded**?		−2	
Is the **sample size** calculation described/ adequate?	+3		Data from at least 60 patients per group were used in calculations giving a statistical power of 80 % to detect an absolute difference in mortality of 20 % between groups
Does it have a hard primary **end point**?	+1		Mortality 30 days and renal recovery
Is the end point surrogate?	0		
Is the follow-up appropriate?	+1		
Was there a **Bias**?	−2		34 patients were withdrawn in course of study due to death during first dialysis session, early mechanical complications, switching to CRRT, and needing surgery
Is the dropout >25 %?	+1		

Parameters	Yes	No	Comment
Is the analysis **ITT**?		−3	Dropped patients during study were excluded from final analysis
Utility/usefulness			
Can the findings be generalized?		−1	Single-center study and small population
Was the NNT <100?			N/A: negative study
Score	**0 %**		Serious methodological limitations, results inconclusive

Summary and Conclusions

In the developed world continuous renal replacement therapy and intermittent hemodialysis are the most commonly used in AKI [57]. However, in recent years there has been a resurgence of interest in the use of peritoneal dialysis in AKI [58]. A single cuff Tenckhoff catheter placed at the bedside by any trained physician can achieve peritoneal access. Acute peritoneal dialysis is widely used in developing countries due to lower costs, availability, ease of administration, hemodynamic stability, and decreased risk of bleeding. PD for treatment of AKI is limited to small children in developed countries. However, PD may play an important role in Western countries during natural catastrophes when hemodialysis is unavailable due to decreased access to power and clean water facilities [57].

A major concern of peritoneal dialysis in AKI is whether it can deliver adequate clearance in hypercatabolic AKI. To date, there is very little data on the optimal dosing of PD in AKI. Based on data from chronic dialysis and CRRT literature, std-Kt/Vurea of 2.1 may be a reasonable "minimum" dose of peritoneal dialysis [59]. This target may need to be higher depending for those patients considered to have higher catabolism. Other limitations of peritoneal dialysis in AKI include requirement for an intact peritoneal cavity, inability to precisely control ultrafiltration, hyperglycemia and peritonitis. Finally, peritoneal dialysis is unable to rapidly correct life-threatening conditions such as severe hyperkalemia, drug intoxications, and acute pulmonary edema.

Gabriel et al. previously showed that high volume PD (HVPD) can adequately treat critically ill patients with AKI without significant complications in a small prospective study [60]. The same group performed a randomized controlled trial in 120 AKI patients comparing the efficacy and safety of HVPD and daily intermittent hemodialysis (dHD). HVPD was performed using a Tenckhoff catheter, 2 l exchanges, and 35- to 50-min dwell time. The prescribed Kt/V value was 0.65 per session (4.5 per week), the duration of each session was 24 h, and the total dialysate volume was 36–44 L/day (18–22 exchanges per day). dHD was performed with a double-lumen central venous catheter and polysulfone filters. Kt/V for each dHD session was 1.2. Both modalities achieved similar metabolic control. The delivered dialysis dose was higher for dHD compared to PD (KtV 4.76 ± 0.65 v 3.59 ± 0.6), but ultrafiltration was similar between both groups. The primary outcome of mortality was similar between dHD and PD (58 % versus 53 %). The mortality rate was very high in both groups and reflected the sickness of the population (mean APACHE II score of 25). The percentage of renal recovery was similar for both modalities, but PD was associated with a significantly shorter time to recovery (7.2 ± 2.6 vs. 10.6 ± 4.7 days). There were no significant differences in the rate of infectious complications between the two groups. Peritonitis occurred in 18 % of HVPD patients, and catheter infection in 13 % of patients of the dHD group. Patients treated with HVPD did not have uncontrolled hyperglycemia. Both modalities had a similar decrease in serum albumin, but the dialysate effluent in PD had significant protein loss of 22 g/day.

However, there are serious flaws in this study, rendering its results inconclusive. Thirty-four patients (22 %) were withdrawn from the final analysis post-randomization for a variety of reasons including change to CRRT, death during first session, mechanical complications, or needing surgery. Notably, nine patients randomized to the PD group were excluded due to early mechanical complications such as leakage. Unfortunately, these exclusions were not counted as adverse events in the final analysis. Also, this is a single-center study with a small sample size. Therefore, the conclusions are not generalizable and the results are not definitive. Furthermore, PD may impair respiratory mechanics due to increased intra-abdominal pressures in mechanically ventilated patients. This study did not evaluate differences in respiratory parameters.

A recent comprehensive systematic review on PD in AKI reported a paucity of high quality data on this topic. Pooled analysis of 11 studies found no difference between PD and extracorporeal blood purification therapies. However, most studies failed to report the dosing of PD, renal recovery, or PD-related complications [58]. Whether PD can adequately achieve solute clearances compared to hemodialysis in AKI remains unresolved. The minimum small solute clearance to achieve comparable outcomes remains undefined. However, if PD is the only available modality, the prescription in AKI should be individualized and higher small-solute clearances may be necessary for patients with more complex catabolic illnesses. This study highlights that future high quality RCTs are required.

General Conclusions and Summary

This chapter has focused on key randomized controlled trials in the area of AKI as of 2014. There are many observational trials and systematic reviews on topics related to those addressed here, which were not the focus of this chapter.

It is clear that the presence of AKI, defined as even small changes in serum creatinine, confers a worse prognosis for both short- and long-term outcomes in patients. The etiologies of AKI remain diverse and are often multifactorial, the diagnosis is often delayed or debated, and optimal prevention or treatment strategies remain unknown. The use of serum creatinine changes as the "definition" of AKI remains controversial, as changes in biomarkers have not conventionally been acceptable to define disease states. However, as a change in serum creatinine is on the causal pathway to CKD, need for dialysis, and other adverse events, we would submit that it is reasonable to accept this as a bonafide definition in certain scenarios. For example, the KDIGO definition of CIAKI is a change of serum creatinine from baseline within 72 h post contrast exposure. Therefore, it may be reasonable for trials examining incidence of CIAKI to use changes in serum creatinine as an end point. However, future studies need to measure harder end points such as progression to ESRD and mortality.

We have increasingly recognized that early identification is essential for improved outcomes, as is true for all other conditions. However, we continue to struggle with the definition of AKI, for the purposes of enrolment into trials. Newer biomarkers, either in urine or serum, may help us to identify early episodes of injury, but fundamentally, if we were to consistently recognize that any rise in serum creatinine and any sustained change in urine output that results in positive fluid balance is AKI, then we may be able to develop a series of clinical trials that address how best to intervene.

Some important questions for the international community include the viability of PD as a real therapeutic option in the acute setting, in both the developed and developing worlds; optimal treatment of CHF; and the impact of interventions which "induce" AKI on short- and long-term outcomes. Studies which could demonstrate that the use of robust measures to better assess volume status improves outcomes (through both earlier identification of AKI and by facilitating institution of appropriate therapy (e.g., diuretics or dialysis)) in a timely manner would be valuable. Whether pre-ischemic conditioning is of value in AKI remains to be seen.

The two main driving questions in the field include: What is the most robust and accurate early method for diagnosing AKI and what is the appropriate time to start dialysis in those with established AKI? Accurate diagnosis and timely intervention have been shown in other conditions to improve outcomes: perhaps the next decade will bring us closer to answering these questions and thus reduce AKI incidence and severity and improve prognosis.

References

1. Tepel M, Aspelin P, Lameire N. Contrast-induced nephropathy: a clinical and evidence-based approach. Circulation. 2006;113(14):1799–806. doi:10.1161/CIRCULATIONAHA.105.595090.

2. Lameire N, Kellum JA. Contrast-induced acute kidney injury and renal support for acute kidney injury: a KDIGO summary (part 2). Crit Care. 2013;17(1):205. doi:10.1186/cc11455.

3. Kshirsagar AV, Poole C, Mottl A, Shoham D, Franceschini N, Tudor G, Agrawal M, Denu-Ciocca C, Magnus Ohman E, Finn WF. N-acetylcysteine for the prevention of radiocontrast induced nephropathy: a meta-analysis of prospective controlled trials. J Am Soc Nephrol. 2004;15(3):761–9.

4. Fishbane S. N-acetylcysteine in the prevention of contrast-induced nephropathy. Clin J Am Soc Nephrol. 2008;3(1):281–7. doi:10.2215/CJN.02590607.

5. Bagshaw SM, McAlister FA, Manns BJ, Ghali WA. Acetylcysteine in the prevention of contrast-induced nephropathy: a case study of the pitfalls in the evolution of evidence. Arch Intern Med. 2006;166(2):161–6. doi:10.1001/archinte.166.2.161.

6. Marenzi G, Assanelli E, Marana I, Lauri G, Campodonico J, Grazi M, De Metrio M, Galli S, Fabbiocchi F, Montorsi P, Veglia F, Bartorelli AL. N-acetylcysteine and contrast-induced nephropathy in primary angioplasty. N Engl J Med. 2006;354(26):2773–82.

7. Group KAGW (2012) KDIGO clinical practice guideline for acute kidney injury. Kidney Int Suppl. 2012;2:83–84

8. Sendeski MM. Pathophysiology of renal tissue damage by iodinated contrast media. Clin Exp Pharmacol Physiol. 2011;38(5):292–9. doi:10.1111/j.1440-1681.2011.05503.x.

9. Heyman SN, Rosen S, Rosenberger C. Renal parenchymal hypoxia, hypoxia adaptation, and the pathogenesis of radiocontrast nephropathy. Clin J Am Soc Nephrol. 2008;3(1):288–96. doi:10.2215/CJN.02600607.

10. Seeliger E, Sendeski M, Rihal CS, Persson PB. Contrast-induced kidney injury: mechanisms, risk factors, and prevention. Eur Heart J. 2012;33(16):2007–15. doi:10.1093/eurheartj/ehr494.

11. Gordon CE, Balk EM, Becker BN, Crooks PA, Jaber BL, Johnson CA, Michael MA, Pereira BJ, Uhlig K, Levin A. KDOQI US commentary on the KDIGO clinical practice guideline for the prevention, diagnosis, evaluation, and treatment of hepatitis C in CKD. Am J Kidney Dis. 2008;52(5):811–25. doi:10.1053/j.ajkd.2008.08.005.

12. Palevsky PM, Liu KD, Brophy PD, Chawla LS, Parikh CR, Thakar CV, Tolwani AJ, Waikar SS, Weisbord SD. KDOQI US commentary on the 2012 KDIGO clinical practice guideline for acute kidney injury. Am J Kidney Dis. 2013;61(5):649–72. doi:10.1053/j.ajkd.2013.02.349.

13. Weisbord SD, Palevsky PM. Prevention of contrast-induced nephropathy with volume expansion. Clin J Am Soc Nephrol. 2008;3(1):273–80. doi:10.2215/CJN.02580607.

14. Mueller C, Buerkle G, Buettner HJ, Petersen J, Perruchoud AP, Eriksson U, Marsch S, Roskamm H. Prevention of contrast media-associated nephropathy: randomized comparison of 2 hydration regimens in 1620 patients undergoing coronary angioplasty. Arch Intern Med. 2002;162(3):329–36.

15. Ozcan EE, Guneri S, Akdeniz B, Akyildiz IZ, Senaslan O, Baris N, Aslan O, Badak O. Sodium bicarbonate, N-acetylcysteine, and saline for prevention of radiocontrast-induced nephropathy. A comparison of 3 regimens for protecting contrast-induced nephropathy in patients undergoing coronary procedures. A single-center prospective controlled trial. Am Heart J. 2007;154(3):539–44. doi:10.1016/j.ahj.2007.05.012.

16. Zoungas S, Ninomiya T, Huxley R, Cass A, Jardine M, Gallagher M, Patel A, Vasheghani-Farahani A, Sadigh G, Perkovic V. Systematic review: sodium bicarbonate treatment regimens for the prevention of contrast-induced nephropathy. Ann Intern Med. 2009;151(9):631–8. doi:10.7326/0003-4819-151-9-200911030-00008.

17. Palevsky PM, Liu KD, Brophy PD, Chawla LS, Parikh CR, Thakar CV, Tolwani AJ, Waikar SS, Weisbord SD. KDOQI US commentary on the 2012 KDIGO clinical practice guideline for acute kidney injury. Am J Kidney Dis. 2013;61(5):649–72. doi:10.1053/j.ajkd.2013.02.349.

18. Heyman SN, Rosen S, Epstein FH, Spokes K, Brezis ML. Loop diuretics reduce hypoxic damage to proximal tubules of the isolated perfused rat kidney. Kidney Int. 1994;45(4):981–5.

19. Ludens JH, Hook JB, Brody MJ, Williamson HE. Enhancement of renal blood flow by furosemide. J Pharmacol Exp Ther. 1968;163(2):456–60.

20. Aravindan N, Aravindan S, Riedel BJ, Weng HR, Shaw AD. Furosemide prevents apoptosis and associated gene expression in a rat model of surgical ischemic acute renal failure. Ren Fail. 2007;29(4):399–407. doi:10.1080/08860220701263671.

21. Morgan DJ, Ho KM. A comparison of nonoliguric and oliguric severe acute kidney injury according to the risk injury failure loss end-stage (RIFLE) criteria. Nephron Clin Pract. 2010;115(1):c59–65. doi:10.1159/000286351.

22. Bagshaw SM, Bellomo R, Kellum JA. Oliguria, volume overload and loop diuretics. Crit Care Med. 2008;36(4 Suppl):S172–8. doi:10.1097/CCM.0b013e318168c92f.

23. Bouchard J, Soroko SB, Chertow GM, Himmelfarb J, Ikizler TA, Paganini EP, Mehta RL. Fluid accumulation, survival and recovery of kidney function in critically ill patients with acute kidney injury. Kidney Int. 2009;76(4):422–7. doi:10.1038/ki.2009.159.

24. Uchino S. Outcome prediction for patients with acute kidney injury. Nephron Clin Pract. 2008;109(4):c217–23. doi:10.1159/000142931

25. Shilliday IR, Quinn KJ, Allison ME. Loop diuretics in the management of acute renal failure: a prospective, double-blind, placebo-controlled, randomized study. Nephrol Dial Transplant. 1997;12(12):2592–6.

26. Nigwekar SU, Waikar SS. Diuretics in acute kidney injury. Semin Nephrol. 2011;31(6):523–34. doi:10.1016/j.semnephrol.2011.09.007.

27. Ho KM, Power BM. Benefits and risks of furosemide in acute kidney injury. Anaesthesia. 2010;65(3):283–93. doi:10.1111/j.1365-2044.2009.06228.x.

28. Dibartola SP. Fluid, electrolyte, and acid–base disorders in small animal practice. 4th ed. Elsevier, St. Louis 2012.

29. Brunkhorst FM, Engel C, Bloos F, Meier-Hellmann A, Ragaller M, Weiler N, Moerer O, Gruendling M, Oppert M, Grond S, Olthoff D, Jaschinski U, John S, Rossaint R, Welte T, Schaefer M, Kern P, Kuhnt E, Kiehntopf M, Hartog C, Natanson C, Loeffler M, Reinhart K, German Competence Network S. Intensive insulin therapy and pentastarch resuscitation in severe sepsis. N Engl J Med. 2008;358(2):125–39.

30. Claus RA, Sossdorf M, Hartog C. The effects of hydroxyethyl starch on cultured renal epithelial cells. Anesth Analg. 2010;110(2):300–1. doi:10.1213/ANE.0b013e3181ca03a4.

31. Steinhausen M, Weis S, Fleming J, Dussel R, Parekh N. Responses of in vivo renal microvessels to dopamine. Kidney Int. 1986;30(3):361–70.

32. Szerlip HM. Renal-dose dopamine: fact and fiction. Ann Intern Med. 1991;115(2):153–4.

33. Denton MD, Chertow GM, Brady HR. "Renal-dose" dopamine for the treatment of acute renal failure: scientific rationale, experimental studies and clinical trials. Kidney Int. 1996;50(1):4–14.

34. Friedrich JO, Adhikari N, Herridge MS, Beyene J. Meta-analysis: low-dose dopamine increases urine output but does not prevent renal dysfunction or death. Ann Intern Med. 2005;142(7):510–24.

35. Group KAGW. KDIGO clinical practice guideline for acute kidney injury. Kidney Int Suppl. 2012;2:50.

36. De Vriese AS, Colardyn FA, Philippe JJ, Vanholder RC, De Sutter JH, Lameire NH. Cytokine removal during continuous hemofiltration in septic patients. J Am Soc Nephrol. 1999;10(4):846–53.

37. Swartz RD, Bustami RT, Daley JM, Gillespie BW, Port FK. Estimating the impact of renal replacement therapy choice on outcome in severe acute renal failure. Clin Nephrol. 2005;63(5):335–45.

38. Cho KC, Himmelfarb J, Paganini E, Ikizler TA, Soroko SH, Mehta RL, Chertow GM. Survival by dialysis modality in critically ill patients with acute kidney injury. J Am Soc Nephrol. 2006;17(11):3132–8. doi:10.1681/ASN.2006030268.

39. Swartz RD, Messana JM, Orzol S, Port FK. Comparing continuous hemofiltration with hemodialysis in patients with severe acute renal failure. Am J Kidney Dis. 1999;34(3):424–32. doi:10.1053/AJKD03400424.

40. Palevsky PM. Renal replacement therapy in acute kidney injury. Adv Chronic Kidney Dis. 2013;20(1):76–84. doi:10.1053/j.ackd.2012.09.004.

41. Group KAGW. KDIGO clinical practice guideline for acute kidney injury. Kidney Int Suppl. 2012;2:107–110.

42. Ronco C, Bellomo R, Homel P, Brendolan A, Dan M, Piccinni P, La Greca G. Effects of different doses in continuous veno-venous haemofiltration on outcomes of acute renal failure: a prospective randomised trial. Lancet. 2000;356(9223):26–30. doi:10.1016/S0140-6736(00)02430-2.

43. Palevsky PM. Renal replacement therapy in acute kidney injury. Adv Chronic Kidney Dis. 2013;20(1):76–84. doi:10.1053/j.ackd.2012.09.004.

44. Group KAGW. KDIGO clinical practice guideline for acute kidney injury. Kidney Int Suppl. 2012;2:113–115.

45. Network VNARFT, Palevsky PM, Zhang JH, O'Connor TZ, Chertow GM, Crowley ST, Choudhury D, Finkel K, Kellum JA, Paganini E, Schein RMH, Smith MW, Swanson KM, Thompson BT, Vijayan A, Watnick S, Star RA, Peduzzi P. Intensity of renal support in critically ill patients with acute kidney injury. N Engl J Med. 2008;359(1):7–20 [Erratum appears in N Engl J Med. 2009;361(24):2391].

46. Prowle JR, Schneider A, Bellomo R. Clinical review: optimal dose of continuous renal replacement therapy in acute kidney injury. Crit Care. 2011;15(2):207. doi:10.1186/cc9415.

47. Van Wert R, Friedrich JO, Scales DC, Wald R, Adhikari NK. High-dose renal replacement therapy for acute kidney injury: systematic review and meta-analysis. Crit Care Med. 2010;38(5):1360–9. doi:10.1097/CCM.0b013e3181d9d912.

48. Jun M, Heerspink HJ, Ninomiya T, Gallagher M, Bellomo R, Myburgh J, Finfer S, Palevsky PM, Kellum JA, Perkovic V, Cass A. Intensities of renal replacement therapy in acute kidney injury: a systematic review and meta-analysis. Clin J Am Soc Nephrol. 2010;5(6):956–63. doi:10.2215/CJN.09111209.

49. Campbell PT, Ryan J. Diuretic dosing in acute decompensated heart failure: lessons from DOSE. Curr Heart Fail Rep. 2012;9(3):260–5. doi:10.1007/s11897-012-0094-8.

50. Munoz D, Felker GM. Approaches to decongestion in patients with acute decompensated heart failure. Curr Cardiol Rep. 2013;15(2):335. doi:10.1007/s11886-012-0335-1.

51. Felker GM, Lee KL, Bull DA, Redfield MM, Stevenson LW, Goldsmith SR, LeWinter MM, Deswal A, Rouleau JL, Ofili EO, Anstrom KJ, Hernandez AF, McNulty SE, Velazquez EJ, Kfoury AG, Chen HH, Givertz MM, Semigran MJ, Bart BA, Mascette AM, Braunwald E, O'Connor CM. Diuretic strategies in patients with acute decompensated heart failure. N Engl J Med. 2011;364(9):797–805. doi:10.1056/NEJMoa1005419.

52. Metra M, Teerlink JR, Felker GM, Greenberg BH, Filippatos G, Ponikowski P, Teichman SL, Unemori E, Voors AA, Weatherley BD, Cotter G. Dyspnoea and worsening heart failure in patients with acute heart failure: results from the Pre-RELAX-AHF study. Eur J Heart Fail. 2010;12(10):1130–9. doi:10.1093/eurjhf/hfq132.

53. Wu MY, Chang NC, Su CL, Hsu YH, Chen TW, Lin YF, Wu CH, Tam KW. Loop diuretic strategies in patients with acute decompensated heart failure: a meta-analysis of randomized controlled trials. J Crit Care. 2014;29(1):2–9. doi:10.1016/j.jcrc.2013.10.009.

54. Felker GM, Mentz RJ. Diuretics and ultrafiltration in acute decompensated heart failure. J Am Coll Cardiol. 2012;59(24):2145–53. doi:10.1016/j.jacc.2011.10.910.

55. Ryan J, Meng S. Is there still a role for ultrafiltration in the management of acute heart failure? CARRESS and beyond. Curr Heart Fail Rep. 2013;10(3):185–9. doi:10.1007/s11897-013-0142-z.

56. Rossi GP, Calo LA, Maiolino G, Zoccali C. Ultrafiltration for the treatment of congestion: a window into the lung for a better caress to the heart. Nephrol Dial Transplant. 2013. doi:10.1093/ndt/gft371.

57. Burdmann EA, Chakravarthi R. Peritoneal dialysis in acute kidney injury: lessons learned and applied. Semin Dial. 2011;24(2):149–56. doi:10.1111/j.1525-139X.2011.00868.x.

58. Chionh CY, Soni SS, Finkelstein FO, Ronco C, Cruz DN. Use of peritoneal dialysis in AKI: a systematic review. Clin J Am Soc Nephrol. 2013;8(10):1649–60. doi:10.2215/CJN.01540213.

59. Chionh CY, Ronco C, Finkelstein FO, Soni SS, Cruz DN. Acute peritoneal dialysis: what is the 'adequate' dose for acute kidney injury? Nephrol Dial Transplant. 2010;25(10):3155–60. doi:10.1093/ndt/gfq178.

60. Gabriel DP, Nascimento GV, Caramori JT, Martim LC, Barretti P, Balbi AL. High volume peritoneal dialysis for acute renal failure. Perit Dial Int. 2007;27(3):277–82.

Chronic Kidney Disease (CKD) Clinical Trials: A Critical Appraisal

Meguid El Nahas

Introduction

For the last three decades, and since the publication of the "Hyperperfusion–Hyperfiltration" hypothesis by Brenner and his colleagues in Boston, USA [1], considerable research has focused on the understanding of the pathophysiology of chronic kidney disease (CKD). Numerous additional hypotheses and theories have been published, focusing on the key role of renal as well as extrarenal cells in the pathogenesis of progressive renal scarring and fibrosis and the consequent decline in kidney function witnessed in CKD. These have been followed by a slow transition from the preclinical world of laboratory investigations to the bedside with a number of key clinical trials.

Clinical trials started with dietary manipulations of protein intake, aimed to reduce renal and glomerular hyperfiltration, followed by inhibition of the renin–angiotensin–aldosterone system (RAAS), also aimed at reducing putative glomerular hypertension as well as the associated proteinuria and progression of glomerulosclerosis. Attention has also been focused on the impact of different levels of blood pressure (BP) control on CKD progression.

The better understanding of mechanisms of renal scarring has opened the way to the manipulation of a range of putative fibrogenic pathways [2]. Most of the latter have been undertaken in randomized control trials (RCTs) targeting patients with diabetic nephropathy (discussed in Chapter...).

Of all the interventions aimed at slowing CKD progression, the inhibition of the RAAS has received most attention over the last 30 years, with thousands of publications reporting the impact of RAAS inhibition on the progression of diabetic and also nondiabetic CKD. Such an approach has become an integral part of the management of patients with CKD, diabetic or otherwise. Most guidelines nowadays recommend the introduction of RAAS inhibitors to control hypertension, reduce proteinuria, and slow the progression of CKD [3, 4]. However, the enthusiasm for the adoption of such an approach has not been tempered by a critical appraisal of the RCTs that informed such a medical trend.

It is the intention of this chapter to have a critical look and appraise key RCTs aimed at slowing the progression of CKD published over the last 25–30 years. It aims to give the reader not only a critical and constructive but also a practical perspective on these key publications in Nephrology that informed medical practice in recent decades.

We have also included in this chapter some RCTs pertaining to the control of progressive CKD through percutaneous interventions, including renal artery angioplasty and stenting of atherosclerotic renal artery stenosis (ARAS), as well arsenal artery sympathetic denervation, aimed at controlling resistant hypertension, as these could also impact CKD and its progression.

Dietary Protein Restriction

The MDRD Trial

N Engl J Med. 1994 Mar 31;330(13):877–84.

The effects of dietary protein restriction and blood pressure control on the progression of chronic renal disease. Modification of Diet in the Renal Disease Study Group

Klahr S, Levey AS, Beck GJ, Caggiula AW, Hunsicker L, Kusek JW, Striker G.

Abstract

Background: Restricting protein intake and controlling hypertension delay the progression of renal disease in animals. We tested these interventions in 840 patients with various chronic renal diseases.

M. El Nahas, MD, PhD, FRCP
Sheffield Kidney Institute, Global Kidney Academy,
Sheffield S17 3NG, UK
e-mail: m.el-nahas@sheffield.ac.uk

M. El Kossi, A. Khwaja, and M. El Nahas (eds.), *Informing Clinical Practice in Nephrology: The Role of RCTs,*
DOI 10.1007/978-3-319-10292-4_5, © Springer International Publishing Switzerland 2015

Methods: In study 1, 585 patients with glomerular filtration rates (GFR) of 25–55 mL/min/1.73 m^2 of body surface area were randomly assigned to a usual protein diet or a low-protein diet (1.3 or 0.58 g of protein/kg body weight/day) and to a usual- or a low-blood-pressure (BP) group (mean arterial pressure, 107 or 92 mmHg). In study 2, 255 patients with GFR of 13–24 mL/min/1.73 m^2 were randomly assigned to a low-protein diet (0.58 g/kg/day) or a very-low-protein diet (0.28 g/kg/day) with a keto-acid–amino acid supplement, and a usual- or a low-BP group (same values as those in study 1). An 18–45-month follow-up was planned, with monthly evaluations of the patients.

Results: The mean follow-up was 2.2 years. In study 1, the projected mean decline in the GFR at 3 years did not differ significantly between the diet groups or between the BP groups. As compared with the usual protein group and the usual BP group, the low-protein group and the low-BP group had a more rapid decline in GFR during the first 4 months after randomization and a slower decline thereafter. In study 2, the very-low-protein group had a marginally slower decline in the GFR than did the low-protein group ($P = 0.07$). There was no delay in the time to the occurrence of end-stage renal disease or death. In both studies, patients in the low-blood-pressure group who had more pronounced proteinuria at baseline had a significantly slower decline in the glomerular filtration rate.

Conclusions: Among patients with moderate renal insufficiency, the slower decline in renal function that started 4 months after the introduction of a low-protein diet suggests a small benefit of this dietary intervention. Among patients with more severe renal insufficiency, a very-low-protein diet, as compared with a low-protein diet, did not significantly slow the progression of renal disease.

Discussion

A number of studies investigated the impact of dietary protein restriction on the progression of CKD in the 1970s and 1980s. While suggesting a beneficial effect, they were largely flawed and consequently inconclusive [6], primarily because of the reliance on changes in serum creatinine parameters to evaluate the impact of the intervention on the progression of CKD; this was clearly unacceptable in view of the fact that a dietary protein restriction impacts serum creatinine levels through other mechanisms, independent of the changes in GFR, not the least a reduction in protein intake, creatine/creatinine intake, and metabolism, as well as possible confounders, such as malnutrition and sarcopenia [6].

The MDRD study was therefore the first and only RCT that investigated the impact of dietary protein restrictions on the progression of CKD, as measured by the clearance of radiolabeled-Iothalamate. MDRD study was a 2 × 2 factorial designed study to investigate the impact of two levels of dietary protein intake and two levels of BP control on the

Critical Appraisal

Parameters	Yes	No	Comment
Validity			
Is the **randomization** procedure well described?	+1		The protocol was fully described in a prior publication [5]
			2 × 2 factorial design aimed at investigating:
			Impact of different [5] low-protein diets
			Low-protein diet (0.58 g/kg/day) and very low protein intake (0.28 g/kg/day) supplemented with keto-amino acids
			And
			Different [5] levels of BP control
			Mean arterial pressure, 92 and 107 mmHg
Double **blinded**?		−2	Blinding dietary interventions is difficult to achieve. But compliance and dietary protein intake were estimated by the measurement of urinary urea nitrogen excretion
Is the **sample size** calculation described/adequate?	+3		Study 1 = 585
			Study 2 = 255
Does it have a hard primary **end point**?	+1		Yes; the decline in measured GFR (radiolabeled-Iothalamate clearance)
Is the end point surrogate?	0		
Is the follow-up appropriate?	+1		36 months
Was there a **Bias**?		+2	
Is the drop out >25 %?		+1	
Is the analysis **ITT**?	+3		
Utility/usefulness			
Can the findings be generalized?	+1		Mainly to CKD 3 and 4
			GFR between 25 and 55 mL/min
			Note that the large percentage (25 %) of ADPKD in the MDRD study population is not representative (overestimate) of their distribution prevalence in CKD
Was NNT <100?			Not applicable, as the study was negative
Score	73 %		

progression of CKD over a 36-month observation period. It proved negative on both outcomes.

An equally large European study had previously also proved negative in terms of the effect of low-protein diet on CKD progression, albeit by measuring changes in serum creatinine and in the face of issues relating to adherence/compliance to the prescribed diet and limited difference in dietary protein intake between the groups [7]. Subsequent meta-analyses, combining a heterogeneous number of studies with different types of dietary protein restrictions and different methods of measuring CKD progression, mostly relying on changes in serum creatinine estimation, continued to claim otherwise and justify the dietary protein restriction to delay the progression of CKD to end-stage renal disease (ESRD) [8].

MDRD also failed to show an impact of lower BP control (MAP=92 mmHg) compared to usual control (MAP=107 mmHg) on the progression of CKD.

Disappointingly, the interpretation of the results of the MDRD studies and outcomes has been confounded by a number of factors:

1. The high percentage of patients with ADPKD (25 %) included in the study; these patients usually have a fast and relentless rate of decline in kidney function. This also impacts the utility of the study as it may be less representative of common CKD populations where the percentage of ADPKD tends to be lower (<10 %).
2. The high rate of prescription of ACE inhibitors, thus potentially impacting independently the rate of GFR decline and thus confounding the predicted differences between the group and consequently the power of the study to detect such a difference.
3. The complicated interpretation and potential impact of the initial, 4 months, faster decline in GFR in patients treated with a low-protein diet and those assigned to the low-BP group. Dietary protein restriction and lower BP, or related increased ACE inhibition, may have had in this study the anticipated early impact on reducing GFR (first 4 months), thus negatively impacting the overall data analysis, while the analysis based on the 4–36 months seemed more positive and potentially protective.
4. The heterogeneity of the CKD population studies, including some with low and others with high levels of proteinuria, leading to different impacts of the lower BP intervention on the different populations; slower rate of GFR decline upon lower BP control in those with high proteinuria levels compared to those with low proteinuria levels. Also, different responses were noted between black and white patients. However, subgroup analyses can only be hypothesis-generating rather than providing conclusive evidence.
5. Blood pressure measurement relied on casual office estimation and not on the preferable daytime and nighttime recordings of BP or its 24 h ambulatory BP monitoring (ABPM). The latter appear to correlate better with outcomes [9].

Finally, this study calls upon investigators to measure GFR when studying the rate of decline of kidney function in CKD and also have a careful preplanned/specified anticipation of possible breakpoints in GFR decline slopes due to the impact of a given intervention on renal physiology and pathophysiology. MDRD led the way in the thorough evaluation of renal function decline in RCTs by iothalamate clearance measurement, but sadly very few studies followed that lead.

Conclusions

It was a well-designed and well-conducted RCT that showed no substantial benefit of dietary protein restriction on the progression of CKD. It also failed to show a benefit of a lower BP compared to usual BP control. This was more or less the end of dietary protein restrictions to slow CKD progression. On the other hand, MDRD was the first to examine the impact of more intensive BP control on CKD progression.

Angiotensin-Converting Enzyme (ACE) Inhibition Studies

AIPRI Trial

N Engl J Med. 1996 Apr 11;334(15):939–45.

Effect of the angiotensin-converting enzyme inhibitor benazepril on the progression of chronic renal insufficiency. The Angiotensin-Converting Enzyme Inhibition in Progressive Renal Insufficiency Study Group.

Maschio G, Alberti D, Janin G, Locatelli F, Mann JF, Motolese M, Ponticelli C, Ritz E, Zucchelli P.

Abstract

Background: Drugs that inhibit angiotensin-converting enzyme slow the progression of renal insufficiency in patients with diabetic neuropathy. Whether these drugs have a similar action in patients with other renal diseases is not known. We conducted a study to determine the effect of the angiotensin-converting enzyme inhibitor benazepril on the progression of renal insufficiency in patients with various underlying renal diseases.

Methods: In a 3-year trial involving 583 patients with renal insufficiency caused by various disorders, 300 patients received benazepril and 283 received placebo. The underlying diseases included glomerulopathies (in 192 patients), interstitial nephritis (in 105), nephrosclerosis (in 97), polycystic kidney disease (in 64), diabetic nephropathy (in 21), and miscellaneous or unknown disorders (in 104). The severity of renal insufficiency was classified according to the baseline creatinine clearance: 227 patients had mild insufficiency (creatinine clearance, 46–60 mL/min), and 356 had moderate insufficiency (creatinine clearance, 30–45 mL/min). The primary end point was a doubling of the baseline serum creatinine concentration or the need for dialysis.

Results: At 3 years, 31 patients in the benazepril group and 57 in the placebo group had reached the primary end point (P<0.001). In the benazepril group, the reduction in the risk of reaching the end point was 53 % overall (95 % CI, 27–70 %), 71 % (95 % CI, 21–90 %) among the patients with mild renal insufficiency, and 46 % (95 % CI, 12–67 %) among those with moderate renal insufficiency. The reduction in risk was greatest among the male patients; those with glomerular diseases, diabetic nephropathy, or miscellaneous or unknown causes of renal disease; and those with baseline urinary protein excretion above 1 g/24 h. Benazepril was not effective in patients with polycystic disease. Diastolic pressure decreased by 3.5–5.0 mmHg in the benazepril group and increased by 0.2–1.5 mmHg in the placebo group.

Conclusions: Benazepril provides protection against the progression of renal insufficiency in patients with various renal diseases.

Critical Appraisal

Parameters	Yes	No	Comment
Validity			
Is the **randomization** procedure well described?		−1	Randomization procedure was not well described beyond the fact that it was aimed to match the control and intervention groups based on the disease severity in each center
Double **blinded**?	+2		
Is the **sample size** calculation described/ adequate?	+3		Not described, but likely to be adequate: Benazepril group: 300 patients Control: 283 patients Subsequently stratified into patients with mild CKD (Creatinine clearance: 60–45 mL/ min) and moderate CKD (CrCl: 44–30 mL/min)
Does it have a hard primary **end point**?		−1	Doubling of serum creatinine or the need for dialysis (the need for dialysis [ESRD] definition not protocolized/prespecified)
Is the end point surrogate?		0	GFR not measured ESRD not defined by a creatinine clearance, but instead by the need for dialysis
Is the follow-up appropriate?	+1		3 years
Was there a **Bias**?		+2	
Is the drop out >25 %?		+1	
Is the analysis **ITT**?	+3		
Utility/usefulness			
Can the findings be generalized?	+1		Nondiabetic CKD with CrCl between 60 and 30 mL/min
Was the NNT <100?	+1		11 treated with benazepril for 3 years to prevent one end point Five patients treated for 3 years if proteinuria >3 g/24 h
Score	81 %		

Discussion

AIPRI was the first large RCT investigating the impact of ACE inhibition (benazepril) on the progression of nondiabetic CKD; <5 % had diabetic nephropathy. It followed the publication of the Captopril study that Lewis et al. undertook and published in 1993 and showed that the rate of progression of diabetic nephropathy in patients with type 1 diabetes mellitus (DM) was significantly slowed down by ACE inhibition [10].

AIPRI is a well-designed and well-conducted RCT that seemed to indicate that benazepril (ACE inhibition) slows the progression of CKD. It also showed a significant reduction in proteinuria. AIPRI led to a huge number of subsequent studies claiming similar beneficial outcomes for ACE inhibitors in nondiabetic CKD.

While plausible, the limitations of this RCT are manifold:

1. Significant differences in systolic and diastolic BP between the treated and placebo groups cannot exclude a beneficial effect being solely due to lower BP and its possible impact on CKD progression. This was addressed in the study by statistical adjustment for changes in BP; however, a statistical correction for the biological effect of lower BP on CKD progression is difficult to achieve in order to exclude this major confounder.

2. Also, differences in BP control between groups were ascertained by casual office BP recordings. This is less than optimal in a trial of an intervention that primarily lowers BP, bearing in mind that more frequent daytime and nighttime recordings as well as 24 h ABPM are nowadays thought to be more reliable and less subject to variability as well as more predictive of outcomes [11].

3. CKD progression was to a very large extent (90 % of participants) evaluated by the doubling of serum creatinine, a commonly used progression parameter. This would be acceptable if ACE inhibition did not impact tubular secretion of creatinine [12, 13], thus confounding the interpretation and the validity of that end point in such trials. GFR was not measured.

Conclusions

This was undoubtedly a seminal trial in the field of CKD progression along with that of Lewis et al. in 1993 in patients with diabetic nephropathy [10]. Along with the REIN study that followed it [14], they set the trend of ACE inhibition in CKD.

Unfortunately, the AIPRI study shares many of the limitations of the entire literature on ACE inhibition in CKD, including the lack of measured GFR and rigor in BP measurements.

REIN Trial

Lancet. 1997 Jun 28;349(9069):1857–63.

Randomized placebo-controlled trial of effect of ramipril on the decline in glomerular filtration rate and risk of terminal renal failure in proteinuric, nondiabetic nephropathy. The GISEN Group (Gruppo Italiano di Studi Epidemiologici in Nefrologia)

Abstract

Background: In diabetic nephropathy, angiotensin-converting-enzyme (ACE) inhibitors have a greater effect than other antihypertensive drugs on proteinuria and the progressive decline in glomerular filtration rate (GFR). Whether this difference applies to the progression of non-diabetic proteinuric nephropathies is not clear. The Ramipril Efficacy in Nephropathy study of chronic nondiabetic nephropathies aimed to address whether glomerular protein traffic influences renal disease progression, and whether an ACE inhibitor was superior to conventional treatment, with the same blood pressure control, in reducing protein-uria, limiting GFR decline, and preventing end-stage renal disease.

Methods: In this prospective double-blind trial, 352 patients were classified according to baseline proteinuria (stratum 1: 1–3 g/24 h; stratum 2: ≥3 g/24 h), and randomly assigned ramipril or placebo plus conventional antihyperten-sive therapy targeted at achieving diastolic BP under 90 mmHg. The primary end point was the rate of GFR decline. Analysis was by intention to treat.

Findings: At the second planned interim analysis, the difference in decline in GFR between the ramipril and pla-cebo groups in stratum 2 was highly significant ($p = 0.001$). The Independent Adjudicating Panel therefore decided to open the randomization code and do the final analysis in this stratum (stratum 1 continued in the trial). Data (at least three GFR measurements including baseline) were available for 56 ramipril-assigned patients and 61 placebo-assigned patients. The decline in GFR per month was sig-nificantly lower in the ramipril group than the placebo group (0.53 [0.08] vs. 0.88 [0.13] mL/min, $p = 0.03$). Among the ramipril-assigned patients, percentage reduction in pro-teinuria was inversely correlated with the decline in GFR ($p = 0.035$) and predicted the reduction in risk of doubling of baseline creatinine or end-stage renal failure (18 ramipril vs. 40 placebo, $p = 0.04$). The risk of progression was still significantly reduced after adjustment for changes in sys-tolic ($p = 0.04$) and diastolic ($p = 0.04$) BP, but not after

Critical Appraisal

Parameters	Yes	No	Comment
Validity			
Is the **randomization** procedure well described?	+1		Randomization code allocated by Hoescht research institute
Double **blinded**?		−2	Study was unblinded at 27 months, in view of publication of a study showing a beneficial effect of ACE inhibition. The study continued unblinded for an additional 3 years as open label
Is the **sample size** calculation described/adequate?		−3	Assumptions of progression and protection by ACE inhibitor were made based on the studies of patients with progressive diabetic nephropathy
			This may not be translatable to nondiabetic CKD
			No, in view of the small number of patients included in the study (50 % of the total randomized: 177 of 352) and the even smaller number of those whose data was analyzed by measured GFR: 117 of 166 in strata 2 (proteinuric)
Does it have a hard primary **end point**?	+1		Rate of decline in measured GFR measured by the clearance of nonradioactive iohexol clearance
Is the end point surrogate?		0	However, GFR was measured in a percentage of patients (117 of 166 = ~70 %) enrolled, and ESRD was not protocolized and well defined. The last point is all the more relevant since the study was unblinded to the investigators from the 27th month and for a duration of the three following years
Is the follow-up appropriate?	+1		42 months
Was there a **Bias**?		+2	
Is the drop out >25 %?	−1		Only 50 % of those enrolled had a GFR-based analysis
Is the analysis **ITT**?		−3	Only those who had measured GFR were analyzed, although the authors state that the study was an ITT-based analysis
Utility/usefulness			
Can the findings be generalized?	+1		To patients with proteinuric CKD3
Was the NNT <100?	+1		
Score	0 %		

adjustment for changes in proteinuria. Blood pressure control and the overall number of cardiovascular events were similar in the two treatment groups.

Interpretation: In chronic nephropathies with proteinuria of 3 g or more per 24 h, ramipril safely reduces proteinuria and the rate of GFR decline to an extent that seems to exceed the reduction expected for the degree of BP lowering.

Discussion

REIN is undoubtedly the single most important RCT on the impact of ACE inhibition (ramipril) on the progression of nondiabetic CKD. It is certainly the most cited. It has led to a tsunami of ACE inhibition prescription to patients with proteinuric CKD and even to those without the same severity of proteinuria (>3–4 g/24 h). It has considerably informed subsequent guidelines on the management of hypertension in patients with CKD [15, 16].

It also claimed that the changes in the measured GFR were independent from comparable BP control in both groups but dependent on the changes in proteinuria that decreased in the ramipril group.

The REIN study has significant limitations:

1. It is undoubtedly underpowered as the sample size of the stratum [16], analyzed in the publication under discussion, is half the total study randomized population (177 of 352); those with lower level proteinuria showed no beneficial effect of ACE inhibition on progression, and had the total population been included in the analysis, there would have been no overall effect of ramipril on CKD progression.

2. Overall, only 177 of 352 patients in the REIN study had measured GFR. The sample of the study population who had the evaluation of the primary end point measured GFR, in the strata/substudy 2 (proteinuric patients), was even smaller – 56 of 78 (ramipril-treated) and 61 of 88 (controls). Consequently, this was a per-protocol study analysis, although the authors state otherwise (ITT).

3. Blood pressure control was comparable in both groups, but it can be argued that measuring casual/office blood pressure is no longer considered an accurate enough reflection of overall blood pressure control; 24 h ambulatory blood pressure monitoring (24 h ABPM) is considered more reliable [17]. In fact, in another study on the impact of ramipril on cardiovascular outcomes, differences in outcome proved to be associated with better nighttime BP control and 24 h BP control in the ramipril group, an effect that would have been overlooked if only office BP was measured [18].

4. The use of ESRD and start of dialysis as an end point without prior defined protocolization with clear specification of the level at which ESRD would be determined is unsatisfactory, all the more so in an unblinded study such as REIN.

Conclusions

Unfortunately, REIN is an underpowered study with an inadequate sample size, insufficiently large to draw firm and irrefutable conclusions.

REIN Follow-Up Trial

Lancet. 1999 Jul 31;354(9176):359–64.

Renoprotective properties of ACE inhibition in nondiabetic nephropathies with nonnephrotic proteinuria

Ruggenenti P, Perna A, Gherardi G, Garini G, Zoccali C, Salvadori M, Scolari F, Schena FP, Remuzzi G.

Abstract

Background: Stratum 2 of the Ramipril Efficacy in Nephropathy (REIN) study has already shown that in patients with chronic nephropathies and proteinuria of 3 g or more per 24 h, angiotensin-converting enzyme (ACE) inhibition reduced the rate of decline in glomerular filtration and halved the combined risk of doubling of serum creatinine or end-stage renal failure (ESRF) found in controls on placebo plus conventional antihypertensives. In REIN stratum 1 reported here, 24 h proteinuria was 1 g or more, but less than 3 g/24 h.

Methods: In stratum 1 of this double-blind trial, 186 patients were randomized to a ramipril or a control (placebo plus conventional antihypertensive therapy) group targeted at achieving a diastolic blood pressure of less than 90 mmHg. The primary end points were changed in glomerular filtration rate (GFR) and time to ESRF or overt proteinuria (≥ 53 g/24 h). Median follow-up was 31 months.

Findings: The decline in GFR per month was not significantly different (ramipril, 0.26 [SE 0.05] mL/min/1.73 m^2; control, 0.29 [0.06]). Progression to ESRF was significantly less common in the ramipril group (9/99 vs. 18/87) for a relative risk (RR) of 2.72 (95 % CI, 1.22–6.08); so was the progression to overt proteinuria (15/99 vs. 27/87, RR 2.40 [1.27–4.52]). Patients with a baseline GFR of 45 mL/min/1.73 m^2 or less and proteinuria of 1.5 g/24 h or more had more rapid progression and gained the most from ramipril treatment. Proteinuria decreased by 13 % in the ramipril group and increased by 15 % in the controls. Cardiovascular events were similar. As expected, the rate of decline in GFR and the frequency of ESRF were much lower in stratum 1 than they had been in stratum 2.

Interpretation: In nondiabetic nephropathies, ACE inhibition confers renoprotection even to patients with nonnephrotic proteinuria.

Critical Appraisal

Parameters	Yes	No	Comment
Validity			
Is the **randomization** procedure well described?	+1		Randomization code allocated by the Hoescht Research Institute
Double **blinded**?		−2	Study was unblinded at 27 months and subsequently pursued for 3 years as open label
Is the **sample size** calculation described/adequate?		−3	Assumptions of progression and protection by ACE inhibitor were made based on the studies of patients with progressive diabetic nephropathy
			This may not be translatable to nondiabetic CKD
			Study likely to be underpowered, in view of the small number of patients included in the study – 186 of 352 (Strata 1 = ~50 % of the total randomized). The number of patients whose data was analyzed by measured GFR is not specified and is likely to be an even smaller number
Does it have a hard primary **end point**?			Rate of decline in measured GFR and ESRD (the latter could be a subjective decision regarding initiation of RRT by investigators who had unblinded information)
Is the end point surrogate?		0	
Is the follow-up appropriate?	+1		Median follow-up = 31 months
Was there a **Bias**?		+2	Baseline GFR was higher in the ramipril group
Is the drop out >25 %?		+1	Number of those who had a measured GFR is unclear but those who reached ESRD is given
Is the analysis **ITT**?			Number of those who had a measured GFR is unclear but those who reached ESRD is given
Utility/usefulness			
Can the findings be generalized?	+1		To nondiabetic patients with CKD3 and proteinuria <3 g/24 hour
Was the NNT <100?	+1		
Score	12.5 %		

Discussion

This is the other half of the REIN study (strata 1) evaluating the impact of ACE inhibition with ramipril on the progression of nondiabetic CKD with nonnephrotic range proteinuria (<3 g/24 h).

It suffers the same limitations as the main REIN study (stratum 2 in nephrotic patients).

But, in addition, it has the following limitations:

1. The overall end point result relating to the decline in the measured GFR, 0.26 mL/min/month, is identical between the two groups, ramipril and placebo. It is only when a subgroup analysis is undertaken of those with GFR lesser or greater than 45 mL/min that those with GFR < 45 mL/min seem to benefit from ramipril treatment. Subgroup analysis is at best hypothesis-generating and not concluding evidence.

2. Intriguingly, while there was no difference in the GFR rate of decline, there was a higher percentage of patients reaching ESRF in the placebo group. Starting RRT was a clinical decision and not one based on reaching a prespecified protocolized cutoff GFR. This was confounded by the fact that the investigators by that stage of the study were no longer blinded, as the study was unblended at 27 months.

Conclusions

Overall, this is a negative albeit underpowered study. Subgroup analysis claims to show a benefit in those with GFR < 45 mL/min, but this would be at best hypothesis-generating, as the study was not powered to answer the question of the level of GFR that responded best to ACE inhibition.

RAS Inhibition in Advanced CKD4–5

N Engl J Med. 2006 Jan 12;354(2):131–40.

Efficacy and safety of benazepril for advanced chronic renal insufficiency.

Hou FF, Zhang X, Zhang GH, Xie D, Chen PY, Zhang WR, Jiang JP, Liang M, Wang GB, Liu ZR, Geng RW.

Abstract

Background: Angiotensin-converting enzyme inhibitors provide renal protection in patients with mild-to-moderate renal insufficiency (serum creatinine level, 3.0 mg/dL or less). We assessed the efficacy and safety of benazepril in patients without diabetes who had advanced renal insufficiency.

Methods: We enrolled 422 patients in a randomized, double-blind study. After an 8-week run-in period, 104 patients with serum creatinine levels of 1.5–3.0 mg/dL (group 1) received 20 mg of benazepril per day, whereas 224 patients with serum creatinine levels of 3.1–5.0 mg/dL (group 2) were randomly assigned to receive 20 mg of benazepril per day (112 patients) or placebo (112 patients) and then followed for a mean of 3.4 years. All patients received conventional antihypertensive therapy. The primary outcome was the composite of a doubling of the serum creatinine level, end-stage renal disease, or death. Secondary end points included changes in the level of proteinuria and the rate of progression of renal disease.

Results: Of 102 patients in group 1, 22 patients (22 %) reached the primary end point, as compared with 44 of 108 patients given benazepril in group 2 (41 %) and 65 of 107 patients given placebo in group 2 (60 %). As compared with placebo, benazepril was associated with a 43 % reduction in the risk of the primary end point in group 2 ($P = 0.005$). This benefit did not appear to be attributable to BP control. Benazepril therapy was associated with a 52 % reduction in the level of proteinuria and a reduction of 23 % in the rate of decline in renal function. The overall incidence of major adverse events in the benazepril and placebo subgroups of group 2 was similar.

Conclusions: Benazepril conferred substantial renal benefits in patients without diabetes who had advanced renal insufficiency. (ClinicalTrials.gov number, NCT00270426.)

Critical Appraisal

Parameters	Yes	No	Comment
Validity			
Is the **randomization** procedure well described?	+1		Computer-generated randomization
Double **blinded**?	+2		
Is the **sample size** calculation described/ adequate?	+3		Although an assumption of 60 % progression to ESRD in the group not treated with ACE inhibitors may be incorrect, the assumption that ACE inhibition would slow progression by 40 % is questionable. The sample size calculation assumption raises concern about the power of the study
Does it have a hard primary **end point**?		−1	Composite end points including doubling of serum creatinine, ESRD, and start of RRT or death GFR was not measured
Is the end point surrogate?		−2	Serum creatinine parameters, and nonprotocolized and prespecified ESRD cutoff point make these end points soft
Is the follow-up appropriate?			3.4 years
Was there a **Bias**?		−2	Only one control group with CKD4 and none for those with higher GFR (group 1)
Is the drop out >25 %?		−1	Large number (>35 %) of randomized, but not analyzed, patients in all groups: 326 of 422 analyzed
Is the analysis **ITT**?		−3	>30 % not analyzed
Utility/usefulness			
Can the findings be generalized?		−1	Applicable to Chinese with CKD4 and 5
Was the NNT <100?	+1		
Score	0 %		

Discussion

This study took the use of ACE inhibitors a step further and into patients with CKD stage 4. This has encouraged a trend of the prescription of this class of antihyperten-sive agents to all CKD patients, even those with GFRs < 20 mL/min.

The study concluded that benazepril treatment was capable of considerably improving outcomes (by 50 %) even in advanced CKD – stage 4.

The study and its design have a number of limitations and inconsistencies:

1. GFR was not measured as a gold standard to evaluate CKD progression at this advanced stage of CKD.
2. A composite end point of interrelated end points, doubling of serum creatinine, ESRD, or death, was used with the serious limitations of such an approach and without clarification of the end point with the highest impact and meaning. This calls for cautious interpretation of results [19].
3. The design of this RCT is complicated, with one placebo group with a lower GFR for two benazepril groups of different GFRs: 26 and 37 mL/min.
4. Blood pressure was claimed to be the same between groups, although one received placebo and the other two benazepril. Also, casual 3-monthly office BP recording leaves a lot to be desired in RCTs, where the intervention is primarily an antihypertensive strategy; day and night BP recordings as well as 24 h ABPM would have been more conclusive [20].
5. Some inconsistencies such as identical values for creatinine clearance and GFR at baseline, when it is well known that at CKD stage 4, creatinine clearance can exceed GFR by as much as 50 % due to increased tubular secretion of creatinine.
6. Study power and sample size as well as benazepril dosage differed in this study from a parallel publication of the same study by the same group in a Chinese journal [21]. This warrants clarification and justification.

Conclusions

Critical appraisal highlights numerous limitations to this RCT, raising concern that such a study has been adopted by many without careful evaluation of data, justifying the prescription of RAS inhibitors to patients with advanced renal insufficiency at the risk of further decline in kidney function.

REIN 2 Trial

Lancet. 2005 Mar 12–18;365(9463):939–46.

Blood pressure control for renoprotection in patients with nondiabetic chronic renal disease (REIN-2): multicenter, randomized controlled trial.

Ruggenenti P, Perna A, Loriga G, Ganeva M, Ene-Iordache B, Turturro M, Lesti M, Perticucci E, Chakarski IN,

Leonardis D, Garini G, Sessa A, Basile C, Alpa M, Scanziani R, Sorba G, Zoccali C, Remuzzi G; REIN-2 Study Group.

Abstract

Background: In chronic nephropathies, inhibition of angiotensin-converting enzyme (ACE) is renoprotective, but can further renoprotection be achieved by reduction of blood pressure (BP) to lower than usual targets? We aimed to assess the effect of intensified versus conventional BP control on progression to end-stage renal disease.

Methods: We undertook a multicenter, randomized controlled trial of patients with nondiabetic proteinuric nephropathies receiving background treatment with the ACE inhibitor ramipril (2.5–5 mg/day). We randomly assigned participants, either conventional (diastolic<90 mmHg; $n = 169$) or intensified (systolic/diastolic<130/80 mmHg; $n = 169$) BP control. To achieve the intensified BP level, patients received add-on therapy with the dihydropyridine calcium channel blocker felodipine (5–10 mg/day). The primary outcome measure was the time to end-stage renal disease over 36 months' follow-up, and analysis was by intention to treat.

Findings: Of 338 patients who were randomized, 3 (2 assigned intensified and 1 allocated conventional BP control) never took study drugs, and they were excluded. Over a median follow-up of 19 months (IQR, 12–35), 38/167 (23 %) patients assigned to intensified BP control and 34/168 (20 %) allocated conventional control progressed to end-stage renal disease (hazard ratio, 1.00 [95 % CI 0.61–1.64]; $p = 0.99$).

Interpretation: In patients with nondiabetic proteinuric nephropathies receiving background ACE inhibitor therapy, no additional benefit from further BP reduction by felodipine could be shown.

Discussion

The emphasis of the REIN 2 study was to evaluate whether more aggressive BP reduction (<130/80 mmHg compared to diastolic BP<90 mmHg), by the addition of a dihydropyridine calcium antagonist (Felodipine) to ramipril, impacted favorably on the progression of nondiabetic CKD.

This is essentially a negative study, whereby lower BP targets achieved throughout the study in the two arms of the study by adding felodipine to an antihypertensive regimen including ramipril failed to reduce the incidence of ESRD.

Randomization and inclusion criteria are complex as patients with proteinuria between 1 and 3 g/24 h were included if their GFR<45 mL/min, while those with heavier and nephrotic range proteinuria (>3 g/24 h) were included up to a GFR of 70 mL/min; having said that, looking at baseline

Parameters	Yes	No	Comment
Validity			
Is the **randomization** procedure well described?	+1		
Double **blinded**?		−2	Patients and investigators were aware of the allocation
Is the **sample size** calculation described/adequate?	+3		Early termination may have affected the study power
Does it have a hard primary **end point**?		−1	Time to ESRD over 36 months, although ESRD was neither protocolized nor specified
Is the end point surrogate?		−2	Time to ESRD in an unblinded study with no prespecified ESRD cutoff point is a soft end point
Is the follow-up appropriate?			Terminated early for futility
Was there a **Bias**?		+2	
Is the drop out >25 %?		+1	
Is the analysis **ITT**?	+3		
Utility/usefulness			
Can the findings be generalized?	+1		CKD3 patients with variable levels of proteinuria
Was the NNT <100?			Negative study
Score	27 %		

characteristics of both groups, no significant difference in GFR between the groups is apparent.

The study managed to sustain a significant difference in the mean arterial BP between the two groups.

However, limitations include the following:

1. GFR was measured in a subgroup (~50 %), thus casting doubt on the power of the analysis in view of the smaller sample size. Also, early termination confounds interpretation and power and precludes any meaningful conclusions.
2. The unblinded nature of the study raises concerns over investigators' bias as well as different attitude to diet and drug compliance among patients.
3. ESRD was not defined by a prespecified GFR cutoff, so time to ESRD as the start of renal replacement therapy (RRT) could be subjectively assigned by unblinded investigators.
4. For a study pertaining to examine the impact of BP control, a more assiduous monitoring of BP would have been justified to ascertain true differences in BP throughout the day/night as well as over 24 h [22]. Casual/office BP measurements do justice to the aim of such a study.
5. It has also been argued that the choice of a dihydropyridine as the agent to further reduce BP may have been counteracted by its potential to increase glomerular hypertension and possibly filtration, at least initially, although this was not reported in the result section of the study. Also, this was not manifested by an increase in

proteinuria in the felodipine arm, although an early and transient increase in proteinuria may have taken place, but again this was not reported in the result section of the study. Such changes took place in another CKD and BP control study, AASK, where a calcium antagonist was used [23].

6. Distinction between acute and chronic intervention changes was not sought in this study as it was in the AASK study where an early (first 3 months), acute reduction in BP may have had a negative impact on progression, followed later by a slower and sustained benefit [23] (see AASK study appraisal); such a biphasic slope effect was also noted in the MDRD study, comparing two levels of BP control [24].

7. Finally, the rate of progression/decline of GFR was rather slow, averaging around 0.20 mL/min/month in those with proteinuria < 3 g/24 h, considered by most as slow decline in GFR and casting doubt on the progressive nature of CKD in a significant proportion of participants. A slow progression rate in patients already treated by an ACE inhibitor may have warranted a higher power and a larger sample size.

Conclusions

No meaningful conclusion can be drawn from this study in view of its design, early termination, and most likely underpowered nature.

AASK Trial

JAMA. 2002 Nov 20;288(19):2421–31.

Effect of blood pressure lowering and antihypertensive drug class on the progression of hypertensive kidney disease: results from the AASK trial.

Wright JT Jr, Bakris G, Greene T, Agodoa LY, Appel LJ, Charleston J, Cheek D, Douglas-Baltimore JG, Gassman J, Glassock R, Hebert L, Jamerson K, Lewis J, Phillips RA, Toto RD, Middleton JP, Rostand SG; African American Study of Kidney Disease and Hypertension Study Group.

Abstract

Context: Hypertension is a leading cause of end-stage renal disease (ESRD) in the United States, with no known treatment to prevent progressive declines leading to ESRD.

Objective: To compare the effects of two levels of blood pressure (BP) control and three antihypertensive drug classes on glomerular filtration rate (GFR) decline in hypertension.

Design: Randomized 3×2 factorial trial, with enrollment from February 1995 to September 1998.

Setting and Participants: A total of 1,094 African Americans aged 18–70 years with hypertensive renal disease (GFR, 20–65 mL/min/1.73 m^2) were recruited from 21 clinical centers throughout the United States and followed up for 3–6.4 years.

Interventions: Participants were randomly assigned to one of two mean arterial pressure goals, 102–107 mmHg (usual; $n=554$) or 92 mmHg or less (lower; $n=540$), and to initial treatment with either a beta-blocker (metoprolol, 50–200 mg/day; $n=441$), an angiotensin-converting enzyme inhibitor (ramipril, 2.5–10 mg/day; $n=436$), or a dihydropyridine calcium channel blocker (amlodipine, 5–10 mg/day; $n=217$). Open-label agents were added to achieve the assigned BP goals.

Main Outcome Measures: Rate of change in GFR (GFR slope): clinical composite outcome of reduction in GFR by 50 % or more (or ≥ 25 mL/min/1.73 m^2) from baseline, ESRD, or death. Three primary treatment comparisons were specified: lower versus usual BP goal; ramipril versus metoprolol; and amlodipine versus metoprolol.

Results: An average of (SD) 128/78 (12/8) mmHg in the lower BP group and 141/85 (12/7) mmHg in the usual BP group was achieved in the study. The mean (SE) GFR slope from baseline through 4 years did not differ significantly between the lower BP group (−2.21 [0.17] mL/min/1.73 m^2/year) and the usual BP group (−1.95 [0.17] mL/min/1.73 m^2/year; $P=.24$), and the lower BP goal did not significantly reduce the rate of the clinical composite outcome (risk reduction for lower BP group=2 %; 95 % CI, -22–21 %; $P=.85$). None of the drug group comparisons showed consistent significant differences in the GFR slope. However, compared with the metoprolol and amlodipine groups, the ramipril group manifested risk reductions in the clinical composite outcome of 22 % (95 % CI, 1–38 %; $P=.04$) and 38 % (95 % CI, 14–56 %; $P=.004$), respectively. There was no significant difference in the clinical composite outcome between the amlodipine and metoprolol groups.

Conclusions: No additional benefit of slowing progression of hypertensive nephrosclerosis was observed with the lower BP goal. Angiotensin-converting enzyme inhibitors appear to be more effective than beta-blockers or dihydropyridine calcium channel blockers in slowing GFR decline.

Discussion

The AASK study was the second large-scale study, after MDRD [25], to investigate the impact of lower BP targets on the progression of CKD; AASK emphasis was on the African-American (AA) population with hypertensive

Critical Appraisal

Parameters	Yes	No	Comment
Validity			
Is the **randomization** procedure well described?	+1		Based on a 3×2 factorial design, participants were randomized equally to a usual mean arterial pressure goal of 102–107 mmHg or to a lower mean goal of 92 mmHg or lower, and to treatment with one of three antihypertensive drugs
Double **blinded**?	+2		
Is the **sample size** calculation described/adequate?	+3		1,094 patients
Does it have a hard primary **end point**?	+1		Changes in measured GFR (radioactive Iothalamate clearance)
Is the end point surrogate?	0		
Is the follow-up appropriate?	+1		Up to 4 years
Was there a **Bias**?		+2	
Is the drop out >25 %?		+1	
Is the analysis **ITT**?	+3		
Utility/usefulness			
Can the findings be generalized?		−1	Applicable to African Americans with hypertensive nephrosclerosis
Was the NNT <100?			Negative study
Score	86 %		

nephrosclerosis. It attempted to build on the MDRD preliminary data showing a possible advantage of lower BP in AA and also explore the true impact of ACE inhibition on the progression of CKD in this population. Assumptions were previously made that AA respond poorly to ACE inhibition, as their hypertension tends to be more volume dependent with a somewhat suppressed RAA system. It was a 2×3 factorial design, also aimed at exploring the different impacts of the levels of blood pressure control as well as that of the classes of antihypertensive agents.

AASK was an extremely well-designed, conducted, and analyzed RCT. It took into consideration not only the short-term and long-term effects of the interventions on GFR slopes, but also BP control and proteinuria. The difference of BP readings between usual (MAP=104 mmHg) and lower BP (MAP=95 mmHg) controls remained sustained at around a difference of 10 mmHg in the MAP throughout the study. In spite of that, there was no overall difference in CKD progression between the groups.

There was no significant difference in the primary outcome of GFR-measured decline between the groups treated with different antihypertensive agents, although

ramipril showed a beneficial effect compared to metoprolol and amlodipine in the secondary composite end point of GFR reduction, ERSD, and death.

A major strength of AASK is the fact that GFR was measured on its participants at regular intervals and not estimated (eGFR).

Another strength is the awareness of the investigators to the potential acute effects of acute BP reduction and calcium antagonist treatment on GFR as well as their evaluation along the chronic long-term effects. This helped explain some of the study findings but added little to the overall long-term outcome of 4 years.

A note of caution is the interpretation of a beneficial effect of ramipril over the other agents when interrelated secondary composite outcomes were used. Such an approach, relying on interrelated composite end points with different important gradients, can easily overestimate the impact of an intervention.

Blood pressure was measured casually and warranted more careful considerations: daytime and nighttime recordings and/or 24 h ABPM.

Conclusions

This cornerstone study shows convincingly that over an observation time of 4 years, more intensive BP control had little impact on the rate of CKD progression. AASK also showed that ACE inhibition was not more effective than metoprolol in slowing the decline in GFR over a 4-year period in AA with hypertensive nephrosclerosis.

Of interest, a cohort follow-up observational study of the AASK study examining the impact of different levels of BP control showed that the intensity of BP control had little overall impact on the rate of progression of CKD, with the possible exception of proteinuric patients who may benefit from lower BP targets [25].

ACCOMPLISH Trial

Lancet. 2010 Apr 3;375(9721):1173–81. doi: 10.1016/S0140-6736(09)62100-0. Epub 2010 Feb 18.

Renal outcomes with different fixed-dose combination therapies in patients with hypertension at high risk for cardiovascular events (ACCOMPLISH): a prespecified secondary analysis of a randomized controlled trial.

Bakris GL, Sarafidis PA, Weir MR, Dahlöf B, Pitt B, Jamerson K, Velazquez EJ, Staikos-Byrne L, Kelly RY, Shi V, Chiang YT, Weber MA; ACCOMPLISH Trial investigators.

Collaborators (554)

Abstract

Background: The Avoiding Cardiovascular Events through Combination Therapy in Patients Living with Systolic Hypertension (ACCOMPLISH) trial showed that initial antihypertensive therapy with benazepril plus amlodipine was superior to that with benazepril plus hydrochlorothiazide in reducing cardiovascular morbidity and mortality. We assessed the effects of these drug combinations on the progression of chronic kidney disease.

Methods: ACCOMPLISH was a double-blind, randomized trial undertaken in five countries (The United States, Sweden, Norway, Denmark, and Finland). About 11,506 patients with hypertension and who were at high risk for cardiovascular events were randomly assigned via a central, telephone-based interactive voice response system in a 1:1 ratio to receive benazepril (20 mg) plus amlodipine (5 mg; $n = 5,744$) or benazepril (20 mg) plus hydrochlorothiazide (12.5 mg; $n = 5,762$), orally once daily. Drug doses were force-titrated for patients to attain the recommended blood pressure goals. Progression of chronic kidney disease, a prespecified end point, was defined as doubling of serum creatinine concentration or end-stage renal disease (estimated glomerular filtration rate < 15 mL/min/1.73 m^2) or need for dialysis. Analysis was by intention to treat (ITT). This trial is registered with ClinicalTrials.gov, number NCT00170950.

Findings: The trial was terminated early (mean follow-up: 2.9 years [SD 0.4]) because of the superior efficacy of benazepril plus amlodipine compared with benazepril plus hydrochlorothiazide. At trial completion, vital status was not known for 143 (1 %) patients who were lost to follow-up (benazepril plus amlodipine, $n = 70$; benazepril plus hydrochlorothiazide, $n = 73$). All randomized patients were included in the ITT analysis. There were 113 (2.0 %) events of chronic kidney disease progression in the benazepril plus amlodipine group compared with 215 (3.7 %) in the benazepril plus hydrochlorothiazide group (HR 0.52, 0.41–0.65, $p < 0.0001$). The most frequent adverse event in patients with chronic kidney disease was peripheral edema (benazepril plus amlodipine, 189 of 561, 33.7 %; benazepril plus hydrochlorothiazide, 85 of 532, 16.0 %). In patients with chronic kidney disease, angio-edema was more frequent in the benazepril plus amlodipine group than in the benazepril plus hydrochlorothiazide group. In patients without chronic kidney disease, dizziness, hypokalemia, and hypotension were more frequent in the benazepril plus hydrochlorothiazide group than in the benazepril plus amlodipine group.

Interpretation: Initial antihypertensive treatment with benazepril plus amlodipine should be considered in preference to benazepril plus hydrochlorothiazide since it slows progression of nephropathy to a greater extent.

Funding: Novartis.

Critical Appraisal

Parameters	Yes	No	Comment
Validity			
Is the **randomization** procedure well described?	+1		
Double **blinded**?	+2		
Is the **sample size** calculation described/ adequate?		−3	Sample size justification explained, but the study is probably underpowered to examine the impact of interventions on CKD progression also in view of the early (~2.9 years) termination of the trial due to higher cardiovascular event rate in the ACE inhibitor + thiazide group
Does it have a hard primary **end point**?		−1	GFR was not measured
Is the end point surrogate?		−2	Serum creatinine parameters including eGFR are soft end points ESRD was prespecified, but it also relied on eGFR GFR was not measured
Is the follow-up appropriate?		−1	Study terminated prematurely, thus impacting the duration of renal follow-up and the renal study power
Was there a **Bias**?	+2		
Is the drop out >25 %?	+1		
Is the analysis **ITT**?	+3		
Utility/usefulness			
Can the findings be generalized?		−1	Proteinuria was minimal in this study Not primarily a CKD progression study; thus, CKD population poorly defined
Was the NNT <100?	+1		
Score	12.5 %		

Discussion

Most guidelines and recommendations related to the use of RAS inhibitors in CKD suggest that optimization of their antihypertensive as well as antiproteinuric effects is facilitated by the addition of either dietary salt restriction or the addition of a diuretic [26]. Also, the beneficial effect of RAS inhibition depends, to a significant extent, on their antiproteinuric effect [27]. ACCOMPLISH intended to question some of these assertions by comparing the combination of an ACE inhibitor with a thiazide diuretic to that of the same ACE inhibitor combined to a calcium antagonist. Of note, ACCOMPLISH was primarily a study on the impact of these different drug combinations on cardiovascular outcomes.

Although the ACCOMPLISH study was not primarily aimed at the investigation of the impact of the interventions on the progression of CKD, but instead at the investigation of CVD outcomes, CKD progression was one of the prespecified end points.

The slower CKD progression rate on the combination of benazepril and amlodipine compared to benazepril and hydrochlorothiazide was somewhat unexpected. Slower progression also occurred in association with a more significant reduction in proteinuria progression in the benazepril + hydrochlorothiazide group.

However, a number of limitations preclude any meaningful conclusion:

1. As stated by the authors, the study was not powered as a CKD progression study. Data interpretation is further limited by the shortened follow-up time (2.9 years) due to early termination of the study.
2. For a study focusing on the impact of antihypertensive agents, it is somewhat surprising that BP was not accurately measured with daytime and nighttime recordings and/or 24 h ABPM. The relationship between casual/office BP recording and CVD outcomes is weak [27, 28]. Therefore, it is impossible to exclude that the difference in outcomes between groups is independent from the differences in blood pressure control. When faced with this criticism, the authors reported in a letter to the editor that subgroups of patients in the ACCOMPLISH study had more thorough evaluation of their BP with daytime, nighttime, and 24 h ABPM recording but failed to show significant differences in BP control between groups [29].
3. GFR was not measured, therefore raising the possibility that changes in serum creatinine and derived eGFR may be affected by changes in tubular secretion of creatinine.

Conclusions

The study seems to imply that a combination of an ACE inhibitor with a calcium antagonist is superior to the combination of the ACE inhibitor with a diuretic in spite of a less efficient antiproteinuric effect. However, the study limitations highlighted above preclude meaningful conclusions.

Bicarbonate Supplementation Trial

J Am Soc Nephrol. 2009 Sep;20(9):2075–84. doi: 10.1681/ASN.2008111205. Epub 2009 Jul 16.

Bicarbonate supplementation slows progression of CKD and improves nutritional status

de Brito-Ashurst I, Varagunam M, Raftery MJ, Yaqoob MM.

Abstract

Bicarbonate supplementation preserves renal function in experimental chronic kidney disease (CKD), but whether the same benefit occurs in humans is unknown. Here, we randomly assigned 134 adult patients with CKD (creatinine clearance [CrCl], 15–30 mL/min/1.73 m^2, and serum bicarbonate, 16–20 mmol/L) to either supplementation with oral sodium bicarbonate or standard care for 2 years. The primary end points were rate of CrCl decline, the proportion of patients with rapid decline of CrCl (>3 mL/min/1.73 m^2/year), and ESRD (CrCl < 10 mL/min). Secondary end points were dietary protein intake, normalized protein nitrogen appearance, serum albumin, and mid-arm muscle circumference. Compared with the control group, decline in CrCl was slower with bicarbonate supplementation (5.93 vs. 1.88 mL/min/1.73 m^2; $P < 0.0001$). Patients supplemented with bicarbonate were significantly less likely to experience rapid progression (9 % vs. 45 %; relative risk, 0.15; 95 % CI, 0.06–0.40; $P < 0.0001$). Similarly, fewer patients supplemented with bicarbonate developed ESRD (6.5 % vs. 33 %; relative

Critical Appraisal

Parameters	Yes	No	Comment
Validity			
Is the **randomization** procedure well described?	+1		
Double **blinded**?		−2	Study was open label. Controls did not receive placebo
Is the **sample size** calculation described/adequate?		−3	Study is likely to be underpowered compared to other comparable CKD progression studies with similar assumptions and comparable end points
			The sample size of 134 patients is justified in view of the single center nature of the study
Does it have a hard primary **end point**?		−1	GFR was not measured
Is the end point surrogate?		−2	Changes in serum creatinine is at best considered a soft end point
			ESRD and start of RRT were not prespecified
Is the follow-up appropriate?	+2		2 years, acceptable for advanced renal insufficiency CKD4–5
Was there a **Bias**?		+2	
Is the drop out >25 %?		+1	
Is the analysis **ITT**?	+3		
Utility/usefulness			
Can the findings be generalized?	+1		To CKD4–5
Was the NNT <100?	+1		
Score	31 %		

risk, 0.13; 95 % CI, 0.04–0.40; $P<0.001$). Nutritional parameters improved significantly with bicarbonate supplementation, which was well tolerated. This study demonstrates that bicarbonate supplementation slows the rate of progression of renal failure to ESRD and improves nutritional status among patients with CKD.

Discussion

A large body of experimental data has suggested that metabolic acidosis exerts a negative and detrimental influence on CKD. Animal experimentation has led to the postulate that CKD is associated with a reduction in renal mass associated with a proximal tubular hyperammoniagenesis aimed at counteracting the metabolic acidosis of renal insufficiency, but that in turn had a potential harmful effect on renal fibrogenesis and scarring [30]. The clinical correlate would be that the correction of CKD-associated metabolic acidosis would attenuate such a potentially harmful process and slow the progression of CKD. While animal experimentation has been somewhat inconclusive, clinical data has been emerging in the last 10 years, supporting such correction and the administration of sodium bicarbonate to slow CKD progression [31].

This study relies entirely on the changes in serum creatinine and the start of RRT as end points to ascertain that sodium bicarbonate supplementation slows the progression of CKD. It also makes the confounded assumption that the standard of care for acidotic CKD patients with stages 4 and 5 does not include sodium bicarbonate supplementation to correct the metabolic acidosis, in spite of the well-known fact that renal metabolic acidosis is associated with negative nutritional and renal osteodystrophy consequences [32].

The study has a number of limitations:

1. The study is likely to be underpowered with a sample size of <100/group.
2. It is unblinded (open label) and not placebo controlled.
3. Duration is relatively short (2 years), although this may be acceptable in advanced renal insufficiency.
4. The renal function trajectory of those recruited in the study was not predetermined to ascertain their rate of functional decline, thus allowing for the assumption of invariable progression rate and hence the relative short observation time.
5. Reliance on serum creatinine/CrCl estimation fails to acknowledge potential confounders such as the effect of correction of metabolic acidosis on creatinine intake (changes were observed in dietary protein intake in the study), metabolism (changes in muscle mass were observed in the study), or tubular secretion (potentially influenced by acidosis and its correction).

6. An additional confounder could be the dilutional effect due to additional sodium intake (sodium bicarbonate group) that might have led to an element of blood volume expansion and serum creatinine dilutional reduction. A sodium chloride control would have been warranted.
7. GFR was not measured.
8. Interdependent composite end points seem to have been used, with the known caution in the interpretation of related assumptions [33].

Conclusions

This study is a hybrid between an observational practice cohort study and a RCT. It therefore falls well short of the quality requirements for the latter.

Daily oral sodium bicarbonate preserves glomerular filtration rate by slowing its decline in early hypertensive nephropathy

Mahajan A, Simoni J, Sheather SJ, Broglio KR, Rajab MH, Wesson DE. J Kidney Int. 2010;78(3):303–9

Abstract

In most patients with hypertensive nephropathy and low glomerular filtration rate (GFR), the kidney function progressively declines despite the adequate control of the hypertension with angiotensin-converting enzyme (ACE) inhibition. Previously, we found that 2 years of oral sodium citrate slowed GFR decline in patients whose estimated GFR (eGFR) was very low (mean 33 mL/min). This treatment also slowed GFR decline in an animal model of surgically reduced nephron mass. Here, we tested if daily oral sodium bicarbonate slowed GFR decline in patients with hypertensive nephropathy with reduced but relatively preserved eGFR (mean, 75 mL/min) in a 5-year, prospective, randomized, placebo-controlled, and blinded interventional study. Patients matched for age, ethnicity, albuminuria, and eGFR received daily placebo or equimolar sodium chloride or bicarbonate while maintaining antihypertensive regimens (including ACE inhibition) aiming for their recommended blood pressure (BP) targets. After 5 years, the rate of eGFR decline, estimated using plasma cystatin C, was slower, and eGFR was higher in patients given sodium bicarbonate than in those given placebo or sodium chloride. Thus, our study shows that in hypertensive nephropathy, daily sodium bicarbonate is an effective kidney protective adjunct to BP control along with ACE inhibition.

Critical Appraisal

Parameters	Yes	No	Comment
Validity			
Is the **randomization** procedure well described?	+1		
Double **blinded**?	+2		
Is the **sample size** calculation described/adequate?	+3		It was estimated that 108 subjects completing the protocol would yield 80 % likelihood to detect a difference in crGFR decline rate among the three groups at 0.05 significance level assuming decline rates of −2.26 mL/min per year in placebo, −1.51 ml/min per year in NaHCO$_3$, and −2.26 ml/min per year in the NaCl group
Does it have a hard primary **end point**?		−1	GFR was not measured
Is the end point surrogate?	−2		Changes in serum creatinine or cystatin C slopes are soft end points, especially at this early stage of CKD
Is the follow-up appropriate?	+2		5 years
Was there a **Bias**?		+2	
Is the drop out >25 %?	−1		>50 %
Is the analysis **ITT**?		−3	Less than 50 % of those randomized completed the 5-year follow-up; only 120 of 349 were analyzed
Utility/usefulness			
Can the findings be generalized?	+1		Only to nonacidotic early CKD
Was the NNT <100?	+1		
Score	31 %		

Discussion

This study intended to investigate the effect of sodium bicarbonate supplementation in patients with CKD2 and overt proteinuria who do not have metabolic acidosis. This was aimed primarily at determining whether sodium bicarbonate supplementation per se, rather than the correction of metabolic acidosis, slowed the rate of decline in early proteinuric CKD (stage 2).

This is a well-designed and well-conducted study with the group supplemented with sodium bicarbonate matched by another group supplemented with sodium chloride and a third matched by placebo tablets. It implies that sodium bicarbonate supplementation in nonacidotic CKD2 individuals slows the decline in eGFR (cystatin C) over 5 years.

The study has limitations:

1. It is likely to be underpowered.
2. It is a per-protocol analysis at 5 years of a small group of patients, who did not seem to show any difference at 3 years.
3. Early CKD (2) individuals with unpredictable CKD progression, with many likely nonprogressors, especially in the absence of significant proteinuria, making the study power and sample size most likely inadequate.
4. Serum creatinine and cystatin C eGFR equations are used to assess progression. GFR was not measured.
5. Of interest, urine ACR did not change in the bicarbonate-supplemented group, while its trajectory increased in the other two groups, raising the suspicion that urinary creatinine excretion might have increased in the bicarbonate group.

Conclusions

It is most likely an underpowered study with no hard end point, such as measured GFR; therefore, it is largely inconclusive. Also, the clinical relevance of such intervention is questionable in nonproteinuric early CKD, which is mostly nonprogressive.

Studies of Renal Revascularization

ASTRAL Trial

N Engl J Med. 2009 Nov 12;361(20):1953–62. doi: 10.1056/NEJMoa0905368.

Revascularization versus medical therapy for renal artery stenosis.

ASTRAL Investigators, Wheatley K, Ives N, Gray R, Kalra PA, Moss JG, Baigent C, Carr S, Chalmers N, Eadington D, Hamilton G, Lipkin G, Nicholson A, Scoble J. Collaborators (475)

Abstract

Background: Percutaneous revascularization of the renal arteries improves patency in atherosclerotic renovascular disease; yet, evidence of a clinical benefit is limited.

Methods: In a randomized, unblinded trial, we assigned 806 patients with atherosclerotic renovascular disease, either to undergo revascularization in addition to receiving medical therapy or to receive medical therapy alone. The primary outcome was renal function, as measured by the reciprocal of the serum creatinine level (a measure that has a linear relationship with creatinine clearance). Secondary outcomes were blood pressure, the time to renal and major cardiovascular events, and mortality. The median follow-up was 34 months.

Results: During a 5-year period, the rate of progression of renal impairment (as shown by the slope of the reciprocal of the serum creatinine level) was $-0.07 \times 10(-3)$ L/mmol/year in the revascularization group, as compared with $-0.13 \times 10(-3)$ L/mmol/year in the medical therapy group, a difference favoring revascularization of $0.06 \times 10(-3)$ L/mmol/year (95 % confidence interval [CI], -0.002 to 0.13; $P=0.06$). Over the same time, the mean serum creatinine level was 1.6 mmol/L (95 % CI, -8.4 to 5.2 [0.02 mg/dL; 95 % CI, -0.10 to 0.06]) lower in the revascularization group than in the medical therapy group. There was no significant between-group difference in systolic blood pressure; the decrease in diastolic blood pressure was smaller in the revascularization group than in the medical therapy group. The two study groups had similar rates of renal events (hazard ratio in the revascularization group, 0.97; 95 % CI, 0.67–1.40; $P=0.88$), major cardiovascular events (hazard ratio, 0.94; 95 % CI, 0.75–1.19; $P=0.61$), and death (hazard ratio, 0.90; 95 % CI, 0.69–1.18; $P=0.46$). Serious complications associated with revascularization occurred in 23 patients, including two deaths and three amputations of toes or limbs.

Conclusions: We found substantial risks but no evidence of a worthwhile clinical benefit from revascularization in patients with atherosclerotic renovascular disease. (Current Controlled Trials number, ISRCTN59586944.)

Critical Appraisal

Parameters	Yes	No	Comment
Validity			
Is the **randomization** procedure well described?	+1		
Double **blinded**?		−2	Unblinded, and without placebo intervention
Is the **sample size** calculation described/adequate?	+3		The sample size was adequate: 385/388 patients per group
Does it have a hard primary **end point**?		−1	GFR was not measured. 1/sCr slopes were used to evaluate CKD progression
Is the end point surrogate?		−1	Serum creatinine, and its changes with time, is a surrogate for GFR decline
Is the follow-up appropriate?	+2		5 years
Was there a **Bias**?		+2	
Is the drop out >25 %?		−1	>50 %
Is the analysis **ITT**?	+3		
Utility/usefulness			
Can the findings be generalized?	+1		Patients with resistant hypertension and ARAD
Was the NNT <100?			Negative study
Score		**40 %**	

Discussion

With the increasing age of CKD patients, a large number presents to Nephrology practitioners with atherosclerotic renal artery disease (ARAD). They are often characterized by older age, severe and often resistant systolic hypertension, as well as slowly declining kidney function. The ASTRAL study examined the impact of renal revascularization (PTCA + stenting in most) on the rate of progression of CKD, most probably CKD4–5. Secondary end points include the control of hypertension as well as CVD events and death.

This is essentially a negative study, but the interpretation of outcomes has been confounded by the following limitations:

1. The study lacked a placebo intervention group.
2. Revascularization success was not ascertained, beyond the fact that it was "deemed" to be a success. The lack of difference in BP between the groups raises the suspicion of ineffective revascularization, although at 1 year, those who underwent revascularization used less antihypertensive medication.
3. The slope of the reciprocal of serum creatinine was used to assess CKD progression; this would cast a shadow over the possible confounding effect of the impact of renal revascularization on the peritubular renal circulation and its impact on renal tubular function including the secretion of creatinine.
4. GFR was not measured.
5. Blood pressure was measured casually at the office, but not appropriately for such a large trial by 24 h ABPM. Therefore, it is difficult to ascertain the lack of difference in BP control between the groups.

Conclusions

This was a negative study that led, at least in the United Kingdom, to a significant change in practice of the management of ARAD. The study has a number of limitations that casts some doubts over its results and interpretations.

CORAL Trial

N Engl J Med. 2014 Jan 2;370(1):13–22. doi: 10.1056/NEJMoa1310753. Epub 2013 Nov 18.

Stenting and medical therapy for atherosclerotic renal artery stenosis.

Cooper CJ, Murphy TP, Cutlip DE, Jamerson K, Henrich W, Reid DM, Cohen DJ, Matsumoto AH, Steffes M, Jaff MR, Prince MR, Lewis EF, Tuttle KR, Shapiro JI, Rundback JH, Massaro JM, D'Agostino RB Sr, Dworkin LD; CORAL Investigators. Collaborators (297)

Abstract

Background: Atherosclerotic renal artery stenosis is a common problem in the elderly. Despite two randomized trials that did not show a benefit of renal artery stenting with respect to kidney function, the usefulness of stenting for the prevention of major adverse renal and cardiovascular events is uncertain.

Methods: We randomly assigned 947 participants who had atherosclerotic renal artery stenosis and either systolic hypertension while taking two or more antihypertensive drugs or chronic kidney disease to medical therapy plus renal artery stenting or medical therapy alone. Participants were followed for the occurrence of adverse cardiovascular and renal events (a composite end point of death from cardiovascular or renal causes, myocardial infarction, stroke, hospitalization for congestive heart failure, progressive renal insufficiency, or the need for renal replacement therapy).

Results: Over a median follow-up period of 43 months (interquartile range, 31–55), the rate of the primary composite end point did not differ significantly between the participants who underwent stenting in addition to receiving medical therapy and those who received medical therapy alone (35.1 and 35.8 %, respectively; hazard ratio with stenting, 0.94; 95 % confidence interval [CI], 0.76–1.17; $P = 0.58$). There were also no significant differences between the treatment groups in the rates of the individual components of the primary end point or in all-cause mortality. During follow-up, there was a consistent modest difference in systolic blood pressure favoring the stent group (−2.3 mmHg; 95 % CI, −4.4 to −0.2; $P = 0.03$).

Conclusions: Renal artery stenting did not confer a significant benefit with respect to the prevention of clinical events when added to comprehensive, multifactorial medical therapy in people with atherosclerotic renal artery stenosis and hypertension or chronic kidney disease. (Funded by the National Heart, Lung and Blood Institute and others; ClinicalTrials.gov number, NCT00081731.).

Critical Appraisal

Parameters	Yes	No	Comment
Validity			
Is the **randomization** procedure well described?	+1		
Double **blinded**?		−2	Unblinded, and without placebo intervention
Is the **sample size** calculation described/adequate?	+3		Sample size was adequate: 467/480 patients per group
Does it have a hard primary **end point**?		−1	GFR was not measured eGFR calculated
Is the end point surrogate?	−1		Serum creatinine, and its changes with time, is a surrogate for GFR decline
Is the follow-up appropriate?	+2		43 months
Was there a **Bias**?		+2	
Is the drop out >25 %?		+1	
Is the analysis **ITT**?	+3		
Utility/usefulness			
Can the findings be generalized?	+1		Of note, not all those included in CORAL had CKD; baseline eGFR ~ 57 mL/min/1.73 m²
Was the NNT <100?			Negative Trial
Score	60 %		

Discussion

This is essentially a negative study, but interpretation of outcomes has been confounded by the following limitations:

1. Revascularization success was not ascertained. Lack of difference in BP and in the number of antihypertensive medication between the groups raises the suspicion of ineffective revascularization.
2. eGFR was used to investigate renal events; this would cast a shadow over the possible confounding effect of the impact of renal revascularization on the peritubular renal circulation and its impact on renal tubular function, including the secretion of creatinine.
3. GFR was not measured.
4. Blood pressure was measured casually at the office, and not appropriately for such a large trial, by 24 h ABPM. Therefore, it is difficult to ascertain the lack of difference in BP control between the groups.

Conclusions

The same limitations as the preceding UK ASTRAL study making firm conclusions difficult to reach.

SIMPLICITY HTN-3 Trial

N Engl J Med. 2014 Apr 10;370(15):1393–401. doi: 10.1056/NEJMoa1402670. Epub 2014 Mar 29.

A controlled trial of renal denervation for resistant hypertension.

Bhatt DL, Kandzari DE, O'Neill WW, D'Agostino R, Flack JM, Katzen BT, Leon MB, Liu M, Mauri L, Negoita M, Cohen SA, Oparil S, Rocha-Singh K, Townsend RR, Bakris GL; SYMPLICITY HTN-3 Investigators.

Collaborators (209)

Abstract

Background: Prior unblinded studies have suggested that catheter-based renal artery denervation reduces blood pressure in patients with resistant hypertension.

Methods: We designed a prospective, single-blind, randomized, sham-controlled trial. Patients with severe resistant hypertension were randomly assigned in a 2:1 ratio to undergo renal denervation or a sham procedure. Before randomization, patients were receiving a stable antihypertensive regimen involving maximally tolerated doses of at least three drugs, including a diuretic. The primary efficacy end point was the change in office systolic blood pressure at 6 months; a secondary efficacy end point was the change in mean 24 h ambulatory systolic blood pressure. The primary safety end point was a composite of death, end-stage renal disease, embolic events resulting in end-organ damage, renovascular complications, or hypertensive crisis at 1 month or new renal artery stenosis of more than 70 % at 6 months.

Results: A total of 535 patients underwent randomization. The mean (±SD) change in systolic blood pressure at 6 months was −14.13±23.93 mmHg in the denervation group as compared with −11.74±25.94 mmHg in the sham procedure group ($P<0.001$ for both comparisons of the change from baseline), for a difference of −2.39 mmHg (95 % confidence interval [CI], −6.89 to 2.12; $P=0.26$) for superiority with a margin of 5 mmHg. The change in 24 h ambulatory systolic blood pressure was −6.75±15.11 mmHg in the denervation group and −4.79±17.25 mmHg in the sham procedure group, for a difference of −1.96 mmHg (95 % CI, −4.97 to 1.06; $P=0.98$) for superiority with a margin of 2 mmHg. There were no significant differences in safety between the two groups.

Conclusions: This blinded trial did not show a significant reduction of systolic blood pressure in patients with resistant hypertension 6 months after renal artery denervation as compared with a sham control. (Funded by Medtronic; SIMPLICITY HTN-3 ClinicalTrials.gov number, NCT01418261.).

Critical Appraisal

Parameters	Yes	No	Comment
Validity			
Is the **randomization** procedure well described?	+1		
Double **blinded**?	+2		Blinded to patients and BP assessors
Is the **sample size** calculation described/adequate?	+3		This trial was powered for the primary safety and efficacy end points and for the change in mean 24 h ambulatory systolic blood pressure at 6 months (secondary efficacy end point). On the basis of the 9.8 % safety performance criterion, 316 patients were required in the renal denervation group to provide 80 % power, with the use of a one-sided significance level of 0.05
			Sample size was adequate: 364 denervations/171 controls
Does it have a hard primary **end point**?	+1		The primary end point was difference in systolic BP between the groups at 6 months, with a superiority margin of 5 mmHg
			Changes in 24 h ABPM was a secondary end point
Is the end point surrogate?	0		
Is the follow-up appropriate?	+2		6 months is appropriate for a BP control end point
Was there a **Bias**?		+2	
Is the drop out >25 %?		+1	
Is the analysis **ITT**?	+3		
Utility/usefulness			
Can the findings be generalized?	+1		Applicable to patients with resistant hypertension
Was the NNT <100?			Negative study
Score	100 %		

Discussion

This study was primarily a RCT, examining the impact of catheter-delivered, radiofrequency-energy-mediated, renal artery (sympathetic) denervation on hypertension control in the short term (6 months). Primary end points included office as well as 24 h ABPM. SIMPLICITY 3 followed two unblinded and poorly controlled renal artery (sympathetic) denervation studies that suggested a beneficial effect of the intervention in patients with resistant hypertension [34, 35].

This is a well-designed and well-conducted RCT. It has addressed the blinding and control issues that the previous SIMPLICITY 1 and 2 overlooked [34, 35] and answered some of the reservations expressed over the initial pilot and proof of concept studies [36].

SIMPLICITY HTN3 included appropriate BP measurement outcomes, including 24 h ABPM.

It is however unclear how the efficacy or success of the renal artery (sympathetic) denervation can be ascertained. There were no detectable differences between heart rates between the groups. The authors state that the SIMPLICITY catheter recording confirmed energy delivery, but they also acknowledge that there is no easy way to ascertain effective sympathetic denervation. Therefore, the absence of significant BP difference between the groups can imply that the procedure was successful but failed to reduce BP, or that the procedure was unsuccessful, thus failing to show a difference between the groups.

The lack of difference in BP control between groups may be due to the progressive BP fall in the placebo intervention group as well as the treatment group. This may be due to the placebo effect of regular follow-up and improved compliance or to the fact that a run-in period of 2 weeks did not allow a steady state to be established in either group before intervention.

Compliance to antihypertensive medication was not ascertained.

A follow-up of 6 months is sufficient for the primary end point of impact of the intervention on blood pressure control. It may be too short to examine the impact of the denervation on long-term renal function, which was not the aim of the study.

There was no difference in renal function between the groups before and after interventions.

Conclusions

This is a well-designed and well-conducted trial that failed to show a short-term advantage of catheter-induced renal artery sympathetic denervation. Limitations confound interpretation and conclusions.

General Discussion of Interventions to Slow CKD Progression

The last 30 years saw a plethora of clinical trials aimed at slowing the progression of CKD. They have to a large extent informed our clinical practice through a number of assumptions based on these trials.

1. *There is no longer an enthusiasm among nephrologists for dietary protein restriction to slow CKD progression.* Although a number of meta-analyses of very heterogeneous trials and populations as well as dietary protein regimens continue to be published, arguing for some benefit for low-protein diets [37, 38]. These publications are mainly from the United States [39], where a high protein intake tends to prevail in the general population, and from Italy [40], where low-protein diets have been initiated in the 1960s and have been a traditional treatment to retard ESRD ever since. These publications invariably suffer from the same shortcomings highlighted some 30 years ago [41], including the reliance on serum creatinine estimations, an inappropriate marker of CKD progression on dietary protein restriction. They never include measure-

ments of GFR, the gold standard for evaluating CKD progression.
2. ACE inhibition remains the cornerstone of the therapy to slow progression in proteinuric CKD. Of note, the cutoff point for defining proteinuric CKD has slipped from >3.5 g/24 h [42] to >1 g/24 h [43] to 0.5 g/24 h in the latest KDIGO guidelines [44]. This is in spite of the lack of strong evidence to support such recommendations. The critical appraisal of some key ACE inhibition RCTs in CKD highlights the weakness of the available evidence. Also, systematic reviews and meta-analyses have failed to show a convincing advantage of ACE inhibitors over other antihypertensive agents in terms of CKD progression [45] or in terms of cardiovascular complications [46], beyond that conferred by good blood pressure control.
3. Early practice argued that the lower the blood pressure the slower the rate of CKD decline [47]. Evidence presented in this chapter from MDRD [48], REIN2 [49], and AASK [50] failed to support such an assumption – an assumption still prominent in the latest hypertension management in CKD guidelines, suggesting different cutoff for treatment of proteinuric and nonproteinuric CKD as well as diabetic and nondiabetic patients [44].
4. Novel interventions based on the manipulations of other putative mediators of CKD progression, such as endothelin antagonists, growth factors, and signaling pathway mediators, have so far not become part of the routine clinical practice in progressive CKD [51].

Clearly among nephrologists, habits die hard even when time shows them to be confounded. Also, dogmas tend to be difficult to dismiss, especially when they are strongly promoted by authorities and single issues fanatics in the field. Finally, the pharmaceutical industry continues to be the major driver of clinical research in Nephrology with its strong financial support to major and multimillion pounds RCTs, thus occasionally casting some shadow over the interpretation and impartiality of the outcomes. It is high time for a rethink of RCTs evaluating CKD progression.

CKD Progression RCTs: Limitations and Recommendations

A critical appraisal of the literature in the field highlights a number of issues:
1. Assumption is often made that CKD progression is linear and predictable in patients recruited into RCTs, in the absence of a prerandomization determination of the renal function trajectory (RFT). Consequently, heterogeneous groups of patients are recruited into these RCTs impacting study power and trial outcomes. It is high time nephrologists come to realize that a significant percentage

of CKD patients, even at advanced stages, do not progress especially in the absence of significant proteinuria.

2. All too often, the evaluation of CKD progression is based on the measurement of serum creatinine and derived GFR (eGFR). These are inappropriate surrogate markers for CKD progression when a given intervention may affect serum creatinine levels independently from the changes in measured GFR. This has been most dramatically noted recently in the BEAM and BEACON trials, where a fall in serum creatinine and rise in eGFR were heralded to be major breakthroughs, when in reality they reflected the side effect of the tested agent, Bardoxolone, on food intake, weight loss, and overall morbidity and mortality [52].

3. It is high time the Nephrology community came to realize that eGFR does not equate measured GFR (mGFR). Relying on eGFR may be misleading [53]. GFR should be measured, and that is feasible, as shown by the MDRD, REIN, and AASK studies.

4. The Nephrology community has uncritically adopted the dogma that treating proteinuria slows CKD progression in the absence of a shred of evidence that such effect is independent of improved blood pressure control.

5. A large number of CKD progression trials are based on interventions that impact blood pressure control. Unfortunately, all too often, BP is inadequately measured with casual office BP readings replacing the more assiduous use of daytime and nighttime BP readings as well as 24 h ABP monitoring, known to be better predictors of outcomes.

6. The Nephrology community is fond of composite end points in RCTs often involving doubling of serum creatinine and decline in eGFR and ESRD. The use of composite end points is not without its limitations, especially when the end points are clearly interrelated and not homogeneously weighted [54]. The combination of soft end points does not make them harder. Also, the use of ESRD and start of RRT, without clear protocol prespecification of the timing and cutoff point for the start of RRT, is a major weakness in most CKD RCTs.

7. A rethink of design and conduct of CKD RCTs is timely and should consider the points made above and expertly highlighted in a recent editorial by Rosansky and Glassock [55].

Acknowledgments The author acknowledges the contribution made by Swami VJ, Okel J, and Bello AM to an initial version of this chapter.

References

1. Brenner BM, Meyer TW, Hostetter TH. Dietary protein intake and the progressive nature of kidney disease: the role of hemodynamically mediated glomerular injury in the pathogenesis of progressive glomerular sclerosis in aging, renal ablation, and intrinsic renal disease. N Engl J Med. 1982;307(11):652–9.

2. Khwaja A, El Kossi M, Floege J, El Nahas M. The management of CKD: a look into the future. Kidney Int. 2007;72:1316–23.

3. http://www.kdigo.org/clinical_practice_guidelines/pdf/KDIGO_BP_GL.pdf.

4. Paul A, James MD, et al. 2014 Evidence-based guideline for the management of high blood pressure in adults report from the panel members appointed to the Eighth Joint National Committee (JNC 8). JAMA. 2014;311(5):507–20. doi:10.1001/jama.2013.284427.

5. Kusek JW, Coyne T, de Velasco A, Drabik MJ, Finlay RA, Gassman JJ, Kiefer S, Powers SN, Steinman TI. Recruitment experience in the full-scale phase of the Modification of Diet in Renal Disease Study. Control Clin Trials. 1993;14(6):538–57.

6. El Nahas AM, Coles GA. Dietary treatment of chronic renal failure: ten unanswered questions. Lancet. 1986;1(8481):597–600.

7. Locatelli F, Alberti D, Graziani G, Buccianti G, Redaelli B, Giangrande A. Prospective, randomised, multicentre trial of effect of protein restriction on progression of chronic renal insufficiency. Northern Italian Cooperative Study Group. Lancet 1991;1(337):1299–304.

8. Kaysen GA, Odabaei G. Dietary protein restriction and preservation of kidney function in chronic kidney disease. Blood Purif 2013;35(1–3):22–5.

9. Agarwal R. Home and ambulatory blood pressure monitoring in chronic kidney disease. Curr Opin Nephrol Hypertens. 2009 18(6):507–12.

10. Lewis EJ, Hunsicker LG, Bain RP, Rohde RD. The effect of angiotensin-converting-enzyme inhibition on diabetic nephropathy. The Collaborative Study Group. N Engl J Med. 1993;329(20):1456–62.

11. Agarwal R. Home and ambulatory blood pressure monitoring in chronic kidney disease. Curr Opin Nephrol Hypertens 2009;18(6):507–12.

12. Thomas MC, Tikellis C, Burns WC, Thallas V, Forbes JM, Cao Z, Osicka TM, Russo LM, Jerums G, Ghabrial H, Cooper ME, Kantharidis P. Reduced tubular cation transport in diabetes: prevented by ACE inhibition. Kidney Int. 2003;63(6):2152–61.

13. Thomas MC, Jerums G, Tsalamandris C, Macisaac R, Panagiotopoulos S, Cooper ME, MDNSG Study Group. Increased tubular organic ion clearance following chronic ACE inhibition in patients with type 1 diabetes. Kidney Int. 2005;67(6):2494–9.

14. Randomised placebo-controlled trial of effect of ramipril on decline in glomerular filtration rate and risk of terminal renal failure in proteinuric, non-diabetic nephropathy. The GISEN Group (Gruppo Italiano di Studi Epidemiologici in Nefrologia). Lancet 1997;349(9069):1857–63.

15. http://www.kdigo.org/clinical_practice_guidelines/pdf/KDIGO_BP_GL.pdf.

16. Paul A, James MD, et al. 2014 evidence-based guideline for the management of high blood pressure in adults report from the panel members appointed to the Eighth Joint National Committee (JNC 8). JAMA. 2014;311(5):507–20. doi:10.1001/jama.2013.284427.

17. Agarwal R. Home and ambulatory blood pressure monitoring in chronic kidney disease. Curr Opin Nephrol Hypertens. 2009; 18(6):507–12.

18. Svensson P, de Faire U, Sleight P, Yusuf S, Ostergren J. Comparative effects of ramipril on ambulatory and office blood pressures: a HOPE Substudy. Hypertension. 2001;38(6):E28–32.

19. http://www.bmj.com/content/334/7597/786.

20. Agarwal R. Home and ambulatory blood pressure monitoring in chronic kidney disease. Curr Opin Nephrol Hypertens. 2009; 18(6):507–12.

21. Zhang GH, Hou FF, Zhang X, Liu QF. Can angiotensin-converting enzyme inhibitor be used in chronic kidney disease patients with serum creatinine level greater than 266 micromol/L? Zhonghua Nei Ke Za Zhi. 2005;44(8):592–6.

22. Agarwal R. Home and ambulatory blood pressure monitoring in chronic kidney disease. Curr Opin Nephrol Hypertens. 2009; 18(6):507–12.

23. Wright Jr JT, Bakris G, Greene T, Agodoa LY, Appel LJ, Charleston J, Cheek D, Douglas-Baltimore JG, Gassman J, Glassock R, Hebert L, Jamerson K, Lewis J, Phillips RA, Toto RD, Middleton JP, Rostand SG, African American Study of Kidney Disease and Hypertension Study Group. Effect of blood pressure lowering and antihypertensive drug class on progression of hypertensive kidney disease: results from the AASK trial. JAMA. 2002;288(19):2421–31.

24. Klahr S, Levey AS, Beck GJ, Caggiula AW, Hunsicker L, Kusek JW, Striker G. The effects of dietary protein restriction and blood-pressure control on the progression of chronic renal disease. Modification of Diet in Renal Disease Study Group. N Engl J Med. 1994;330(13):877–84.

25. Appel LJ, Wright Jr JT, Greene T, Agodoa LY, Astor BC, Bakris GL, Cleveland WH, Charleston J, Contreras G, Faulkner ML, Gabbai FB, Gassman JJ, Hebert LA, Jamerson KA, Kopple JD, Kusek JW, Lash JP, Lea JP, Lewis JB, Lipkowitz MS, Massry SG, Miller ER, Norris K, Phillips RA, Pogue VA, Randall OS, Rostand SG, Smogorzewski MJ, Toto RD, Wang X, AASK Collaborative Research Group. Intensive blood-pressure control in hypertensive chronic kidney disease. N Engl J Med. 2010;363(10):918–29.

26. Praga M. Therapeutic measures in proteinuric nephropathy. Kidney Int Suppl. 2005;99:S137–41.

27. Agarwal R. Home and ambulatory blood pressure monitoring in chronic kidney disease. Curr Opin Nephrol Hypertens. 2009;18(6):507–12.

28. Angeli F, Reboldi G, Poltronieri C, Bartolini C, D'Ambrosio C, de Filippo V, Verdecchia P. Clinical utility of ambulatory blood pressure monitoring in the management of hypertension. Expert Rev Cardiovasc Ther. 2014;12:623–34.

29. Jamerson KA, Bakris GL, Weber MA. 24-hour ambulatory blood pressure in the ACCOMPLISH trial. N Engl J Med. 2010;363(1):98.

30. Clark EC, Nath KA, Hostetter MK, Hostetter TH. Role of ammonia in tubulointerstitial injury. Miner Electrolyte Metab. 1990;16(5):315–21.

31. Łoniewski I, Wesson DE. Bicarbonate therapy for prevention of chronic kidney disease progression. Kidney Int. 2014;85(3):529–35.

32. Chen W, Abramowitz MK. Treatment of metabolic acidosis in patients with CKD. Am J Kidney Dis. 2014;63(2):311–7.

33. http://www.bmj.com/content/334/7597/786.

34. Krum H, Schlaich M, Whitbourn R, Sobotka PA, Sadowski J, Bartus K, Kapelak B, Walton A, Sievert H, Thambar S, Abraham WT, Esler M. Catheter-based renal sympathetic denervation for resistant hypertension: a multicentre safety and proof-of-principle cohort study. Lancet. 2009;373(9671):1275–81.

35. Esler MD, Krum H, Sobotka PA, Schlaich MP, Schmieder RE, Böhm M, Symplicity HTN-2 Investigators. Renal sympathetic denervation in patients with treatment-resistant hypertension (The Symplicity HTN-2 Trial): a randomised controlled trial. Lancet. 2010;376(9756):1903–9.

36. Parati G, Ochoa JE, Bilo G. Renal sympathetic denervation and daily life blood pressure in resistant hypertension: simplicity or complexity? Circulation. 2013;128(4):315–7.

37. Pedrini MT, Levey AS, Lau J, Chalmers TC, Wang PH. The effect of dietary protein restriction on the progression of diabetic and nondiabetic renal diseases: a meta-analysis. Ann Intern Med. 1996;124(7):627–32.

38. Fouque D, Laville M. Low protein diets for chronic kidney disease in non diabetic adults. Cochrane Database Syst Rev. 2009;(3):CD001892.

39. Kaysen GA, Odabaei G. Dietary protein restriction and preservation of kidney function in chronic kidney disease. Blood Purif. 2013;35(1–3):22–5.

40. Piccoli GB, Ferraresi M, Deagostini MC, Vigotti FN, Consiglio V, Scognamiglio S, Moro I, Clari R, Fassio F, Biolcati M, Porpiglia F. Vegetarian low-protein diets supplemented with keto analogues:

41. el Nahas AM, Coles GA. Dietary treatment of chronic renal failure: ten unanswered questions. Lancet. 1986;1(8481):597–600.

42. Ruggenenti P, Perna A, Gherardi G, Gaspari F, Benini R, Remuzzi G. Renal function and requirement for dialysis in chronic nephropathy patients on long-term ramipril: REIN follow-up trial. Gruppo Italiano di Studi Epidemiologici in Nefrologia (GISEN). Ramipril Efficacy in Nephropathy. Lancet. 1998;352(9136):1252–6.

43. Kent DM, Jafar TH, Hayward RA, Tighiouart H, Landa M, de Jong P, de Zeeuw D, Remuzzi G, Kamper AL, Levey AS. Progression risk, urinary protein excretion, and treatment effects of angiotensin-converting enzyme inhibitors in nondiabetic kidney disease. J Am Soc Nephrol. 2007;18(6):1959–65.

44. http://www.kdigo.org/clinical_practice_guidelines/pdf/KDIGO_BP_GL.pdf.

45. Sharma P, Blackburn RC, Parke CL, McCullough K, Marks A, Black C. Angiotensin-converting enzyme inhibitors and angiotensin receptor blockers for adults with early (stage 1 to 3) non-diabetic chronic kidney disease. Cochrane Database Syst Rev. 2011;(10):CD007751.

46. Blood Pressure Lowering Treatment Trialists' Collaboration, Ninomiya T, Perkovic V, Turnbull F, Neal B, Barzi F, Cass A, Baigent C, Chalmers J, Li N, Woodward M, MacMahon S. Blood pressure lowering and major cardiovascular events in people with and without chronic kidney disease: meta-analysis of randomised controlled trials. BMJ. 2013;347:f5680.

47. Bakris GL, Williams M, Dworkin L, Elliott WJ, Epstein M, Toto R, Tuttle K, Douglas J, Hsueh W, Sowers J. Preserving renal function in adults with hypertension and diabetes: a consensus approach. National Kidney Foundation Hypertension and Diabetes Executive Committees Working Group. Am J Kidney Dis. 2000;36(3):646–61.

48. Klahr S, Levey AS, Beck GJ, Caggiula AW, Hunsicker L, Kusek JW, Striker G. The effects of dietary protein restriction and blood-pressure control on the progression of chronic renal disease. Modification of Diet in Renal Disease Study Group. N Engl J Med. 1994;330(13):877–84.

49. Ruggenenti P, Perna A, Loriga G, Ganeva M, Ene-Iordache B, Turturro M, Lesti M, Perticucci E, Chakarski IN, Leonardis D, Garini G, Sessa A, Basile C, Alpa M, Scanziani R, Sorba G, Zoccali C, Remuzzi G, REIN-2 Study Group. Blood-pressure control for renoprotection in patients with non-diabetic chronic renal disease (REIN-2): multicentre, randomised controlled trial. Lancet. 2005;365(9463):939–46.

50. Wright Jr JT, Bakris G, Greene T, Agodoa LY, Appel LJ, Charleston J, Cheek D, Douglas-Baltimore JG, Gassman J, Glassock R, Hebert L, Jamerson K, Lewis J, Phillips RA, Toto RD, Middleton JP, Rostand SG, African American Study of Kidney Disease and Hypertension Study Group. Effect of blood pressure lowering and antihypertensive drug class on progression of hypertensive kidney disease: results from the AASK trial. JAMA. 2002;288(19):2421–31.

51. Khwaja A, El Kossi M, Floege J, El Nahas M. The management of CKD: a look into the future. Kidney Int. 2007;72(11):1316–23.

52. Tayek JA, Kalantar-Zadeh K. The extinguished BEACON of bardoxolone: not a Monday morning quarterback story. Am J Nephrol. 2013;37(3):208–11.

53. Ruggenenti P, Gaspari F, Cannata A, Carrara F, Cella C, Ferrari S, Stucchi N, Prandini S, Ene-Iordache B, Diadei O, Perico N, Ondei P, Pisani A, Buongiorno E, Messa P, Dugo M, Remuzzi G, GFR-ADPKD Study Group. Measuring and estimating GFR and treatment effect in ADPKD patients: results and implications of a longitudinal cohort study. PLoS One. 2012;7(2):e32533.

54. http://www.bmj.com/content/334/7597/786.

55. Rosansky SJ, Glassock RJ. Is a decline in estimated GFR an appropriate surrogate end point for renoprotection drug trials? Kidney Int. 2014;85(4):723–7.

Mohsen El Kossi

Introduction

The pivotal role of hemoglobin as one of the targets in the holistic management of dialysis patients was the focus of the first published anemia guidelines by KDOQI in 1997. Since the introduction of erythropoietin to anemia management in chronic kidney disease, there has been a continuous debate on the optimal hemoglobin target required to achieve the desirable clinical outcome whether in survival or quality of life. With the unequivocal evidence of the impact of these agents on relatively better quality of life and reduced need for red-cell transfusion with the anticipated potential complications attached to it, there is an element of uncertainty about the exact risk of these agents on chronic kidney disease patients. Iron deficiency is the other area that attracts a lot of interest in anemia management in chronic kidney disease. Absolute and relative iron deficiencies are recognized for a long time as important contributing factors for anemia development in different stages of chronic kidney disease. More importantly, response to erythropoiesis-stimulating agents (ESAs) is suboptimal in the presence of iron deficiency. Most of the up-to-date anemia guidelines emphasize on the central role of iron in anemia management. Disappointing enough, iron treatment recommendations are either not graded or scored low. This emphasizes the unmet need for better quality evidence to address a confusing dilemma in iron treatment in this group of patients. Disproportionately, a large number of high-quality and well-designed studies became available in ESA treatment area which allowed for high-rank quality of evidence. Questions that remain without clear answers are: When to start iron treatment? Which route of administration to use? What are the targets of iron treatment? What are the best biochemical variables that reflect iron status? A very limited number of reasonable quality studies have tried to answer

some of these questions. I included only one of those trials that attracted a lot of debate in this area and have remarkable impact on anemia management in nondialysis chronic kidney disease patients. I also included some of the landmark ESA trials at different levels of chronic kidney disease.

Iron Treatment in Chronic Kidney Disease

The US Sucrose Clinical Trial

Title: A randomized, controlled trial comparing IV iron sucrose to oral iron in anemic patients with nondialysis-dependent CKD

Authors: Van Wyck DB, Roppolo M, Martinez CO, Mazey RM, and Mcmurray S, for the US Sucrose (Venofer) Clinical Trials Group

Journal: *Kidney Int.* 2005;68:2846–56

Abstract

Background: Although iron deficiency frequently complicates anemia in patients with nondialysis-dependent CKD (ND-CKD), the comparative treatment value of IV iron infusion and oral iron supplementation has not been established.

Methods: In a randomized, controlled multicenter trial, we compared the efficacy of iron sucrose, given as 1 g in divided IV doses over 14 days, with that of ferrous sulphate, given 325 mg orally thrice daily for 56 days in patients with ND-CKD stages 3–5, Hb < or =11 g/dL, TSAT < or =25 %, and ferritin < or =300 ng/mL. Epoetin/darbepoetin therapy, if any, was not changed for 8 weeks prior to or during the study.

Results: The proportion of patients achieving the primary outcome (Hb increase > or =1 g/dL) was greater in the IV iron treatment group than in the oral iron treatment group (44.3 % vs. 28.0 %, $P=0.0344$), as was the mean increase in Hb by day 42 (0.7 vs. 0.4 g/dL, $P=0.0298$). Compared to those in the IV iron group, patients in the oral iron treatment group showed a greater decline in GFR during the study (-4.40 vs. -1.45 mL/min/1.73 m^2, $P=0.0100$). No serious

M. El Kossi, MBBCh, MSc, MD, FRCP
Doncaster Renal Unit, Doncaster Royal Infirmary Hospital,
Armthorpe Road, DN2 5LT Doncaster, UK
e-mail: elkossi@gmail.com

adverse drug events (ADE) were seen in patients administered IV iron sucrose as 200 mg IV over 2–5 min, but drug-related hypotension, including one event considered serious, occurred in two females weighing less than 65 kg after 500 mg doses were given over 4 h.

Conclusion: IV iron administration using 1,000 mg iron sucrose in divided doses is superior to oral iron therapy in the management of ND-CKD patients with anemia and low iron indices.

Critical Appraisal

Parameters	Yes	No	Comment
Validity			
Is the **Randomization** Procedure well described?		−1	Method of randomization was not clearly described
			Group stratification prior to randomization was explained in detail
Double **blinded**?	+2		Open-labeled, phase III, randomized, controlled trial. The outcome measure is a laboratory result which is unlikely to be affected by unblinding
Is the **sample size** calculation described/ adequate?		−1	It was based on 25 % event rate difference between both arms (40 % vs. 15 %). In reality, the difference was around 16 %, which should require bigger sample size. This is to achieve two-sided significance level at 0.05 and a power of 90 % with expected 10 % failure rate during observation. This requires 160 subjects in total for both arms. There was no account for dropout rate (22 %)
Does it have a hard primary **endpoint**?	+1		Increase in Hb of at least 1.0 g/ dL at any time between baseline and either the end of study or withdrawal
Is the endpoint surrogate?		0	
Is the follow-up appropriate?		−1	8 weeks which may be appropriate for efficacy but not for safety?
Was there a **Bias**?		−1	The inherent nature of open-labeled design without clear explanation of randomization method raises the risk of selection and performance bias
Is the dropout >25 %?	+1		
Is the analysis **ITT**?	+3		
Utility/usefulness			
Can the findings be generalized?		−1	Relatively short follow-up period and small sample size question the power of the study and outcome results. The study was restricted on predialysis patients and Hb <11 g/dL
Score	**13 %**		

Comments and Discussion

Iron deficiency is one of the main causes of resistance to erythropoietin treatment in CKD patients [1]. These patients have a unique feature of poor gastrointestinal iron absorption due to various reasons including the use of gastric acid-lowering tablets, common use of phosphate binders, and the persistent inflammatory state characteristic of CKD [2]. Therefore, this study was designed to address the important question whether intravenous iron is superior to oral iron therapy in this group of patients and whether it is safe or not. It also downgraded the value of serum ferritin and transferring saturation as predictors of bone marrow iron stores [3].

The study has a number of limitations:

1. The study design was open-labeled, thus raising the potential of observer: selection and performance bias.
2. The primary outcome in this trial was a laboratory result (increase in Hb concentration by 1 g/dL). While this satisfies the purpose of the clinical trial, it does not necessarily translate to patient's improved quality of life, morbidity or mortality.
3. The study may well be underpowered due to a small sample size (anticipated difference was 25 % and actual difference was 16 % between arms) with no account or allowance for the dropout rate (22 %). Participants who completed the study and actually received the study intervention were around 66 %; hence, it would be of interest to know the difference between ITT and per protocol analyses.
4. Follow-up period was too short (56 days) to assess safety and effect on eGFR. Cumulative hemoglobin response curve was on steady rise until the end of the study for both arms. Increasing the study duration to 12 weeks rather than 8 weeks might have increased the number of participants in the oral arm who achieved the target hemoglobin; it seems that the 56-day study duration was chosen arbitrarily. Of relevance, serum ferritin levels in the oral arm were still rising until the end of the study, albeit to a lesser extent than the IV iron arm.
5. Multiple subgroup analyses for such a small sample size are inconclusive and at best hypothesis generating.

It was hard to explain the significant decline of eGFR (-4.4 ml/min/1.73 m^2) based only on two readings within the relatively very short interval of 2 months [4] with patients receiving a drug (oral iron) routinely used in daily practice without such huge detrimental effect.

Conclusion

It has become acceptable practice in CKD4-5 to administer iron intravenously, rather than orally, to correct iron-deficiency anemia. There is little doubt that the US trial described above had a major influence on such practice. However, it is worth noting its limitations and also the fact that those given oral iron supplementation had a progressive improvement of their serum ferritin levels, albeit at a lower and slower rate than those who received parenteral iron.

Target Hemoglobin Level with Erythropoietin Treatment in CKD

CREATE study

Title: Normalization of hemoglobin level in patients with chronic kidney disease and anemia

Title Acronym: Cardiovascular Risk Reduction by Early Anemia Treatment with Epoetin Beta (CREATE)

Authors: Drüeke TB, Locatelli F, Clyne N, Eckardt K, Macdougall IC, Tsakiris D, Burger H, and Scherhag A, for the CREATE Investigators

Journal: *NEJM*. 2006;355(20):2071–84

Abstract

Background: Whether correction of anemia in patients with stage 3 or 4 chronic kidney disease improves cardiovascular outcomes is not established.

Methods: We randomly assigned 603 patients with an estimated glomerular filtration rate (GFR) of 15.0–35.0 ml per minute per 1.73 m^2 of body surface area and mild-to-moderate anemia (hemoglobin level, 11.0–12.5 g/dL) to a target hemoglobin value in the normal range (13.0–15.0 g/dL, group 1) or the subnormal range (10.5–11.5 g/dL, group 2). Subcutaneous erythropoietin (epoetin beta) was initiated at randomization (group 1) or only after the hemoglobin level fell below 10.5 g/dL (group 2). The primary endpoint was a composite of eight cardiovascular events; secondary endpoints included left ventricular mass index, quality-of-life scores, and the progression of chronic kidney disease.

Results: During the 3-year study, complete correction of anemia did not affect the likelihood of a first cardiovascular event (58 events in group 1 vs. 47 events in group 2; hazard ratio, 0.78; 95 % confidence interval, 0.53–1.14; $P=0.20$). Left ventricular mass index remained stable in both groups. The mean estimated GFR was 24.9 ml per minute in group 1 and 24.2 ml per minute in group 2 at baseline and decreased by 3.6 and 3.1 ml per minute per year, respectively ($P=0.40$). Dialysis was required in more patients in group 1 than in group 2 (127 vs. 111, $P=0.03$). General health and physical function improved significantly ($P=0.003$ and $P<0.001$, respectively, in group 1, as compared with group 2). There was no significant difference in the combined incidence of adverse events between the two groups, but hypertensive episodes and headaches were more prevalent in group 1.

Conclusions: In patients with chronic kidney disease, early complete correction of anemia does not reduce the risk of cardiovascular events.

ClinicalTrials.gov number, NCT00321919

Critical Appraisal

Parameters	Yes	No	Comment
Validity			
Is the **Randomization** Procedure well described?	+1		Randomization method was described in detail. There was no statistical difference between baseline variables of both groups
Double **blinded**?		−2	Open-labeled, randomized, controlled trial
Is the **sample size** calculation described/adequate?	+3		It is an event-driven trial, based on an event rate of 15 % in the control group to achieve 80 % power and 5 % significance with a projected reduction in the hazard ratio for a first cardiovascular event by one-third. This requires 200 events to happen within the recruitment and follow-up period
Does it have a hard primary **endpoint**?	+1		Time to a composite of eight cardiovascular events including sudden death, fatal or nonfatal myocardial infarction, acute heart failure, angina pectoris or cardiac arrhythmias requiring hospitalization for 24 h or more, fatal or nonfatal stroke, transient ischemic attack, peripheral vascular disease (amputation, necrosis)
Is the endpoint surrogate?		0	
Is the follow-up appropriate?	+1		Recruitment period of 2 years and follow-up 2 years after enrollment of the last patient
Was there a **Bias**?	−1		There is a potential risk of selection and performance bias with the open-labeled design. This is particularly important with the primary hard endpoint
Is the dropout >25 %?		+1	
Is the analysis **ITT**?	+3		
Utility/usefulness			
Can the findings be generalized?	+1		It was a multicenter study including participants from 94 renal units in 22 European, Asian, and Latin American countries
Score	53 %		

Comments and Discussion

Hemoglobin target is one of the controversial areas in anemia management in chronic kidney disease [5]. In conjunction with CHOIR, both studies were the first efforts to identify the appropriate hemoglobin levels in chronic kidney disease patients not yet on dialysis. Their results were long-awaited by the guideline working groups to provide them with robust evidence [6]. The study has had a clear design with hard endpoints.

The study has some limitations:

1. A number of factors reduced its power. For instance, sample size calculation relied on a single reference from a population with an event rate far higher than actual event rate (15 % vs. 6 %). The reasons behind the low event rate they encountered in their cohort were due to improved patient care for cardiovascular risks and the better-than-usual performance of participants in control arm of clinical trials [7]. This obviously resulted in a smaller sample size. This was further compromised when it was not clear whether they accounted for the dropout rate in the initial calculation or not (25 and 17 % in both arms).

2. The number of participants who left the study to start dialysis was high (238). This should be expected when the lower limit of eGFR accepted for participation was 15 ml/min and study duration was expected to last for 2 years after the last randomized patient. The relatively higher number of patients who required dialysis in the higher-hemoglobin arm should be understood in the context of dialysis initiation which was not protocolized (controlled) and the study was not powered for this outcome.

3. The risk of performance and selection bias cannot be ignored with the open-labeled design of this trial.

4. The use of composite endpoint is usually justified by the assumption that the effect on each of the components will be similar and that patients will attach similar importance to each component. This is not necessarily the case with the eight cardiovascular endpoints chosen. The validity of composite endpoints depends to a large extent on similarity in patients' importance (weighting), treatment effect, and number of events across components [8]. This may not be the case with those chosen in this trial.

Conclusion

CREATE was primarily a negative study that shaped subsequent practice of hemoglobin correction and related guidelines [9] in CKD. It showed no advantage of normalization of hemoglobin levels beyond a hemoglobin level >12 g/dl.

CHOIR Study

Title: Correction of anemia with epoetin alfa in chronic kidney disease

Title Acronym: Correction of Hemogloblin and Outcomes in Renal Insufficiency (CHOIR)

Authors: Singh AK, Szczech L, Tang KL, Barnhart H, Sapp S, Wolfson M, and Reddan D, for the CHOIR Investigators
Journal: *NEJM*. 2006;355(20):2085–98

Abstract

Background: Anemia, a common complication of chronic kidney disease, usually develops as a consequence of erythropoietin deficiency. Recombinant human erythropoietin (epoetin alfa) is indicated for the correction of anemia associated with this condition. However, the optimal level of hemoglobin correction is not defined.

Methods: In this open-labeled trial, we studied 1,432 patients with chronic kidney disease, 715 of whom were randomly assigned to receive a dose of epoetin alfa targeted to achieve a hemoglobin level of 13.5 g/dL and 717 of whom were assigned to receive a dose targeted to achieve a level of 11.3 g/dL. The median study duration was 16 months. The primary endpoint was a composite of death, myocardial infarction, hospitalization for congestive heart failure (without renal replacement therapy), and stroke.

Results: A total of 222 composite events occurred: 125 events in the high-hemoglobin group, as compared with 97 events in the low-hemoglobin group (hazard ratio, 1.34; 95 % confidence interval, 1.03–1.74; $P=0.03$). There were 65 deaths (29.3 %), 101 hospitalizations for congestive heart failure (45.5 %), 25 myocardial infarctions (11.3 %), and 23 strokes (10.4 %). Seven patients (3.2 %) were hospitalized for congestive heart failure and myocardial infarction combined, and one patient (0.5 %) died after having a stroke. Improvements in the quality of life were similar in the two groups. More patients in the high-hemoglobin group had at least one serious adverse event.

Conclusions: The use of a target hemoglobin level of 13.5 g/dL (as compared with 11.3 g/dL) was associated with increased risk and no incremental improvement in the quality of life (ClinicalTrials.gov number, NCT00211120 [ClinicalTrials.gov].

Critical Appraisal

Parameters	Yes	No	Comment
Validity			
Is the **Randomization** Procedure well described?	+1		Randomization method was described in detail. There was no difference between baseline variables except for higher number of cases with history of hypertension and coronary artery bypass grafting in the high-hemoglobin group
Double **blinded**?		−2	Open-labeled, phase IV, randomized, controlled, multi-center trial

Parameters	Yes	No	Comment
Is the **sample size** calculation described/adequate?	+3		It is an event-driven trial; 1,352 patients in both groups required to achieve type I error of 0.05 and a power of 80 % to detect a 25 % reduction in the composite event rate in the high-hemoglobin arm over a period of 3 years, assuming a 30 % event rate in the low-hemoglobin arm
Does it have a hard primary **endpoint**?	+1		Time to the composite of all-cause mortality, myocardial infarction, hospitalization for congestive heart failure (excluding renal replacement therapy), or stroke
Is the endpoint surrogate?		0	No
Is the follow-up appropriate?		−1	Mean duration of follow-up was 16 months and study was terminated earlier than planned after data and safety monitoring board recommendation after second interim analysis
			The original plan was to give epoetin alfa until start of renal replacement therapy or for 36 months
Was there a **Bias**?	−1		Open-labeled design carries risk of selection and performance bias
Is the dropout >25 %?	−1		
Is the analysis **ITT**?	+3		Intention to treat but high dropout rate and premature study termination. ITT analysis was no different from per protocol analysis
Utility/usefulness			
Can the findings be generalized?		−1	Participants were only from the USA. The study was terminated prematurely
Score	....%		Not scored as the study was terminated earlier than planned

Comments and Discussion

This study was published in the same issue of *NEJM* with CREATE (discussed above). Both trials addressed the same question about the value of hemoglobin normalization in nondialysis chronic kidney disease (CKD) patients, but with many variations in the study design, conduct, and analysis. In CREATE, the sample size was adequate initially and took into account the dropout rate, particularly those who would leave to start dialysis treatment.

The study had some limitations including:

1. There was a high dropout rate in CHOIR due in part to the start of dialysis. Nearly half of the participants were lost in each group with relatively more in the low-hemoglobin arm of the study.

2. The early study termination, along with the high dropout rate, makes any assumptions from the results difficult to interpret with confidence in view of the decreased study power.

3. In addition, there are other areas of concern in CHOIR, such as the unusually high Epo dose used in the protocol; 10,000 units of Epo were used weekly during the first 3 weeks of the study, regardless of patient's weight. This was challenged by some authors [7, 10, 11] and investigators response reflected the routine use of high Epo dose in clinical practice in the states. It is all the more surprising that only 75 % of the high-hemoglobin arm reached the target Hb level (12.6 g/dl), in spite of such high dose.

4. Also, baseline variables including the history of hypertension and coronary artery bypass surgery were statistically higher in the group with higher event rate. This imbalance, while possibly due to chance, could influence the outcome as it is closely linked to some of the outcome measures. The authors did adjust for these variables in a regression analysis (not published in the initial report) and results have not been affected [12].

5. There were a high proportion of patients with heart failure in both arms of the study (24.4 % versus 22.9 %), but no clarification was given regarding the NYHA class of these patients in each arm. This is of relevance bearing in mind that congestive cardiac failure contributed significantly to the worse outcome measures in the high-hemoglobin arm.

6. A protocol amendment took place after 24 % of participants were already enrolled, with different baseline hemoglobin levels, and it is unclear how many of those patients were included in the final analysis or why such protocol amendment took place.

7. Composite endpoint analyses make a number of assumptions and it is unclear whether those chosen for this trial meet the requirements and justifications of composite endpoints [8].

Conclusion

CHOIR, like CREATE, has shaped current practice of anemia management and informed recent anemia guidelines [9].

TREAT Trial

Title: A trial of darbepoetin alfa in type 2 diabetes and chronic kidney disease

Title Acronym: Trial to Reduce cardiovascular Events with Aranesp Therapy (TREAT)

Authors: Pfeffer MA, Burdmann EA, Chen C-Y, Cooper ME, de Zeeuw D, Eckardt K-U, Feyzi JM, Ivanovich P,

Kewalramani R, Levey AS, Lewis EF, McGill JB, McMurray J, Parfrey P, Parving H-H, Remuzzi G, Singh AK, Solomon SD, and Toto R, for the TREAT Investigators

Journal: *NEJM*. 2009;361(21):2019–32

Abstract

Background: Anemia is associated with an increased risk of cardiovascular and renal events among patients with type 2 diabetes and chronic kidney disease. Although darbepoetin alfa can effectively increase hemoglobin levels, its effect on clinical outcomes in these patients has not been adequately tested.

Methods: In this study involving 4,038 patients with diabetes, chronic kidney disease, and anemia, we randomly assigned 2,012 patients to darbepoetin alfa to achieve a hemoglobin level of approximately 13 g per deciliter and 2,026 patients to placebo, with rescue darbepoetin alfa when the hemoglobin level was less than 9.0 g per deciliter. The primary endpoints were the composite outcomes of death or a cardiovascular event (nonfatal myocardial infarction, congestive heart failure, stroke, or hospitalization for myocardial ischemia) and of death or end-stage renal disease.

Results: Death or a cardiovascular event occurred in 632 patients assigned to darbepoetin alfa and 602 patients assigned to placebo (hazard ratio for darbepoetin alfa vs. placebo, 1.05; 95 % confidence interval [CI], 0.94–1.17; P=0.41). Death or end-stage renal disease occurred in 652 patients assigned to darbepoetin alfa and 618 patients assigned to placebo (hazard ratio, 1.06; 95 % CI, 0.95–1.19; P=0.29). Fatal or nonfatal stroke occurred in 101 patients assigned to darbepoetin alfa and 53 patients assigned to placebo (hazard ratio, 1.92; 95 % CI, 1.38–2.68; P<0.001). Red cell transfusions were administered to 297 patients assigned to darbepoetin alfa and 496 patients assigned to placebo (P<0.001). There was only a modest improvement in patient-reported fatigue in the darbepoetin alfa group as compared with the placebo group.

Conclusions: The use of darbepoetin alfa in patients with diabetes, chronic kidney disease, and moderate anemia who were not undergoing dialysis did not reduce the risk of either of the two primary composite outcomes (either death or a cardiovascular event or death or a renal event) and was associated with an increased risk of stroke. For many persons involved in clinical decision-making, this risk will outweigh the potential benefits (ClinicalTrials.gov number, NCT00093015).

Critical Appraisal

Parameters	Yes	No	Comment
Validity			
Is the **Randomization** Procedure well described?	+1		Randomization method was described in detail. More importantly, randomization was stratified further according to study site, level of proteinuria, and history of cardiovascular disease. Both arms were well balanced at baseline with no statistical difference

Parameters	Yes	No	Comment
Double **blinded**?	+2		Double-blind, phase III, randomized, placebo-controlled, multicenter trial
Is the **sample size** calculation described/ adequate?	+3		It is an event-driven trial that required 1,203 cardiovascular composite events to achieve 80 % statistical power to detect a 20 % risk reduction for this outcome, with a two-sided type I error of 0.048. This required sample size of 4,000 participants in both arms, accounting for an incidence of event rate of 12.5 %/year in the placebo arm and 15 % dropout rate
Does it have a hard primary **endpoint**?	+1		Time to composite of death from any cause or cardiovascular event including nonfatal MI, congestive heart failure, stroke or hospitalization from myocardial ischemia. Time to composite outcome also of death or end-stage renal disease
Is the endpoint surrogate?		0	
Is the follow-up appropriate?	+1		Median follow-up was reasonable (29.1 month/patient)
Was there a **Bias**?		+2	
Is the dropout >25 %?		+1	
Is the analysis **ITT**?	+3		
Utility/usefulness			
Can the findings be generalized?		−1	Restricted to diabetics with non dialysis chronic kidney disease
Score	**80 %**		

Comments and Discussion

It is one of the best designed and executed trials in renal medicine, showing no advantage of high hemoglobin levels in patients with CKD and diabetes. In fact, there was an increased risk of stroke in the high-hemoglobin arm as well as cancer in those with a previous predisposition [13].

The increased risk of thrombotic stroke confirmed previous observations in CHOIR and CREATE [14–16]. Out of 188 patients with history of cancer, 14 died in the high-hemoglobin arm compared to only one from 160 in the low-hemoglobin arm. These observations are of interest; however, it is important to bear in mind that the study was not powered to detect differences in these event rates.

With the use of double-blind placebo design, they avoided the potential risk of bias surrounding the open-labeled trials. The two major predecessor trials for the same clinical question were open labeled (CREATE and CHOIR). The choice of placebo arm in an area with well-established therapeutic benefits of Epo was considered by some as unethical. The unexpected results of the previous trials made the placebo arm in the design more acceptable in order to read the results as the sole effect of Epo intervention.

However, the study warrants some comments:

1. The nature of the placebo arm was challenged because of the rescue therapy with darbepoetin alfa in this arm. Nearly half of these patients received darbepoetin alfa [17]. Such crossover from one arm of the study to the other confounds interpretation.
2. There was an imbalance between some of the baseline variables despite the large sample size and thorough randomization process. This problem was minimized by the further stratification of randomization particularly for the variable of history of cardiovascular disease.
3. Dropout rate was very close to the anticipated figure (13 vs. 15 %). Wisely enough, drug safety and monitoring (DSM) committee did not stop the trial prematurely despite CHOIR trial negative results. Moreover, the executive committee requested a more cautious stopping rule from the DSM who did not see the need to stop the trial prematurely. This decision allowed generation of more reliable evidence against high hemoglobin level in anemia management in CKD.
4. One of the composite endpoints, the start of dialysis, was not protocolized or prespecified, leaving the likelihood of considerable practice variability between centers and between countries.
5. The heterogeneity of the composite endpoints ranging from CV events, hospitalization, ESRD/requirement of renal replacement therapy, and death and their different relevance to patients and outcomes warrant questioning [8].

Conclusion

TREAT has shaped the current practice of anemia correction in CKD. It has also raised concern about the indiscriminate administration of high doses of Epo, in poor responders including those with cancer [18]. It remains unclear whether the higher morbidity noted in the high-hemoglobin arm is primarily due to the raised hematocrit/hemoglobin level or rather to the very high doses of Epo administered to reach targets and overcome Epo resistance in some with underlying comorbidities.

Target Hemoglobin Level with Erythropoietin Treatment in Hemodialysis

Title: The effects of normal as compared with low hematocrit values in patients with cardiac disease who are receiving hemodialysis and epoetin

Authors: Besarab A, Bolton WK, Browne JK, Egrie JC, Nissenson AR, Okamoto DM, Schwab SJ, and Goodkin DA

Journal: *NEJM*. 1998;339(9):584–90

Abstract

Background: In patients with end-stage renal disease, anemia develops as a result of erythropoietin deficiency, and recombinant human erythropoietin (epoetin) is prescribed to correct the anemia partially. We examined the risks and benefits of normalizing the hematocrit in patients with cardiac disease who were undergoing hemodialysis.

Methods: We studied 1,233 patients with clinical evidence of congestive heart failure or ischemic heart disease who were undergoing hemodialysis: 618 patients were assigned to receive increasing doses of epoetin to achieve and maintain a hematocrit of 42 %, and 615 were assigned to receive doses of epoetin sufficient to maintain a hematocrit of 30 % throughout the study. The median duration of treatment was 14 months. The primary endpoint was the length of time to death or a first nonfatal myocardial infarction.

Results: After 29 months, there were 183 deaths and 19 first nonfatal myocardial infarctions among the patients in the normal-hematocrit group and 150 deaths and 14 nonfatal myocardial infarctions among those in the low-hematocrit group (risk ratio for the normal-hematocrit group as compared with the low-hematocrit group, 1.3; 95 % confidence interval, 0.9–1.9). Although the difference in event-free survival between the two groups did not reach the prespecified statistical stopping boundary, the study was halted. The causes of death in the two groups were similar. The mortality rates decreased with increasing hematocrit values in both groups. The patients in the normal-hematocrit group had a decline in the adequacy of dialysis and received intravenous iron dextran more often than those in the low-hematocrit group.

Conclusions: In patients with clinically evident congestive heart failure or ischemic heart disease who are receiving hemodialysis, administration of epoetin to raise their hematocrit to 42 % is not recommended.

Critical Appraisal

Parameters	Yes	No	Comment
Validity			
Is the **Randomization** Procedure well described?		−1	It was not clear, although baseline variables were well balanced, raising the confidence in the method used
Double **blinded**?		−2	Open-labeled, phase III, randomized, controlled, multicenter trial
Is the **sample size** calculation described/ adequate?	+3		1,233 participants recruited on both arms with estimated sample size of 1,000 based on 90 % power to detect a difference of 20 % in primary event-free survival after 3 years at an overall alpha level of 0.05
Does it have a hard primary **endpoint**?	+1		The length of time to death or a first nonfatal myocardial infarction
Is the endpoint surrogate?		0	
Is the follow-up appropriate?		−1	Median 14 months with a range between 4 days and 30 months

Parameters	Yes	No	Comment
Was there a **Bias**?	−1		Open-labeled design for hard primary endpoint carries the risk of selection and performance bias. Early study termination without reaching prespecified stopping boundary and absence of blinded central adjudication process for the outcome measure carried high risk of inconsistence and bias
Is the dropout >25 %?	−1		Unclear
Is the analysis **ITT**?	+3		It was ITT analysis although study was terminated earlier than planned. This means that the protocol itself has not been completed
Utility/usefulness			
Can the findings be generalized?		−1	Participants were only those with history of ischemic heart disease or congestive cardiac failure. More than 50 % of participants in both arms were diabetics and mean age was 65 years. The premature termination of the study precludes its generalization
Score	….%		Not scored as study terminated earlier than planned

Comments and Discussion

This study was the earliest study to warn about erythropoietin (Epo) use to achieve normal hematocrit level in CKD patients with an emphasis on those treated by hemodialysis.

However, the characteristics of the included participants with high cardiovascular morbidity and high rate of diabetics make any generalization from the study difficult.

Further, the premature termination of the study with the consequent impact on its power to detect endpoints differences precludes definitive conclusions. Interestingly, the authors provided further analysis 1 year following the study termination and they retained the same conclusion [19]; clearly, such post hoc analysis provides little supporting evidence but instead support the hypothesis raised by the study that normalization of hematocrit in a high cardiovascular risk HD population may cause more harm than benefit.

The potential link between higher mortality rate and higher iron doses raises the recurring question as to whether those who required the higher iron doses prior to death might be the same who required higher Epo doses and whether it is their underlying and preexisting comorbidity that determined outcome rather than the treatment itself or the target hemoglobin level [20, 21].

Conclusion

The normalization of hematocrit study has defined the target hemoglobin/hematocrit levels in ESRD. These have been adopted subsequently by most anemia in CKD guidelines [9] that reiterated the warning against normalization of hematocrit in HD patients. This may have led to an unnecessary caution and an unwarranted generalization, not fully justifiable by the trial patient selection criteria.

General Discussion

The management of anemia in CKD has been shaped by the key clinical trials discussed in this chapter. It has led to clear and concerted reservation about normalization or even high hemoglobin levels in CKD/ESRD patients. However, it is clear from this review that many of the trials had considerable biases that question their generalization to the entire CKD and ESRD population. This is all the more questionable since the CKD and ESRD populations are very heterogeneous with considerable differences in underlying comorbidities and risk profile. A 20-year-old with rapidly progressive glomerulonephritis recently started on HD does not have the same CVD risk profile as a 70-year-old patient with type 2 diabetes mellitus who has been on dialysis for 10 years. Depriving the former from higher hemoglobin levels based on observations made in studies and RCTs such as TREAT and the normalization of hematocrit trial is questionable to say the least.

Also, the question of underlying comorbidity and risk profile may confound issues related to high or low hemoglobin levels but instead highlight those related to Epo sensitivity or resistance as a function of patients' risk profile and comorbidities.

Recommendations

Further studies are required with narrow and well-defined, low- and high-risk CKD and ESRD patients to define best treatment options. Thus, a better definition of the patients included in anemia correction studies may bear variable results and tolerability to different doses of Epo but also different levels of hemoglobin.

In the meanwhile, it would be advisable to individualize anemia management in CKD to avoid undertreating some and overtreating others.

References

1. Sunder-Plassmann G, Horl WH. Importance of iron supply for erythropoietin therapy. Nephrol Dial Transplant. 1995;10:2070–6.
2. Fishbane S, Maesaka JK. Iron management in end-stage renal disease. Am J Kidney Dis. 1997;29:319–33.
3. Drüeke TB, Parfrey PS. Summary of the KDIGO guideline on anemia and comment: reading between the (guide) line(s). Kidney Int. 2012;82(9):952–60.

4. Agarwal R. Is i.v. iron really superior in CKD patients not on dialysis? Kidney Int. 2006;70(6):1188.

5. Valliant A, Hofmann RM. Managing dialysis patients who develop anemia caused by chronic kidney disease: focus on peginesatide. Int J Nanomedicine. 2013;8:3297–307.

6. KDOQI; National Kidney Foundation. II. KDOQI Clinical practice guidelines and clinical practice recommendations for anemia in chronic kidney disease in adults. Am J Kidney Dis. 2006;47(5 Suppl 3):S16–85.

7. Levin A. Understanding recent hemoglobin trials in CKD: methods and lesson learned from CREATE and CHOIR. Nephrol Dial Transplant. 2007;22(2):309–12.

8. Montori VM, Permanyer-Miralda G, Ferreira-González I, Busse JW, Pacheco-Huergo V, Bryant D, Alonso J, Akl EA, Domingo-Salvany A, Mills E, Wu P, Schünemann HJ, Jaeschke R, Guyatt GH. Validity of composite end points in clinical trials. BMJ. 2005;330(7491):594–6.

9. KDIGO Clinical Practice Guideline for Anemia in Chronic Kidney Disease. Kidney Int. 2012;suppl 2(4):279–335.

10. Roger SD. Chronic kidney disease, anemia, and epoetin. N Engl J Med. 2007;356(9):958; author reply 958–9.

11. Mikhail A, Goldsmith D. Chronic kidney disease, anemia, and epoetin. N Engl J Med. 2007;356(9):956–7.

12. Singh AK, Szczech L, Tang KL, Barnhart H, Sapp S, Wolfson M, Reddan D. Anemia of CKD—the CHOIR study revisited. Nephrol Dial Transplant. 2007;22(7):1806–10.

13. Goldsmith D, Covic A. Time to Reconsider Evidence for Anemia Treatment (TREAT) = Essential Safety Arguments (ESA). Nephrol Dial Transplant. 2010;25(6):1734–7.

14. Wright RJ, Kanagasundaram NS, Quinton R. Darbepoetin alfa and chronic kidney disease. N Engl J Med. 2010;362(7):653; author reply 655.

15. Minnerup J, Schäbitz WR. Darbepoetin alfa and chronic kidney disease. N Engl J Med. 2010;362(7):653–4; author reply 655.

16. Skali H, Parving HH, Parfrey PS, Burdmann EA, Lewis EF, Ivanovich P, Keithi-Reddy SR, McGill JB, McMurray JJ, Singh AK, Solomon SD, Uno H, Pfeffer MA, TREAT Investigators. Stroke in patients with type 2 diabetes mellitus, chronic kidney disease, and anemia treated with Darbepoetin Alfa: the trial to reduce cardiovascular events with Aranesp therapy (TREAT) experience. Circulation. 2011;124(25):2903–8.

17. Locatelli F, Del Vecchio L, Casartelli D. Darbepoetin alfa and chronic kidney disease. N Engl J Med. 2010;362(7):654–5; author reply 655.

18. Solomon SD, Uno H, Lewis EF, Eckardt KU, Lin J, Burdmann EA, de Zeeuw D, Ivanovich P, Levey AS, Parfrey P, Remuzzi G, Singh AK, Toto R, Huang F, Rossert J, McMurray JJ, Pfeffer MA. Trial to reduce cardiovascular events with aranesp therapy (TREAT) Investigators. Erythropoietic response and outcomes in kidney disease and type 2 diabetes. N Engl J Med. 2010;363(12):1146–55.

19. Besarab A, Goodkin DA, Nissenson AR, Normal Hematocrit Cardiac Trial Authors. The normal hematocrit study – follow-up. N Engl J Med. 2008;358(4):433–4.

20. Sklar AH, Narsipur S. Effects of normal as compared with low hematocrit values in patients with cardiac disease undergoing hemodialysis and receiving epoetin. N Engl J Med. 1998;339(27):2023; author reply 2023–4.

21. Gonzales F. Effects of normal as compared with low hematocrit values in patients with cardiac disease undergoing hemodialysis and receiving epoetin. N Engl J Med. 1998;339(27):2023; author reply 2023–4.

Lipids and Chronic Kidney Disease Clinical Trials: A Critical Appraisal

Mohsen El Kossi

Cardiovascular disease is the leading cause of mortality and morbidity in patients with different stages of chronic kidney disease (CKD). The phenotypic picture of cardiovascular disease differs between those on dialysis and patients with early stages of chronic kidney disease. While atherosclerotic coronary artery disease is common in the early stages of CKD, arrhythmias, congestive cardiac failure, and sudden cardiac death (SCD) prevail in patients on dialysis, thus confounding interventions. Lipid profile also differs between both stages with high cholesterol levels being common at early CKD stages with relatively well-nourished patients compared to normal or low cholesterol levels in end-stage renal disease (ESRD) patients treated by dialysis who are usually under- or malnourished. Lipid profiles also differ between hemodialysis and peritoneal dialysis patients; due to the high caloric content of peritoneal dialysis fluids, patient treated by this modality have higher triglycerides levels.

Hyperlipidemia is a well-known risk factor for cardiovascular disease in the general population with established protective effect of statins on cardiovascular morbidity and mortality. There are also some observational studies suggesting a link between hyperlipidemia and CKD progression. This was prompted by the lipid hypothesis put forward in 1982 by Moorhead and his colleagues, postulating a link between dyslipidemia and the pathogenesis of CKD [1]. Following the limited recommendations endorsed by the ATP III guidelines (Adult Treatment Panel III) for patients with CKD [2], the only major development was the publication by KDOQI (Kidney Disease Outcomes Quality Initiative) in 2003 of the Practice Guidelines for Managing Dyslipidemias in Chronic Kidney Disease [3]. These guidelines relied largely on assumptions made from clinical trials undertaken in the general population and assumed that their translation to CKD/ESRD patients would be protective.

Situation has changed over the last decade, when a number of high-quality randomized controlled trials were published pertaining to CKD patients. They shaped the most recent guidelines of lipid management in CKD [4].

Trial (1): 4D

Title: Atorvastatin in patients with type 2 diabetes mellitus undergoing hemodialysis

Title Acronym: Die Deutsche Diabetes Dialyze (4D)

Authors: Wanner C, Krane V, März W, Olschewski M, Mann JF, Ruf G, and Ritz E; German Diabetes and Dialysis Study Investigators

Journal: *NEJM* 2005 21;353(3):238–48

Abstract

Background: Statins reduce the incidence of cardiovascular events in persons with type 2 diabetes mellitus. However, the benefit of statins in such patients receiving hemodialysis, who are at high risk for cardiovascular disease and death, has not been examined.

Methods: We conducted a multicenter, randomized, double-blind, prospective study of 1,255 subjects with type 2 diabetes mellitus receiving maintenance hemodialysis who were randomly assigned to receive 20 mg of atorvastatin per day or matching placebo. The primary endpoint was a composite of death from cardiac causes, nonfatal myocardial infarction, and stroke. Secondary endpoints included death from all causes and all cardiac and cerebrovascular events combined.

Results: After 4 weeks of treatment, the median level of low-density lipoprotein cholesterol was reduced by 42 % among patients receiving atorvastatin, and among those receiving placebo, it was reduced by 1.3 %. During a median follow-up period of 4 years, 469 patients (37 %) reached the primary endpoint, of whom 226 were assigned to atorvastatin and 243 to placebo (relative risk, 0.92; 95 % confidence

M. El Kossi, MBBCh, MSc, MD, FRCP
Doncaster Renal Unit, Doncaster Royal Infirmary Hospital,
Armthorpe Road, DN2 5LT Doncaster, UK
e-mail: elkossi@gmail.com

M. El Kossi, A. Khwaja, and M. El Nahas (eds.), *Informing Clinical Practice in Nephrology: The Role of RCTs*,
DOI 10.1007/978-3-319-10292-4_7, © Springer International Publishing Switzerland 2015

interval, 0.77–1.10; $P=0.37$). Atorvastatin had no significant effect on the individual components of the primary endpoint, except that the relative risk of fatal stroke among those receiving the drug was 2.03 (95 % confidence interval, 1.05–3.93; $P=0.04$). Atorvastatin reduced the rate of all cardiac events combined (relative risk, 0.82; 95 % confidence interval, 0.68–0.99; $P=0.03$, nominally significant) but not all cerebrovascular events combined (relative risk, 1.12; 95 % confidence interval, 0.81–1.55; $P=0.49$) or total mortality (relative risk, 0.93; 95 % confidence interval, 0.79–1.08; $P=0.33$).

Conclusions: Atorvastatin had no statistically significant effect on the composite primary endpoint of cardiovascular death, nonfatal myocardial infarction, and stroke in patients with diabetes receiving hemodialysis.

Critical Appraisal

Parameters	Yes	No	Comment
Validity			
Is the **Randomization** Procedure well described?	+1		A computer-generated randomization method was used. Baseline variables were well balanced without any significant difference
Double **blinded**?	+2		
Is the **sample size** calculation described/adequate?	+3		It is an event-driven study requiring 1,200 participants in both arms to have 424 events of primary endpoints over 2.5 years to achieve 90 % power, with alpha level of 0.05 in two-sided test with risk reduction of 27 % of the composite primary endpoint
Does it have a hard primary **endpoint**?	+1		A composite of death from cardiac causes, fatal stroke, nonfatal myocardial infarction, or nonfatal stroke
Is the endpoint surrogate?		0	
Is the follow-up appropriate?	+1		The mean length of follow-up was 3.96 years in the atorvastatin group and 3.91 years in the placebo group
Was there a **Bias**?		+2	None
Is the dropout >25 %?		+1	
Is the analysis **ITT**?	+3		
Utility/usefulness			
Can the findings be generalized?		−1	It included hemodialysis participants from Germany only with renal failure secondary to diabetes
Score	**87 %**		

Comments and Discussion

This trial with its unexpected results has challenged the views held in the ATP III and KDOQI guidelines about the protective value of statins in CKD. Clearly, it did not recommend initiation of statins in diabetic patients on hemodialysis who do not have a specific cardiovascular indication. It also raised the awareness about other pathogenic mechanisms for cardiovascular mortality and morbidity in dialysis patients compared to the general population, hence the lack of statins benefit.

It was the first randomized controlled trial with proper sample size and study power to examine the effect of statins in hemodialysis patients. The study was well designed and conducted. The primary composite endpoints were mortality and morbidity outcomes that were clearly defined and centrally adjudicated. These measures reduced the risk of bias and maintained the consistency of the study. There was no difference in the primary endpoint of composite mortality. Of note, there was a reduction by statins of the secondary endpoint of major adverse cardiovascular events. However the trial was not powered to detect differences in secondary endpoints.

The study became an excellent reference for any future study in this group of patients for event rate and appropriate sample size calculation. It raised a serious concern about the unexpected increased risk of fatal ischemic stroke in this group of patients using atorvastatin and whether this result was by chance or a genuine reason for concern remains unclear [5].

The clear limitation of the study was restricting participants to only diabetics making any generalization of the results to other hemodialysis patients difficult.

Other limitations include the heterogeneity of the population studied with patients included from the age of 18–80 years, average around 65 years. Also, the duration of diabetes varied considerably ranging from less than 5 years since diagnosis to over 25 years. The cardiovascular disease (CVD) risk profile of these patients may therefore vary considerably. Clearly, the age range and duration of diabetes variability may lead to different susceptibilities to major adverse cardiovascular events (MACE), thus risking to confound the effect of an intervention aimed to prevent atherosclerotic vascular disease. This would impact the study power as assumptions made in the older HD patients may not be applicable to the younger ones with short dialysis duration.

Another concern is the use of composite of interrelated endpoints, linked to hypercholesterolemia, that raise concern about a statistical bias [6].

Conclusion

In a large and heterogeneous population of HD patients with diabetes in Germany, it seems as if statins therapy with atorvastatin had little impact on CVD morbidity and mortality. It may have had a beneficial effect on MACE, to be tested subsequently by trials designed to test this hypothesis.

Trial (2): AURORA

Title: Rosuvastatin and cardiovascular events in patients undergoing hemodialysis

Title Acronym: A Study to Evaluate the Use of rosuvastatin in Subjects on Regular Hemodialysis: An Assessment of Survival and Cardiovascular Events (AURORA).

Authors: Fellström BC, Jardine AG, Schmieder RE, Holdaas H, Bannister K, Beutler J, Chae DW, Chevaile A, Cobbe SM, Grönhagen-Riska C, De Lima JJ, Lins R, Mayer G, McMahon AW, Parving HH, Remuzzi G, Samuelsson O, Sonkodi S, Sci D, Süleymanlar G, Tsakiris D, Tesar V, Todorov V, Wiecek A, Wüthrich RP, Gottlow M, Johnsson E, and Zannad F; AURORA Study Group

Journal: *NEJM* 2009;360(14):1395–407

Abstract

Background: Statins reduce the incidence of cardiovascular events in patients at high cardiovascular risk. However, a benefit of statins in such patients who are undergoing hemodialysis has not been proved.

Methods: We conducted an international, multicenter, randomized, double-blind, prospective trial involving 2,776 patients, 50–80 years of age, who were undergoing maintenance hemodialysis. We randomly assigned patients to receive rosuvastatin, 10 mg daily, or placebo. The combined primary endpoint was death from cardiovascular causes, nonfatal myocardial infarction, or nonfatal stroke. Secondary endpoints included death from all causes and individual cardiac and vascular events.

Results: After 3 months, the mean reduction in low-density lipoprotein (LDL) cholesterol levels was 43 % in patients receiving rosuvastatin, from a mean baseline level of 100 mg/dL (2.6 mmol/L). During a median follow-up period of 3.8 years, 396 patients in the rosuvastatin group and 408 patients in the placebo group reached the primary endpoint (9.2 and 9.5 events per 100 patient-years, respectively; hazard ratio for the combined endpoint in the rosuvastatin group vs. the placebo group, 0.96; 95 % confidence interval [CI], 0.84–1.11; $P=0.59$). Rosuvastatin had no effect on individual components of the primary endpoint. There was also no significant effect on all-cause mortality (13.5 vs. 14.0 events per 100 patient-years; hazard ratio, 0.96; 95 % CI, 0.86–1.07; $P=0.51$).

Conclusions: In patients undergoing hemodialysis, the initiation of treatment with rosuvastatin lowered the LDL cholesterol level but had no significant effect on the composite primary endpoint of death from cardiovascular causes, nonfatal myocardial infarction, or nonfatal stroke (ClinicalTrials.gov number, NCT0024033).

Critical Appraisal

Parameters	Yes	No	Comment
Validity			
Is the **Randomization** Procedure well described?	+1		Eligible patients were randomly assigned (in blocks of four in a 1:1 ratio) to receive either rosuvastatin, 10 mg daily, or matching placebo
Double **blinded**?	+2		Yes
Is the **sample size** calculation described/adequate?	+3		It was an event-driven study, requiring 620 composite primary endpoints to achieve two-sided 0.05 significance and 90 % power at an event rate of 11 %/year in the placebo arm with anticipated 25 % reduction in the primary endpoint in the intervention arm. Following 4D result with negative effect of statins in hemodialysis diabetic patients, estimate was readjusted for an intervention benefit of 19.5 %, with the number of events required increased to 805 events to get the same level of significance
Does it have a hard primary **endpoint**?	+1		A composite of death from cardiac causes, nonfatal myocardial infarction, or nonfatal stroke
Is the endpoint surrogate?		0	No
Is the follow-up appropriate?	+1		Median follow-up was 3.8 years (range from 1 day to 5.6 years)
Was there a **Bias**?		+2	
Is the dropout >25 %?	−1		
Is the analysis **ITT**?	+3		
Utility/usefulness			
Can the findings be generalized?	+1		It was a global trial that recruited participants from 280 centers from 25 countries all over the world. The cause of renal failure was a mix of the common causes
Score	**87 %**		

Comments and Discussion

This study complemented the 4D study by expanding participants to include hemodialysis patients secondary to any cause not limiting them to patients with DM only. The negative outcome of 4D prompted AURORA investigators to readjust sample size and reduced the anticipated benefit of statins' intervention. This was reflected as an increase in the number of primary outcome events required to reach the same level of significance. The investigators avoided the relatively young age in their participants, which is appropriate for the composite endpoint of cardiovascular death and nonfatal MI or stroke.

The active intervention achieved a significant drop of serum total and LDL cholesterol after 3 months of randomization. This reduction should have sufficed to show the anticipated clinical benefit. Convergence of the lipid level curves in both arms toward the end of the study might imply more patients on the placebo arm discontinued their placebo to start different statins (not reported in the study). Such lack of desired difference between both arms in any case would question the intervention value.

It was interesting to see no difference between intention to treat and per protocol analyses. However, the high dropout rate (50 %) [7] and lack of precise definition of cardiovascular death endpoint, even though it was centrally adjudicated, put the study power at risk.

There was a heterogeneity in the duration of time on HD with some patients treated for less than 1 year while others more than 7 years. This may confound the CVD risk profile of these patients and impact power. Also, the inclusion of around 20–25 % of patients with DM may introduce another risk confounder. In fact, a post hoc analysis of AURORA suggested a beneficial and protective effect against CV events and death in diabetic patients treated with rosuvastatin [8]. This observation was at odds with the 4D data that showed no beneficial effect in HD patients with diabetes and even an increased risk of ischemic stroke in those treated with atorvastatin [9].

The variable duration of follow-up is a limitation as some patients were followed up for over 5 years while others less than 12 months. This would clearly impact the risks of dialysis-related events.

The use of composite endpoint is not without its problems, when such endpoints are interrelated and easily overlapping [6].

Conclusion

AURORA was another negative trial of lipid-lowering intervention in patients on hemodialysis.

Trial (3): SHARP

Title: The effects of lowering LDL cholesterol with simvastatin plus ezetimibe in patients with chronic kidney disease (Study of Heart and Renal Protection): a randomized placebo-controlled trial.

Title Acronym: Study of Heart and Renal Protection *(SHARP)*

Authors: Baigent C, Landray MJ, Reith C, Emberson J, Wheeler DC, Tomson C, Wanner C, Krane V, Cass A, Craig J, Neal B, Jiang L, Hooi LS, Levin A, Agodoa L, Gaziano M, Kasiske B, Walker R, Massy ZA, Feldt-Rasmussen B, Krairittichai U, Ophascharoensuk V, Fellström B, Holdaas H, Tesar V, Wiecek A, Grobbee D, de Zeeuw D, Grönhagen-Riska C, Dasgupta T, Lewis D, Herrington W, Mafham M, Majoni W, Wallendszus K, Grimm R, Pedersen T, Tobert J, Armitage J, Baxter A, Bray C, Chen Y, Chen Z, Hill M, Knott C, Parish S, Simpson D, Sleight P, Young A, and Collins R SHARP Investigators. Collaborators (2,079)

Journal: *Lancet* 2011. (25); 377 (9784):2181–92

Abstract

Background: Lowering LDL cholesterol with statin regimens reduces the risk of myocardial infarction, ischemic stroke, and the need for coronary revascularization in people without kidney disease, but its effects in people with moderate-to-severe kidney disease are uncertain. The SHARP trial aimed to assess the efficacy and safety of the combination of simvastatin plus ezetimibe in such patients.

Methods: This randomized double-blind trial included 9,270 patients with chronic kidney disease (3,023 on dialysis and 6,247 not) with no known history of myocardial infarction or coronary revascularization. Patients were randomly assigned to simvastatin 20 mg plus ezetimibe 10 mg daily versus matching placebo. The key prespecified outcome was the first major atherosclerotic event (nonfatal myocardial infarction or coronary death, nonhemorrhagic stroke, or any arterial revascularization procedure). All analyses were by intention to treat. This trial is registered at ClinicalTrials.gov NCT00125593, and ISRCTN54137607.

Findings: A total of 4,650 patients were assigned to receive simvastatin plus ezetimibe and 4,620 to placebo. Allocation to simvastatin plus ezetimibe yielded an average LDL cholesterol difference of 0.85 mmol/L (SE 0.02; with about two-thirds compliance) during a median follow-up of 4.9 years and produced a 17 % proportional reduction in major atherosclerotic events (526 [11.3 %] simvastatin plus ezetimibe vs. 619 [13.4 %] placebo; rate ratio [RR] 0.83, 95 % CI 0.74–0.94; log-rank $p=0.0021$). Nonsignificantly fewer patients allocated to simvastatin plus ezetimibe had a nonfatal myocardial infarction or died from coronary heart disease (213 [4.6 %] vs. 230 [5.0 %]; RR 0.92; 95 % CI 0.76–1.11; $p=0.37$) and there were significant reductions in nonhemorrhagic stroke (131 [2.8 %] vs. 174 [3.8 %]; RR 0.75; 95 % CI 0.60–0.94; $p=0.01$) and arterial revascularization procedures (284 [6.1 %] vs. 352 [7.6 %]; RR 0.79; 95 % CI 0.68–0.93; $p=0.0036$). After weighting for subgroup-specific reductions in LDL cholesterol, there was no good evidence that the proportional effects on major atherosclerotic events differed from the summary rate ratio in any subgroup examined, and, in particular, they were similar in patients on dialysis and those who were not. The excess risk of myopathy was only 2 per 10,000 patients per year of treatment with this combination (9 [0.2 %] vs. 5 [0.1 %]). There was no evidence of excess risks of hepatitis (21 [0.5 %] vs. 18 [0.4 %]), gallstones (106 [2.3 %] vs. 106 [2.3 %]), or cancer (438 [9.4 %] vs. 439 [9.5 %], $p=0.89$) and there was no significant excess of death from any nonvascular cause (668 [14.4 %] vs. 612 [13.2 %], $p=0.13$).

Interpretation: Reduction of LDL cholesterol with simvastatin 20 mg plus ezetimibe 10 mg daily safely reduced the incidence of major atherosclerotic events in a wide range of patients with advanced chronic kidney disease.

Critical Appraisal

Parameters	Yes	No	Comment
Validity			
Is the **Randomization** Procedure well described?	+1		Well described with balancing of the baseline variables that could affect outcome through minimized randomization. There was no significant difference between baseline variables
Double **blinded**?	+2		
Is the **sample size** calculation described?	+3		Adequate sample size (9,270), with adequate power (90 %) and two-sided significance of 0.01. Due to less than expected event rate, primary endpoint was changed from major vascular event into major atherosclerotic event to maintain the study power
Does it have a hard primary **endpoint**?	+1		Major atherosclerotic event including nonfatal MI, coronary death, nonhemorrhagic stroke, arterial revascularization other than dialysis access

Parameters	Yes	No	Comment
Is the endpoint surrogate?		0	
Is the follow-up appropriate?	+1		4.9 years with minimum of 4 years
Was there a **Bias**?		+1	Authors did not refer to renal outcome in their discussion
Is the dropout >25 %?		+1	
Is the analysis **ITT**?	+3		
Utility/usefulness			
Can the findings be generalized?	+1		The study involved a wide mix of CKD patients and was a global study involving 380 hospitals in 18 countries
Score	**94 %**		

Comments and Discussion

This is one of the important nephrology clinical trials if not the best from the design, conduct, results, and impact on renal medicine. Authors designed a study with a balanced mix of CKD patients at different stages of CKD including those who are on dialysis (ESRD). They involved patients with peritoneal dialysis, which was not the case in any of the previous major lipid trials.

Sample size calculation was reviewed when the event rate was less than expected and the outcome measure changed to keep the power of the study as planned. There was a change in the outcome measure for the first time to reflect the therapeutic value of statins and LDL lowering by choosing only major atherosclerotic cardiovascular events (MACE), hence the bigger sample size characteristic of this study.

There was a statistically significant (17 %) reduction in the composite MACE; this reduction was significant only for nonhemorrhagic stroke and arterial revascularization [10], but not other components – in particular, no difference was detected in coronary artery-related events. There was no difference in cardiovascular or all-cause mortality. There was no impact on the rate of CKD progression, although GFR was not measured in SHARP.

The lack of benefit in the peritoneal dialysis population generated the hypothesis of no significant effect of this intervention on atherosclerotic events in peritoneal dialysis patients who might in theory be more amenable to the statins' effect in view of the relatively high serum lipid levels compared to hemodialysis. This will require adequately powered study to look into this hypothesis, as SHARP was not powered to detect difference in the CAPD population.

Authors concluded that the outcome was mainly due to LDL cholesterol reduction as in the meta-analysis of cholesterol treatment trialist (CTT) results [11]. This to a large extent could be true except for a major difference when the intervention of the meta-analysis was mainly HMG-CO reductase inhibitors not like in SHARP when it was a combination of statin and ezetimibe. Whether ezetimibe has any additional effect beyond cholesterol LDL lowering is unclear. This also raises the question as to why SHARP failed to incorporate a "statins only" arm in its long-term study design.

The use of composite endpoints in SHARP, as in other studies, gives the false impression that statins + ezetimibe reduce MACE in ESRD when in reality it failed to impact most, including hospitalizations and death, with the exception of nonhemorrhagic, ischemic strokes.

Finally, the very fact that the study was so large and so comprehensive may have generated a number of confounders from the inclusion of patients with CKD4 and CKD5 as well as those on hemodialysis and peritoneal dialysis. It assumed that the morbidity and mortality at all stages of CKD were comparable, thus overlooking the causes of specific dialysis-related morbidity, hospitalization, as well as death.

Conclusion

There is little doubt that SHARP is the most comprehensive and best conducted study on lipids management in CKD/ESRD. It showed some benefit on reduction of ischemic strokes but no impact on cardiovascular, coronary, or all-cause mortality. It has considerably influenced subsequent guidelines, KDIGO, on the management of dyslipidemia in CKD [4].

Trial (4): ALERT

Title: Effect of fluvastatin on cardiac outcomes in renal transplant recipients: a multicenter, randomized, placebo-controlled trial

Title Acronym: Assessment of LEscol in Renal Transplantation (ALERT)

Authors: Holdaas H., Fellström B., Jardine AG., Holme I., Nyberg G., Fauchald P., Jardine A., Grönhagen-Riska C., Madsen S, Neumayer HH, Cole E, Maes B, Weinreich T, Olsson AG, Pedersen TR, Benghozi R, and Hartmann A; ALERT Study Group. Assessment of Lescol in Renal Transplantation.

Journal: *Lancet*. 2003 14; 361(9374):2024–31

Abstract

Background: Renal transplant recipients are at increased risk of premature cardiovascular disease. Although statins reduce cardiovascular risk in the general population, their efficacy and safety in renal transplant recipients have not been established. We investigated the effects of fluvastatin on cardiac and renal endpoints in this population.

Methods: We did a multicenter, randomized, double-blind, placebo-controlled trial in 2,102 renal transplant recipients with total cholesterol 4.0–9.0 mmol/L. We randomly assigned patients fluvastatin (n = 1.050) or placebo (n = 1.052) and follow-up was for 5–6 years. The primary endpoint was the occurrence of a major adverse cardiac event, defined as cardiac death, nonfatal myocardial infarction (MI), or coronary intervention procedure. Secondary endpoints were individual cardiac events, combined cardiac death or nonfatal MI, cerebrovascular events, noncardiovascular death, all-cause mortality, and graft loss or doubling of serum creatinine. Analysis was by intention to treat.

Findings: After a mean follow-up of 5.1 years, fluvastatin lowered LDL cholesterol concentrations by 32 %. Risk reduction with fluvastatin for the primary endpoint (risk ratio 0.83 [95 % CI 0.64–1.06], $p = 0.139$) was not significant, although there were fewer cardiac deaths or nonfatal MI (70 vs. 104, 0.65 [0.48–0.88] $p = 0.005$) in the fluvastatin group than in the placebo group. Coronary intervention procedures and other secondary endpoints did not differ significantly between groups.

Interpretation: Although cardiac deaths and nonfatal MI seemed to be reduced, fluvastatin did not generally reduce rates of coronary intervention procedures or mortality. Overall effects of fluvastatin were similar to those of statins in other populations.

Critical Appraisal

Parameters	Yes	No	Comment
Validity			
Is the **Randomization** Procedure well described?	+1		Mentioned in detail with well-balanced variables at baseline in both arms
Double **blinded**?	+2		Open-label prescribing of fluvastatin to the placebo group may confound results
Is the **sample size** calculation described/ adequate?	+3		Based on event rate of 25 % over 5 years, 25 % size effect, 80 % power, and 0.05 two-sided significance. 738 participants were required for each arm. This number was readjusted to accommodate dropout rate to 1,800 for both arms. The sample size was wisely recalculated after a year because of less-than-expected event rate and the number was increased further by 250
Does it have a hard primary **endpoint**?	+1		The occurrence of first major cardiac event including cardiac death, nonfatal MI, or coronary revascularization
Is the endpoint surrogate?		0	

Parameters	Yes	No	Comment
Is the follow-up appropriate?	+1		Mean follow-up 5.1 years
Was there a **Bias**?		+1	Open-label fluvastatin prescribing in the placebo arm might mask the fluvastatin effect in the active treatment arm
Is the dropout >25 %?	−1		
Is the analysis **ITT**?	+3		
Utility/usefulness			
Can the findings be generalized?	+1		It was a multicenter trial, involving participants with different levels of graft function
Score	80 %		

Comments and Discussion

The study was the first evidence about safety and efficacy of statins in kidney transplant recipients, a group of patients with well-known high cardiovascular morbidity and mortality.

The study provides an excellent reference for the cardiovascular event rate in this group of patients with the magnitude of the potential risk reduction with statins in future studies of similar nature. Authors did stratify for coronary heart disease at randomization, which avoided the confounding effect of this variable on outcomes.

What was clear from the study results is that significant reduction of LDL was not associated with a significant impact on the primary cardiovascular outcomes [12].

Unfortunately, ALERT encountered protocol problems, sample size underestimation and reevaluation, and protocol amendments including changes in the fluvastatin dose. Protocol amendment with doubling fluvastatin dose after 2 years would make the active arm heterogeneous with 35 % of participants already having received the smaller dose of 40 mg. More importantly, this would affect the sample size as the effective follow-up with the new dose became 3 years rather than the preplanned 5 years, which would affect the number of event rate.

Of interest, doubling of fluvastatin dose from the outset might have had a more pronounced effect as shown when the investigators' extension of the study, albeit on an open-label basis, showed a clear statistical advantage in favor of the fluvastatin arm [13]. Clearly, such post hoc extension, and the open-label nature of the follow-up period, makes this observation inconclusive and, at best, hypothesis generating.

ALERT was also underpowered due to the high dropout rate; 665 participants completed the study and were assigned medication out of 1,050 randomized to fluvastatin. The difference between the ITT and per protocol analysis would have been informative.

Study protocol blinded serum total cholesterol levels except for predefined high levels (10 mmol/L) for all patients and (8 mmol/L) for patients with previous MI. These levels are relatively high for such high cardiovascular risk groups including also diabetics and patients with history of angina (around 7 % in each arm) and MI (3 % in each arm).

Protocol allowed prescribing open-labeled fluvastatin of 40 mg in addition to the masked medication for cardiac events and for unacceptably high cholesterol levels. This raises a concern about the potential risk of some patients in the active treatment arm to receive a total dose of fluvastatin as high as 120 mg/day and relatively low dose of 40 mg for the placebo arm with major cardiac event. The investigators admitted that the high rate of open-label fluvastatin prescribing in the placebo arm may have mitigated the differences between treated and "placebo" arms.

A subsequent post hoc analysis of ALERT suggested a close association between CVD events and inflammatory markers such as CRP and interleukin-6 (IL-6) [14].

Conclusion

ALERT negative results may have reflected the problems with the study protocol including statin dosing and distinction between active treatment and placebo groups. It remains that the role of statins for the management of renal transplant recipients is debatable. A Cochrane review of 22 studies and 3,465 patients showed that statins may reduce cardiovascular events in renal transplant recipient but that the effect was imprecise and warranted more studies to improve confidence in the treatment benefits and potential harm of statin therapy in that group of renal patients [15].

General Discussion

The trials discussed above raise a number of issues with lipid-lowering strategy to improve cardiovascular morbidity and mortality outcomes in hemodialysis (HD) patients. As mentioned in the introduction, assumptions are made that patients on HD have the same CVD risk profile when compared to the general population. This remains to be proven. In fact, reverse epidemiology observations tend to confound such impression. For instance, obesity, known to be a major CVD risk factor in the general population, is a protective variable in patients on HD [16], this in spite of the associated metabolic syndrome, glucose intolerance, and dyslipidemia characteristics of those with obesity treated by HD. Of relevance, a post hoc analysis of the 4D trial suggested that it was patients with muscle wasting who were at higher CVD risk [17] and suggesting personalized risk assessment on HD and targeted treatment of those at higher risk [18].

The cause of deaths in the HD population may also not be directly related to lipids or their levels; in fact, analysis of the cause of death in the 4D study revealed the majority to be due to infection (22 %), sudden cardiac death (26 %), and others (22 %), with a very small proportion dying from acute coronary event (6 %) or stroke (9 %) [19].

Also, assumptions were made in the clinical trial design that it would be the lipid-lowering effect of statins that confers benefit in terms of a reduction of CVD events, morbidity, and mortality. This may not be the case as a number of subsequent analyses of 4D, ALERT, and other trials suggested that a reduction in inflammatory markers such as CRP and interleukin-6 (IL-6) [14] may be more relevant to CVD outcomes than lipids levels. This was noted in the JUPITER study of CVD outcomes in patients at high cardiovascular risk where the beneficial effect of rosuvastatin was apparent in patients with high CRP levels regardless of their serum cholesterol levels; in fact, most had low cholesterol levels, suggesting that the combinations of possible wasting associated with inflammation are more significant CVD prognostic factors than hypercholesterolemia per se [20].

Recent KDIGO lipid guidelines [4] take such observations into consideration when they recommend blanket statins treatment in advanced CKD on the assumption of increased CVD risk regardless of serum lipids levels, thus putting little emphasis on dyslipidemia for the indication for starting treatment with statins, and subsequent monitoring, in CKD.

It is most unlikely that further RCTs will be conducted in CKD patients to study the impact of lipid lowering and/or statins on CVD outcomes. The KDIGO guidelines mentioned above [4], albeit with little supporting evidence as discussed in this chapter, have taken the side of statins and their prescription in CKD patients on the assumption of higher CVD. This shows that guidelines do not always take on board the negative outcomes of RCTs such as 4D, AURORA, ALERT, or SHARP. Questions have to be asked as to why this is the case.

References

1. Moorhead JF, Chan MK, El-Nahas M, Varghese Z. Lipid nephrotoxicity in chronic progressive glomerular and tubulo-interstitial disease. Lancet. 1982;2(8311):1309–11.
2. Expert Panel on Detection Evaluation, Treatment of High Blood Cholesterol in Adults. Executive summary of the third report of the National Cholesterol Education Program (NCEP) expert panel on detection, evaluation, and treatment of high blood cholesterol in adults (adult treatment panel III). JAMA. 2001;285:2486–97.
3. National Kidney Foundation. K/DOQI clinical practice guidelines for management of dyslipidemias in patients with kidney disease. Am J Kidney Dis. 2003;41:S1–92.
4. KDIGO Clinical Practice Guideline for Lipid Management in Chronic Kidney Disease. Kidney Int. 2013;suppl 3(3):259–305.
5. Jaber BL, Madias NE. Atorvastatin in patients with type 2 diabetes mellitus undergoing dialysis. N Engl J Med. 2005;353(17):1858–60.
6. Montori VM, Permanyer-Miralda G, Ferreira-González I, Buss JW, Pacheco-Huergo V, Bryant D, Alonso J, Akl EA, Domingo Salvany A, Mills E, Wu P, Schünemann HJ, Jaeschke R, Guyatt GH. Validity of composite end points in clinical trials. BMJ 2005;330(7491):594–6.
7. Shurraw S, Tonelli M. AURORA: is there a role for statin therapy in dialysis patients? Am J Kidney Dis. 2010;55(2):237–40.
8. Holdaas H, Holme I, Schmieder RE, Jardine AG, Zannad F, Norby GE, Fellström BC, AURORA Study Group. Rosuvastatin in diabetic hemodialysis patients. J Am Soc Nephrol 2011;22(7):1335–41.
9. Wanner C, Krane V, März W, Olschewski M, Mann JF, Ruf G, Ritz E, German Diabetes and Dialysis Study Investigators. Atorvastatin in patients with type 2 diabetes mellitus undergoing hemodialysis. NEJM. 2005;353(3):238–48.
10. Upadhyay A, Weiner DE. Lipid lowering therapy in individual with CKD: lessons learned from SHARP. Am J Kidney Dis 2012;59(2):170–3.
11. Baigent C, Keech A, Kearney PM, Blackwell L, Buck G, Pollicino C, Kirby A, Sourjina T, Peto R, Collins R, Simes R, Cholesterol Treatment Trialists' (CTT) Collaborators. Efficacy and safety of cholesterol-lowering treatment: prospective meta-analysis of data from 90,056 participants in 14 randomized trials of statins. Lancet 2005;366(9493):1267–78.
12. Kasiske BL, K/DOQI Dyslipidemia Work Group. Clinical practice guidelines for managing dyslipidemias in kidney transplant patients. Am J Transplant. 2005;5(6):1576.
13. Fellström B, Holdaas H, Jardine AG, Holme I, Nyberg G, Fauchald P, Grönhagen-Riska C, Madsen S, Neumayer HH, Cole E, Maes B, Ambühl P, Olsson AG, Hartmann A, Logan JO, Pedersen TR Assessment of Lescol in Renal Transplantation Study Investigators. Effect of fluvastatin on renal end points in the Assessment of Lescol in Renal Transplant (ALERT) trial. Kidney Int 2004;66(4):1549–55.
14. Abedini S, Holme I, März W, Weihrauch G, Fellström B, Jardine A, Cole E, Maes B, Neumayer HH, Grønhagen-Riska C, Ambühl P, Holdaas H, ALERT Study Group. Inflammation in renal transplantation. Clin J Am Soc Nephrol. 2009;4(7):1246–54.
15. Palmer SC, Navaneethan SD, Craig JC, Perkovic V, Johnson DW, Nigwekar SU, Hegbrant J, Strippoli GF. HMG CoA reductase inhibitors (statins) for kidney transplant recipients. Cochrane Database Syst Rev. 2014;28:1.
16. Vashistha T, Mehrotra R, Park J, Streja E, Dukkipati R, Nissenson AR, Ma JZ, Kovesdy CP, Kalantar-Zadeh K. Effect of age and dialysis vintage on obesity paradox in long-term hemodialysis patients. Am J Kidney Dis. 2014;63(4):612–22.
17. Drechsler C, Grootendorst DC, Pilz S, Tomaschitz A, Krane V, Dekker F, März W, Ritz E, Wanner C. Wasting and sudden cardiac death in hemodialysis patients: a post hoc analysis of 4D (Die Deutsche Diabetes Dialyse Studie). Am J Kidney Dis 2011;58(4):599–607.
18. Wanner C, Tonelli M, Kidney Disease: Improving Global Outcomes Lipid Guideline Development Work Group Members. KDIGO Clinical Practice Guideline for Lipid Management in CKD: summary of recommendation statements and clinical approach to the patient. Kidney Int. 2014;85(6):1303–9.
19. Ritz E, Wanner C. Lipid abnormalities and cardiovascular risk in renal disease. J Am Soc Nephrol. 2008;19(6):1065–70.
20. Ridker PM, Danielson E, Fonseca FA, Genest J, Gotto Jr AM, Kastelein JJ, Koenig W, Libby P, Lorenzatti AJ, MacFadyen JG, Nordestgaard BG, Shepherd J, Willerson JT, Glynn RJ, JUPITER Study Group. Rosuvastatin to prevent vascular events in men and women with elevated C-reactive protein. N Engl J Med 2008;359(21):2195–207.

Chronic Kidney Disease Mineral and Bone Disorder (CKD-MBD) Clinical Trials: A Critical Appraisal

Mohsen El Kossi and Arif Khwaja

Introduction

Chronic kidney disease-mineral bone disorder (CKD-MBD) refers to a triad of mineral, bone, and vascular disorders that are associated with an increased risk of morbidity and mortality in CKD. The last 15 years have seen a huge increase in research activity in this field as a result of better understanding of pathogenesis of bone disease and its inter-relationship with cardiovascular disease. Furthermore epidemiological data indicate that disturbances in mineral metabolism have been associated with an increased risk of vascular calcification, left ventricular hypertrophy, cardiovascular mortality, as well as an increased risk of fractures [1]. It is clear that the pathogenesis of bone and vascular disease is not simply dependent on calcium, phosphorus, vitamin D, and parathyroid hormone (PTH) but a host of other factors, most notably the fibroblast growth factor 23 (FGF-23)-Klotho axis [2]. FGF-23 acts as a potent phosphatonin increasing the expression of the sodium-phosphate co-transporter in the proximal tubule with elevated levels of FGF-23 being closely associated with mortality.

Given the strong association between deranged serum phosphorus, PTH, and vitamin D and adverse outcomes, randomized controlled trials have tended to focus on isolated correction of one of these risk factors. However, given the lack of clear understanding of the exact role of CKD-MBD on bone histology and fractures, CKD progression, and cardiovascular morbidity and mortality, the design of RCTs with hard clinical endpoints (as opposed to surrogate, biochemical endpoints) is extremely challenging.

It is worth noting that the treatment targets outlined by the Kidney Disease Improving Global Outcomes (KDIGO) guidelines [3] were largely based on observational data rather than interventional data that had been demonstrated to improve outcomes. For example, there has been no placebo-controlled trial in either dialysis or pre-dialysis CKD patients that has demonstrated that lowering serum phosphorus per se leads to improved, patient-centered outcomes, and furthermore, there are no interventional data to inform clinicians what the optimal serum phosphorus or PTH levels should be in CKD patients. In the limited space of this chapter, we have focused on clinical trials that have shaped contemporary clinical practice in the management of CKD-MBD. In essence, these are RCTs targeting individual biochemical components of CKD-MBD including secondary hyperparathyroidism and the use of calcium and non-calcium phosphate binders in the management of hyperphosphatemia.

Treat to Goal (TTG) Trial

Publication: *Sevelamer attenuates the progression of coronary and aortic calcification in hemodialysis patients*

Authors: Chertow GM, Burke SK, Raggi P; Treat to Goal Working Group.

Reference: *Kidney Int.* 2002;62(1):245–52

Title Acronym: Treat to Goal

Abstract

Background: Cardiovascular disease is frequent and severe in patients with end-stage renal disease. Disorders of mineral metabolism may contribute by promoting cardiovascular calcification.

Methods: We conducted a randomized clinical trial comparing sevelamer, a non-absorbed polymer, with calcium-based phosphate binders in 200 hemodialysis patients. Study outcomes included the targeted concentrations

M. El Kossi, MBBCh, MSc, MD, FRCP (✉)
Doncaster Renal Unit, Doncaster Royal Infirmary Hospital,
Armthorpe Road, DN2 5LT Doncaster, UK
e-mail: elkossi@gmail.com

A. Khwaja, FRCP, PhD
Sheffield Kidney Institute, Northern General Hospital,
Herries Road, Sheffield, South Yorkshire S57AU, England, UK
e-mail: Arif.khwaja@sth.nhs.uk

M. El Kossi, A. Khwaja, and M. El Nahas (eds.), *Informing Clinical Practice in Nephrology: The Role of RCTs*,
DOI 10.1007/978-3-319-10292-4_8, © Springer International Publishing Switzerland 2015

of serum phosphorus, calcium, and intact parathyroid hormone (PTH) and calcification of the coronary arteries and thoracic aorta using a calcification score derived from electron beam tomography.

Results: Sevelamer and calcium provided equivalent control of serum phosphorus (end-of-study values 5.1 ± 1.2 and 5.1 ± 1.4 mg/dL, respectively, $P=0.33$). Serum calcium concentration was significantly higher in the calcium-treated group ($P=0.002$), and hypercalcemia was more common (16 % vs. 5 % with sevelamer, $P=0.04$). More subjects in the calcium group had end-of-study intact PTH below the target of 150–300 pg/mL (57 % vs. 30 %, $P=0.001$). At study completion, the median absolute calcium score in the coronary arteries and aorta increased significantly in the calcium-treated subjects but not in the sevelamer-treated subjects (coronary arteries 36.6 vs. 0, $P=0.03$ and aorta 75.1 vs. 0, $P=0.01$, respectively). The median percent change in coronary artery (25 % vs. 6 %, $P=0.02$) and aortic (28 % vs. 5 %, $P=0.02$) calcium score also was significantly greater with calcium than with sevelamer.

Conclusions: Compared with calcium-based phosphate binders, sevelamer is less likely to cause hypercalcemia, low levels of PTH, and progressive coronary and aortic calcification in hemodialysis patients.

Critical Appraisal

Parameters	Yes	No	Comment
Validity			
Is the **randomization** procedure well described?	+1		It was well described. Baseline characteristics were well balanced
Double **blinded**?		−1	Open label
Is the **sample size** calculation described/adequate?		−1	The main objective of this study was unclear although assessment of vascular calcification was one of the major study outcomes. Power was based on a projected difference of 10 mg^2/dL^2 in calcium × phosphorus product, and the study achieved only 3 mg^2/dL^2 difference
Does it have a hard primary **endpoint**?		−1	Primary endpoint was unclear
Is the endpoint surrogate?		−1	Laboratory result with vascular calcification
Is the follow-up appropriate?	+1		Yes
Was there a **bias**?		−1	The open-label design, the mix of calcium carbonate and calcium acetate in the calcium intervention arm with different elemental calcium load, the absence of reporting on drug intake of relevance to the outcome as vitamin D sterols, lipid lowering, and calcium dialysate concentration

Parameters	Yes	No	Comment
Is the dropout >25 %?		−1	Dropout rate particularly for vascular calcification was higher than 25 % at 52 weeks
Is the analysis **ITT**?	+3		
Utility/usefulness			
Can the findings be generalized?		−1	Essentially negative and inconclusive trial
Score	**0 %**		TTG has serious limitations

Comments and Discussion

The association between hyperphosphatemia and vascular calcification (VC) has been substantiated by many experimental and observational studies. VC and adverse cardiovascular outcomes are also closely linked whether in the general population [4] or in patients with chronic kidney disease (CKD) [5, 6].

This study was one of the earliest that examined the differential impact of calcium- and non-calcium-containing phosphate binders on vascular calcifications. More significantly, it was one of the landmark studies that looked at VC in prevalent dialysis patients. It suggests that compared to calcium-containing phosphate binders, sevelamer (Renagel) was less likely to cause VC.

The study has major limitations:

1. Its open-label design makes it liable to observer selection and management bias.
2. The study is likely to be underpowered to detect a meaningful clinical difference in the severity of coronary and/or thoracic aorta calcification. Power was based on a projected difference of 10 mg^2/dL^2 in serum calcium × phosphorus product, and the study achieved only a 3 mg^2/dL^2 difference.
3. The calcium-containing phosphate binder-treated group was not homogeneous [7–9]; participants were on either calcium acetate or calcium carbonate with different elemental calcium content/intake and variable phosphate-lowering effects.
4. The outcomes are mainly surrogate including biochemistry and VC detected by electron beam tomography. Changes in these surrogate markers do not necessarily translate into better cardiovascular outcomes and survival in the hemodialysis population. Also, the use of serum calcium × phosphorus product as one of the study endpoint is dubious to say the least. Most recent CKD-MBD guidelines questioned the clinical value of serum calcium × phosphorus product (Ca × Pi) in determining the prognosis and outcomes in CKD.
5. There was no control of other factors known to affect serum calcium and/or VC such as vitamin D intake or blood levels, calcium concentrations in the dialysis bath [7], and lipid-lowering drugs in both arms. This is likely to confound the outcome results, more especially in an unblinded, open-label study.

Conclusion

While the TTG trial attempted to draw attention to the risks associated with calcium-containing phosphate binders and the potential advantage of sevelamer, it is at best inconclusive due to the significant shortcomings listed above.

Over reliance on surrogate markers to determine the efficacy of interventions in the area of mineral and bone disorders (MBD) has been one of the major flaws of clinical investigation in this field.

Renagel in New Dialysis Study (RIND)

Publication: *Effects of sevelamer and calcium on coronary artery calcification in patients new to hemodialysis*

Authors: Block GA, Spiegel DM, Ehrlich J, Mehta R, Lindbergh J, Dreisbach A, Raggi P

Reference: *Kidney Int.* 2005;68(4):1815–24

Abstract

Background: Hemodialysis patients are at increased risk for progressive coronary artery calcification; however, the development and progression of this disease process in patients new to hemodialysis is unknown.

Method: One hundred and twenty-nine patients new to hemodialysis were randomized to receive calcium-containing phosphate binders or the non-calcium phosphate binder sevelamer hydrochloride. Subjects underwent electron beam computed tomography scanning (EBCT) at entry into the study and again at 6, 12, and 18 months.

Results: One hundred and nine patients underwent baseline and at least one additional assessment of coronary calcification. At baseline, 37 % of sevelamer-treated and 31 % of calcium-treated patients had no evidence of coronary calcification. No subject with a zero coronary artery calcium score (CACS) at baseline progressed to a CACS >30 over 18 months. Subjects with a CACS >30 at baseline showed progressive increases in CACS in both treatment arms ($P < 0.05$ for each time point in both groups). Subjects treated with calcium-containing phosphate binders showed more rapid and more severe increases in CACS when compared with those receiving sevelamer hydrochloride ($P = 0.056$ at 12 months, $P = 0.01$ at 18 months).

Conclusion: New hemodialysis patients with no evidence of coronary calcification showed little evidence of disease development over 18 months independent of phosphate binder therapy. However, subjects with evidence of at least mild coronary calcification had significant progression at 6, 12, and 18 months. Use of calcium-containing phosphate binders resulted in more rapid progression of coronary calcification than did use of sevelamer hydrochloride.

Critical Appraisal

Parameters	Yes	No	Comment
Validity			
Is the **randomization** procedure well described?	+1		Well described with balanced baseline variables
Double **blinded**?		−2	Open label
Is the **sample size** calculation described/adequate?		−3	It was "estimated" that 50 patients in each arm would have only 80 % power to detect a significant difference in coronary artery calcification score. However, the basis of such an estimation was not specified in the methodology
Does it have a hard primary **endpoint**?		−1	The primary endpoint was a change in coronary artery calcification score. Mortality was a prespecified secondary endpoint published in a later study
Is the endpoint surrogate?	−2		
Is the follow-up appropriate?	+1		18 months
Was there a **bias**?		+2	
Is the dropout >25 %?		+1	No
Is the analysis **ITT**?	+3		Yes
Utility/usefulness			
Can the findings be generalized?		−1	The surrogate endpoint, the lack of a specified protocol, and the use of different calcium-based binders limit the clinical utility of the study
Are the findings easily translatable?	+1		
Was the NNT <100?			Not applicable
Score	0 %		

Comments and Discussion

The RIND study [10] was one of the first studies to demonstrate the possible adverse effect of calcium-based binders on VC in a hemodialysis population. The results of the RIND study were similar to the earlier Treat To Goal study [11] in that both studies challenged the widespread use of calcium-based binders and suggested that they may adversely affect a well-validated surrogate endpoint, namely, VC. Furthermore, in a preplanned secondary endpoint analysis of the RIND study with a median follow-up of 44 months, patients randomized to sevelamer had a significantly lower mortality rate compared to those randomized to calcium-based binders [12]. However, it is important to recognize that RIND was simply not powered to detect mortality differences given its small sample size. Furthermore, a fundamental problem with both the RIND and Treat To Goal studies was a lack of a specified treatment protocol in the calcium- and sevelamer-based arms with use of different doses and types of calcium-based binders. This clearly undermines the utility of the data generated. However, both RIND and Treat to Goal were, at the time of publication, hypothesis-generating studies challenging the paradigm of phosphorus control based on the ubiquitous use of calcium-containing binders.

Calcium Acetate Renagel Evaluation-2 (CARE-2)

Publication: *A 1-year randomized trial of calcium acetate versus sevelamer on progression of coronary artery calcification in hemodialysis patients with comparable lipid control: the Calcium Acetate Renagel Evaluation-2 (CARE-2) study*

    Authors: Qunibi W, Moustafa M, Muenz LR, He DY, Kessler PD, Diaz-Buxo JA, Budoff M

    Reference: *Am J Kidney Dis*. 2008 Jun;51(6):952–65

Abstract

Background: Previous clinical trials showed that progression of coronary artery calcification (CAC) may be slower in hemodialysis patients treated with sevelamer than those treated with calcium-based phosphate binders. Because sevelamer decreases low-density lipoprotein cholesterol (LDL-C) levels, we hypothesized that intensive lowering of LDL-C levels with atorvastatin in hemodialysis patients treated with calcium acetate would result in CAC progression rates similar to those in sevelamer-treated patients.

    Study Design: Randomized, controlled, open-label, non-inferiority trial with an upper bound for the non-inferiority margin of 1.8.

    Setting and Participants: A total of 203 prevalent hemodialysis patients at 26 dialysis centers with serum phosphorus levels greater than 5.5 mg/dL, LDL-C levels greater than 80 mg/dL, and baseline CAC scores of 30–7,000 units assessed by means of electron beam computed tomography.

    Interventions: 103 patients were randomly assigned to calcium acetate and 100 patients to sevelamer for 12 months to achieve phosphorus levels of 3.5–5.5 mg/dL. Atorvastatin was added to achieve serum LDL-C levels less than 70 mg/dL in both groups.

    Outcomes and Measurements: The primary endpoint was change in CAC score assessed by means of electron beam computed tomography.

    Results: After 12 months, mean serum LDL-C levels decreased to 68.8±22.0 mg/dL in the calcium acetate group and 62.4±23.0 mg/dL in the sevelamer group ($P=0.3$) Geometric mean increases in CAC scores were 35 % in th calcium acetate group and 39 % in the sevelamer group, wit a covariate-adjusted calcium acetate–sevelamer ratio o 0.994 (95 % confidence interval, 0.851–1.161).

    Limitations: Treatment assignment was not blinded. Th 1.8 a priori margin is large, CAC is a surrogate outcome duration of treatment was short, and dropout rate was high.

    Conclusions: With intensive lowering of LDL-C level for 1 year, hemodialysis patients treated with either calcium acetate or sevelamer experienced similar progression o CAC.

Critical Appraisal

Parameters	Yes	No	Comment
Validity			
Is the **randomization** procedure well described?	+1		
Double **blinded**?		−2	Open label
Is the **sample size** calculation described/adequate?	+3		The statistical test power was 80 %
Does it have a hard primary **endpoint**?		−1	Change in coronary artery calcification
Is the endpoint surrogate?	−2		
Is the follow-up appropriate?		−1	12 months may not represent sufficient "time" to detect significant changes in calcification
Was there a **bias**?		+2	
Is the dropout >25 %?	−1		High dropout rate of 42.7 % in calcium acetate arm
Is the analysis **ITT**?	+3		
Utility/usefulness			
Can the findings be generalized?		−1	High dropout rates in both arms limit the utility of the study
Are the findings easily translatable?	+1		
Was the NNT <100?			Not applicable as this was a non-inferiority study
Score	12.5 %		

Comments and Discussion

The original CARE study [13] was an 8-week, blinded RC1 that randomized patients to sevelamer or calcium acetate Unlike RIND or Treat to Goal, there was a specified protoco for the management of hyperphosphatemia in the study

CARE demonstrated that patients allocated to calcium acetate had significantly lower serum phosphorus levels than those allocated to sevelamer, though transient hypercalcemia occurred in 16.7 % of patients randomized to calcium acetate. The data from CARE suggested that calcium acetate provided better biochemical control of serum phosphorus as well as being more effective.

CARE-2 [14] was designed to control for the lipid-lowering effect of sevelamer by determining the risk of VC in patients on sevelamer and calcium acetate who had comparable lipid control. This was achieved by using atorvastatin to lower LDL cholesterol to less than 70 mg/dl in both groups. The headline data demonstrated a comparable increase in coronary artery calcification in both groups. The short duration of the study coupled with the high dropout rate means that data should be interpreted with caution. Furthermore, virtually all the patients in the calcium acetate arm received atorvastatin, whereas 21 % of patients in the sevelamer arm did not receive any atorvastatin. Notwithstanding these significant limitations, both the CARE studies provide an important counterbalance to the heavily pharma-supported narrative that cheaper, calcium-containing binders lead to adverse outcomes by aggravating VC. It is based on the hypothesis that VC is highly predictive of mortality in the dialysis population and that VC can be further aggravated by the use of calcium-based binders. This is perhaps an oversimplistic model of the pathogenesis of VC, which is not a result of passive deposition of calcium and phosphorus in the vessel wall but rather a complex process tightly regulated by inhibitors of VC such as fetuin A and matrix gla protein [15].

Dialysis Clinical Outcomes Revisited (DCOR)

Publication: *Effects of sevelamer and calcium-based phosphate binders on mortality in hemodialysis patients*

Authors: Suki WN, Zabaneh R, Cangiano JL, Reed J, Fischer D, Garrett L, Ling BN, Chasan-Taber S, Dillon MA, Blair AT, Burke SK

Reference: *Kidney Int*. 2007;72(9):1130–7

Abstract

Elevated serum phosphorus and calcium are associated with arterial calcification and mortality in dialysis patients. Unlike calcium-based binders, sevelamer attenuates arterial calcification, but it is unknown whether sevelamer affects mortality or morbidity. In a multicenter, randomized, open-label, parallel design trial, we compared sevelamer and calcium-based

binders on all-cause and cause-specific mortality (cardiovascular, infection, and other) in prevalent hemodialysis patients. A total of 2,103 patients were initially randomized to treatment, and 1,068 patients completed the study. All-cause mortality rates and cause-specific mortality rates were not significantly different. There was a significant age interaction on the treatment effect. Only in patients over 65 years of age was there a significant effect of sevelamer in lowering the mortality rate. There was a suggestion that sevelamer was associated with lower overall, but not cardiovascular-linked, mortality in older patients. We suggest that further research is needed to confirm these findings.

Critical Appraisal

Parameters	Yes	No	Comment
Validity			
Is the **randomization** procedure well described?	+1		Well-balanced baseline variables
Double **blinded**?		−2	Open label
Is the **sample size** calculation described/adequate?	+2		It was designed to have 80 % power to detect a 22 % decrease in all-cause mortality, assuming a mortality rate of 20 per 100 patient-years in the calcium group and a two-sided α of 0.05
Does it have a hard primary **endpoint**?	+1		All-cause mortality, cause-specific mortality (cardiovascular, infection, other), and all-cause hospitalization
Is the endpoint surrogate?		0	No
Is the follow-up appropriate?	+1		Mean follow-up was around 20 months
Was there a **bias**?		+2	
Is the dropout >25 %?	−1		It was >25 %. The dropout rate was high (49 %), and the event rate was lower than expected, and therefore the study was extended for a further year
Is the analysis **ITT**?		−3	In the case of early termination, patients were followed up for 90 days only following discontinuation of the study drug. Statistical plan specified analysis of outcomes during this follow-up period rather than an intent to treat period

Parameters	Yes	No	Comment
Utility/usefulness			
Can the findings be generalized?	+1		Although the study only involved dialysis centers from the USA, this is a powerful study with a large sample size and therefore is highly relevant to current practice
Are the findings easily translatable?	+1		Yes
Was the NNT <100?			Not applicable as it was a negative outcome study
Score	18.75 %		

Comments and Discussion

DCOR [16] in essence is a negative outcome study with no beneficial effect of sevelamer hydrochloride on mortality. Although there appeared to be a survival benefit in patients over the age of 65 years, the "real world" clinical significance of this is not clear. Furthermore, this benefit was not associated with a reduction in cardiovascular mortality, which is somewhat surprising given that the putative benefits of sevelamer hydrochloride have been postulated to be due to a reduction in VC. DCOR is a large, adequately powered study, with a hard primary outcome (mortality) and adequately balanced baseline variables between both groups. The flaws of this study reside in the unusually high dropout rate (49 %), the absence of intention to treat analysis, and the inherent biased nature of an open-label design. A preplanned intention to treat analysis was later published and again showed no beneficial effect of sevelamer on mortality [17]. The high dropout rate may reflect in part issues with the tolerability of sevelamer.

DCOR remains a landmark study in the management of hyperphosphatemia in dialysis patients and again challenged expert, opinion-based guidelines that had promoted the use of sevelamer on the basis of beneficial effects on surrogate endpoints such as VC.

DCOR highlights the difficulty in conducting outcome studies on mortality targeting only one variable (such as phosphorus) in complex, comorbid dialysis patients where the risk of death is likely to be multifactorial. One plausible explanation for the difference between DCOR and the previously positive outcomes seen in the RIND study is that DCOR was conducted in a prevalent dialysis population, and therefore many of the subjects will already have established VC, thereby attenuating any potential impact of sevelamer on VC progression. However, it is clear that from this large, well-powered study that there is no hard evidence to support the use of sevelamer over cheaper calcium-based binders in a prevalent hemodialysis population in the absence of hypercalcemia.

INDEPENDENT Study Investigators – CKD

Publication: *Mortality in kidney disease patients treated with phosphate binders: a randomized study*
    Authors: Di Iorio B, Bellasi A, Russo D
    Reference: *Clin J Am Soc Nephrol.* 2012;7:487–93

Abstract

Background and Objectives: Dietary phosphorus overload and excessive calcium intake from calcium-containing phosphate binders promote coronary artery calcification (CAC) that may contribute to high mortality of dialysis patients. CAC has been found in patients in early stages of non-dialysis-dependent CKD. In this population, no study has evaluated the potential role of phosphorus binders on mortality. This study aimed to evaluate all-cause mortality as the primary endpoint in non-dialysis-dependent CKD patients randomized to different phosphate binders; secondary endpoints were dialysis inception and the composite endpoint of all-cause mortality and dialysis inception.

Design, Setting, Participants, and Measurements: This is a randomized, multicenter, non-blinded pilot study. Consecutive outpatients ($n=212$; stage 3–4 CKD) were randomized to either sevelamer ($n=107$) or calcium carbonate ($n=105$). Phosphorus concentration was maintained between 2.7 and 4.6 mg/dl for patients with stage 3–4 CKD and between 3.5 and 5.5 mg/dl for patients with stage 5 CKD. The CAC score was assessed by computed tomography at study entry and after 6, 12, 18, and 24 months. All-cause mortality, dialysis inception, and the composite endpoint were recorded for up to 36 months.

Results: In patients randomized to sevelamer, all-cause mortality and the composite endpoint were lower; a non significant trend was noted for dialysis inception.

Conclusions: Sevelamer provided benefits in all-cause mortality and in the composite endpoint of death or dialysis inception but not advantages in dialysis inception. Larger studies are needed to confirm these results.

Critical Appraisal

Parameters	Yes	No	Comment
Validity			
Is the **randomization** procedure well described?	+1		
Double **blinded**?		−2	Open label

Parameters	Yes	No	Comment
Is the **sample size** calculation described/adequate?		−3	Unlikely that the sample size is adequate. The authors state that the study had an 80 % power to detect a 60 % reduction in mortality and used a sample size of 240 based on local "historical" data. Given that cardiovascular studies such as SHARP recruited nearly 9,000 patients to detect differences in CV mortality, such a sample size calculation does not seem credible
Does it have a hard primary **endpoint**?	+1		Mortality
Is the endpoint surrogate?		0	No
Is the follow-up appropriate?	+1		36 months
Was there a **bias**?		+2	Interestingly, the coronary artery calcification score at baseline was higher in the sevelamer group. This could not explain the positive impact of sevelamer
Is the dropout >25 %?		+1	
Is the analysis **ITT**?	+3		
Utility/usefulness			
Can the findings be generalized?		−1	Final and on-treatment phosphorus levels were lower in the sevelamer group, therefore making it impossible to determine whether positive outcomes were related to phosphorus lowering per se or the allocated binder
Are the findings easily translatable?	+1		
Was the NNT <100?	+1		
Score	29.4 %		

Comments and Discussion

Given the strong epidemiological data associating high phosphorus levels (independent of GFR) with VC and mortality in the non-dialysis CKD population [18], and previous data suggesting that sevelamer reduced the risk of progression of coronary artery calcification in pre-dialysis patients [19], the INDEPENDENT study investigators are to be commended for attempting to evaluate the role of phosphorus binders on a hard endpoint such as mortality [20]. The headline data are impressive, with a significant reduction in all-cause mortality and a significant reduction in the

development of de novo coronary artery calcification in subjects allocated to sevelamer. Furthermore, there was a delay in inception of dialysis in those allocated to sevelamer, but the criteria for starting dialysis were not clearly specified in the methodology and therefore may be subject to bias. As with the INDEPENDENT study in the dialysis population, the real problem with this study is that time-average phosphorus levels were lower in the sevelamer group and time-average calcium concentrations were significantly higher in the calcium carbonate group. Therefore, it is impossible to delineate whether the positive outcomes are due to phosphorus reduction or sevelamer per se. Furthermore, the choice of calcium carbonate may not be an appropriate control as it has a relatively high calcium content compared to calcium acetate. In summary, this is an interesting, hypothesis-generating study, but one cannot recommend the use of sevelamer over calcium-containing binders on the data in this study.

INDEPENDENT Study Investigators: Incident Hemodialysis Patients

Publication: *Sevelamer versus calcium carbonate in incident hemodialysis patients: results of an open-label 24-month randomized clinical trial*
Authors: Di Iorio B, Molony D, Bell C, Cucciniello E, Bellizzi V, Russo D, Bellasi A
Reference: *Am J Kidney Dis*. 2013 Oct;62(4):771–8

Abstract

Background: Whether the use of sevelamer rather than a calcium-containing phosphate binder improves cardiovascular (CV) survival in patients receiving dialysis remains to be elucidated.

Study Design: Open-label randomized controlled trial with parallel groups.

Settings and Participants: A total of 466 incident hemodialysis patients recruited from 18 centers in Italy.

Intervention: Study participants were randomly assigned in a 1:1 fashion to receive either sevelamer or a calcium-containing phosphate binder (although not required by the protocol, all patients in this group received calcium carbonate) for 24 months.

Outcomes: All individuals were followed up until completion of 36 months of follow-up or censoring. CV death due to cardiac arrhythmias was regarded as the primary endpoint.

Measurements: Blind event adjudication.

Results: At baseline, patients allocated to sevelamer had higher serum phosphorus (mean, 5.6 ± 1.7 [SD] vs. 4.8 ± 1.4 mg/dL) and C-reactive protein levels (mean, 8.8 ± 13.4 vs. 5.9 ± 6.8 mg/dL) and lower coronary artery calcification scores (median, 19 [IQR, 0–30] vs. 30 [IQR, 7–180]). At study completion, serum phosphate levels were lower in the sevelamer arm (median dosages, 4,800 and 2,000 mg/day for sevelamer and calcium carbonate, respectively). After a mean follow-up of 28 ± 10 months, 128 deaths were recorded (29 and 88 due to cardiac arrhythmias and all-cause CV death). Sevelamer-treated patients experienced lower CV mortality due to cardiac arrhythmias compared with patients treated with calcium carbonate (HR, 0.06; 95 % CI, 0.01–0.25; $P < 0.001$). Similar results were noted for all-cause CV mortality and all-cause mortality, but not for non-CV mortality. Adjustments for potential confounders did not affect results.

Limitations: Open-label design, higher baseline coronary artery calcification burden in calcium carbonate-treated patients, different mineral metabolism control in sevelamer-treated patients, overall lower than expected mortality.

Conclusions: These results show that sevelamer compared to a calcium-containing phosphate binder improves survival in a cohort of incident hemodialysis patients. However, the better outcomes in the sevelamer group may be due to better phosphate control rather than reduction in calcium load.

Critical Appraisal

Parameters	Yes	No	Comment
Validity			
Is the **randomization** procedure well described?	+1		
Double **blinded**?		−2	Open label
Is the **sample size** calculation described/adequate?		−3	Although the sample size calculations are well described, it is not clear what data the sample size calculations are made upon. The calculated sample size of 360 to detect differences in cardiovascular mortality is in striking contrast to the much larger trials designed to impact on cardiovascular (CV) mortality in dialysis patients such as DCOR, 4D, and AURORA studies
Does it have a hard primary **endpoint**?	+1		CV deaths due cardiac arrhythmias
Is the endpoint surrogate?		0	
Is the follow-up appropriate?	+1		36 months

Parameters	Yes	No	Comment
Was there a **bias**?		−2	Although baseline characteristics were corrected for in the statistical analysis, there are a number of differences in the laboratory characteristics including a lower weight and serum albumin concentration in the calcium carbonate group, implying that this group was "sicker" and more malnourished when compared to the sevelamer group Furthermore, there was higher baseline coronary artery calcification in the calcium carbonate group, which clearly could account for the higher CV events
Is the dropout >25 %?		+1	
Is the analysis **ITT**?	+3		
Utility/usefulness			
Can the findings be generalized?	+1		
Are the findings easily translatable?		−1	The serum phosphorus levels were significantly higher after 24 months in the calcium carbonate group as compared to the sevelamer group. It is therefore impossible to know whether the beneficial outcome mediated the use of sevelamer or by more aggressive control of hyperphosphatemia
Was the NNT <100?	+1		
Score	11.76 %		

Comments and Discussion

Although DCOR was a negative outcome study, concerns over the high dropout rate, the lower-than-expected event rate, and the study population of prevalent rather than incident dialysis led the INDEPENDENT investigators [21] to evaluate whether sevelamer could have a positive impact on mortality in incident dialysis patients. Data from the RIND study suggesting that sevelamer use was associated with a threefold reduction in mortality in incident dialysis patients was significantly limited by the small sample size. While this INDEPENDENT study is a much larger study, randomizing 466 patients, it is still not clear whether the study is adequately powered. The results of the study are intriguing with a significant reduction in arrhythmias, CV mortality, and all-cause mortality. The authors postulate that sevelamer may have a direct anti-arrhythmogenic effect or may attenuate prolongation of the QT interval due to inhibition of coronary artery calcification. However, there are a number of significant problems with the study that limit the generalizability of its findings. Given the higher baseline coronary artery calcification in the calcium carbonate group coupled with the suggestion that the calcium carbonate group was more malnourished suggests that the positive impact of the study may simply have been due to baseline differences between the two groups. Furthermore, the serum phosphorus was significantly lower at the end of the study in the sevelamer arm versus the calcium carbonate arm, making it impossible to delineate whether the positive outcomes on CV events were mediated by the use of sevelamer itself or by a lower phosphorus level. In summary, there are significant confounders in this study which make its interpretation difficult.

Publication: *Effects of phosphate binders in moderate CKD*

Authors: Block GA, Wheeler DC, Persky MS, Kestenbaum B, Ketteler M, Spiegel DM, Allison MA, Asplin J, Smits G, Hoofnagle AN, Kooienga L, Thadhani R, Mannstadt M, Wolf M, Chertow GM

Reference: *J Am Soc Nephrol*. 2012;23(8):1407–15

Abstract

Background: Some propose using phosphate binders in the CKD population, given the association between higher levels of phosphorus and mortality, but their safety and efficacy in this population are not well understood. Here, we aimed to determine the effects of phosphate binders on parameters of mineral metabolism and vascular calcification among patients with moderate-to-advanced CKD.

Methods: We randomly assigned 148 patients with estimated GFR = 20–45 ml/min/1.73 m² to calcium acetate, lanthanum carbonate, sevelamer carbonate, or placebo. The primary endpoint was change in mean serum phosphorus from baseline to the average of months 3, 6, and 9.

Results: Serum phosphorus decreased from a baseline mean of 4.2 mg/dl in both active and placebo arms to 3.9 mg/dl with active therapy and 4.1 mg/dl with placebo ($P = 0.03$). Phosphate binders, but not placebo, decreased mean 24-h urine phosphorus by 22 %. Median serum intact parathyroid hormone remained stable with active therapy and increased with placebo ($P = 0.002$). Active therapy did not significantly affect plasma C-terminal fibroblast growth factor 23 levels. Active therapy did, however, significantly increase calcification of the coronary arteries and abdominal aorta (coronary: median increases of 18.1 % vs. 0.6 %, $P = 0.05$; abdominal aorta: median increases of 15.4 % vs. 3.4 %, $P = 0.03$).

Conclusion: In conclusion, phosphate binders significantly lower serum and urinary phosphorus and attenuate progression of secondary hyperparathyroidism among patients with CKD who have normal or near-normal levels of

serum phosphorus; however, they also promote the progression of vascular calcification. The safety and efficacy of phosphate binders in CKD remain uncertain.

Critical Appraisal

Parameters	Yes	No	Comment
Validity			
Is the **randomization** procedure well described?	+1		
Double **blinded**?	+2		Yes
Is the **sample size** calculation described/adequate?		−3	The authors estimated that a sample size of 150 would have 80 % power to detect a change in serum phosphorus of .4 mg/dl. The actual difference was 0.3 mg/dl, and the study was not powered to detect differences between different phosphate binders
Does it have a hard primary **endpoint**?		−1	Primary endpoint was change in serum phosphorus
Is the endpoint surrogate?	−2		Biochemical endpoint
Is the follow-up appropriate?	+1		Appropriate for the primary endpoint
Was there a **bias**?		+2	
Is the dropout >25 %?	+1		Dropout rate less than 25 %
Is the analysis **ITT**?	+3		Yes
Utility/usefulness			
Can the findings be generalized?		−1	No. Single-center participants. Active treatment arm was heterogeneous, comprising three different phosphate binders
Are the findings easily translatable?		−1	No, results were inconclusive. Vascular calcification was also a secondary endpoint for which the study was not powered
Was NNT <100			Not applicable
Score	12.5 %		

Comments and Discussion

Given the association between both high phosphorus and elevated FGF-23 levels and mortality in CKD patients [22], many have proposed the use of phosphate binders in earlier stages of CKD when serum phosphorus levels are near normal. The rationale for this approach is that lowering phosphorus levels would in theory reduce the risk of VC. Furthermore, it has been postulated that lowering phosphorus levels even in patients with normal serum phosphorus would lower serum FGF-23 levels, which in turn may have a beneficial effect on mortality. This study demonstrated that phosphate binder therapy leads to a modest reduction in serum phosphorus levels in CKD 3 and 4 subjects [23]. However, active therapy had no impact on FGF-23 levels, and, furthermore, the use of phosphate binders was actually associated with a statistically significant *increased* risk of calcification of both coronary arteries and the abdominal aorta. Although this increased risk of VC appeared to be more pronounced in the group allocated to calcium-based binders, the study was not powered to detect differences between the three different binders used. As a result, the authors rightly conclude that the safety of phosphate binders in moderate CKD remains uncertain. The key importance of this study is that it (a) challenges the notion that phosphate binders need to be given earlier in the natural history of CKD to prevent vascular calcification and (b) suggests that this approach may actually be harmful by actually increasing the risk of VC. Again, the study challenges the dogma strongly promoted by the pharmaceutical industry that VC arises from excessive use of calcium-based phosphate binders.

The ADVANCE Study

Publication: *A randomized study to evaluate the effects of cinacalcet plus low-dose vitamin D on vascular calcification in patients on hemodialysis*

Authors: Raggi P, Chertow GM, Torres PU, Csiky B, Naso A, Nossuli K, Moustafa M, Goodman WG, Lopez N, Downey G, Dehmel B, Floege J; ADVANCE Study Group
Collaborators (92)
Reference: *Nephrol Dial Transplant*. 2011;26(4):1327–39
Title Acronym: ADVANCE

Abstract

Background: This prospective, randomized, controlled trial compared the progression of vascular and cardiac valve calcification in 360 prevalent adult hemodialysis patients with secondary hyperparathyroidism treated with either cinacalcet plus low-dose vitamin D sterols or flexible doses of vitamin D sterols alone.

Methods: Eligible subjects were on hemodialysis for ≥ 3 months with parathyroid hormone (PTH) >300 pg/mL or PTH 150–300 pg/mL with calcium–phosphorus product >50 mg^2/dL^2 while receiving vitamin D. All subjects received calcium-based phosphate binders. Coronary artery calcification (CAC) and aorta and cardiac valve calcium scores were determined both by Agatston and volume scoring using multi-detector computed tomography.

Subjects with Agatston CAC scores ≥ 30 were randomized to cinacalcet (30–180 mg/day) plus low-dose calcitriol or vitamin D analogue (≤ 2 μg paricalcitol equivalent/dialysis) or flexible vitamin D therapy. The primary endpoint was percentage change in Agatston CAC score from baseline to week 52.

Results: Median (P10, P90) Agatston CAC scores increased 24 % (−22, 119 %) in the cinacalcet group and 31 % (−9, 179 %) in the flexible vitamin D group ($P=0.073$). Corresponding changes in volume CAC scores were 22 % (−12, 105 %) and 30 % (−6, 133 %; $P=0.009$). Increases in calcification scores were consistently less in the aorta, aortic valve, and mitral valve among subjects treated with cinacalcet plus low-dose vitamin D sterols, and the differences between groups were significant at the aortic valve.

Conclusions: In hemodialysis patients with moderate-to-severe secondary hyperparathyroidism, cinacalcet plus low-dose vitamin D sterols may attenuate vascular and cardiac valve calcifications.

Critical Appraisal

Parameters	Yes	No	Comment
Validity			
Is the **randomization** procedure well described?		−1	No [24]
Double **blinded**?		−2	Open label
Is the **sample size** calculation described/adequate?	+3		Yes, but the dropout rate was higher than expected
Does it have a hard primary **endpoint**?		−1	
Is the endpoint surrogate?	−2		Yes. Vascular and valvular calcification
Is the follow-up appropriate?		−1	Not for the primary or secondary outcome (only 52 weeks)
Was there a **bias**?		+2	Only subjects with relatively high coronary artery calcification (CAC) score at baseline were enrolled to enhance detection of interval changes in calcification within the time frame studied
Is the dropout >25 %?	−1		
Is the analysis **ITT**?		−3	Per protocol analysis
Utility/usefulness			
Can the findings be generalized?		−1	Essentially negative and inconclusive trial
Score	0 %		ADVANCE trial has serious limitations

Comments and Discussion

The ADVANCE was a hypothesis-generating study that attempted to determine whether improved biochemical control of calcium, phosphorus, and PTH with the calcimimetic cinacalcet could attenuate the progression of VC with an underlying assumption that therapies that ameliorated VC had the potential to improve morbidity and mortality. The ADVANCE study was essentially a negative study as the only significant difference between those receiving cinacalcet and those receiving paricalcitol was related to aortic valve calcification. There was no difference in the primary outcome of coronary artery calcification (CAC) when using the Agatston score, but there was a significant difference when CAC was evaluated using volumetric calcification.

The ADVANCE study has a number of limitations including the open-label design with the inherent subject and observer bias. The follow up period was relatively short to pick up meaningful significant changes in VC [25]. The detected difference in aortic valve calcification is questionable as the study was not powered for this secondary outcome; it is at best hypothesis generating. The control arm was not controlled for confounders as calcitriol analogues with different forms and different modes of administration. The risk of bias is even increased by the exclusive use of calcium-based binders which will be potentially higher in the control arm because of the high doses of vitamin D analogues with the consequence of hyperphosphatemia. It's interesting to see that the median dose of calcium did not differ between the two groups despite of the well-known hypocalcemic effect of cinacalcet. This study does not give any information about the effect of cinacalcet on the de novo development of VC as all participants had significant VC at baseline. This may limit the applicability of the data to a wider dialysis population.

Conclusion

ADVANCE has a number of serious limitations that preclude any meaningful conclusion.

The IMPACT Study

Publication: *Paricalcitol versus cinacalcet plus low-dose vitamin D therapy for the treatment of secondary hyperparathyroidism in patients receiving hemodialysis: results of the IMPACT SHPT study.*

Authors: Ketteler M, Martin KJ, Wolf M, Amdahl M, Cozzolino M, Goldsmith D, Sharma A, Marx S, Khan S

Reference: *Nephrol Dial Transplant.* 2012;27(8):3270–8

Abstract

Background: Optimal treatment for secondary hyperparathyroidism (SHPT) has not been defined. The IMPACT SHPT (ClinicalTrials.gov identifier: NCT00977080) study assessed whether dose-titrated paricalcitol plus supplemental cinacalcet only for hypercalcemia is superior to cinacalcet plus low-dose vitamin D in controlling intact parathyroid hormone (iPTH) levels in patients with SHPT on hemodialysis.

Methods: In this 28-week, multicenter, open-label phase 4 study, participants were randomly selected to receive paricalcitol or cinacalcet plus low-dose vitamin D. Randomization and analyses were stratified by mode of paricalcitol administration [intravenous (IV) or oral]. The primary efficacy endpoint was the proportion of subjects who achieved a mean iPTH value of 150–300 pg/mL during weeks 21–28.

Results: Of the 272 subjects randomized, 268 received one or more dose of study drug; 101 in the IV and 110 in the oral stratum with two or more values during weeks 21–28 were included in the primary analysis. In the IV stratum, 57.7 % of subjects in the paricalcitol versus 32.7 % in the cinacalcet group ($P=0.016$) achieved the primary endpoint. In the oral stratum, the corresponding proportions of subjects were 54.4 % for paricalcitol and 43.4 % for cinacalcet ($P=0.260$). Cochran–Mantel–Haenszel analysis, controlling for stratum, revealed overall superiority of paricalcitol (56.0 %) over cinacalcet (38.2 %; $P=0.010$) in achieving iPTH 150–300 pg/mL during weeks 21–28. Hypercalcemia occurred in 4 (7.7 %) and 0 (0 %) of paricalcitol-treated subjects in the IV and oral strata, respectively. Hypocalcemia occurred in 46.9 and 54.7 % of cinacalcet-treated subjects in the IV and oral strata, respectively.

Conclusion: Paricalcitol versus cinacalcet plus low-dose vitamin D provided superior control of iPTH, with low incidence of hypercalcemia.

Critical Appraisal

Parameters	Yes	No	Comment
Validity			
Is the **randomization** procedure well described?	+1		Yes
Double **blinded**?		−2	Open-label study However, the primary endpoint is a biochemical variable and is unlikely to be biased by unblinding
Is the **sample size** calculation described/ adequate?	+3		There was underestimation of the comparator response (control 36 %) with a resultant smaller sample size

Parameters	Yes	No	Comment
Does it have a hard primary **endpoint**?		−1	Proportion of patients who achieve an iPTH between 150 and 300 pg/ml
Is the endpoint surrogate?		−2	Yes – iPTH range
Is the follow-up appropriate?	+1		28 weeks – appropriate for a biochemical outcome
Was there a **bias**?		−2	The study design "favored" paricalcitol in two ways. Firstly, it allowed the paricalcitol patients who became hypercalcemic to receive the comparator drug cinacalcet. Secondly, low-dose vitamin D dosing was fixed in the cinacalcet arm increasing the risk of hypocalcemia in that arm
Is the dropout >25 %?	+1		Around 23 % (estimated to be 20 % on sample size calculation)
Is the analysis **ITT**?	+3		Yes
Utility/usefulness			
Can the findings be generalized?		−1	The fixed low-dose vitamin D dosing does not reflect "real world" clinical practice
Are the findings easily translatable?	+1		Yes
NNT <100			Not applicable
Score	12.5 %		

Comments and Discussion

This study compared the efficacy and safety of the two commonly used drugs for the treatment of secondary hyperparathyroidism: cinacalcet and paricalcitol [26, 27]. Paricalcitol is a selective vitamin D receptor activator (VDRA) that is licensed for the treatment of secondary hyperparathyroidism (SHPT). Paricalcitol may be less likely to induce hypercalcemia and hyperphosphatemia when compared to non-selective vitamin D agonists such as calcitriol [28]. The IMPACT study attempts to define its role in the management of SHPT when compared to the calcimimetic agent cinacalcet. There are, however, a number of flaws in the study that limit its clinical utility. Firstly, the primary endpoint of a PTH between 150 and 300 pg/ml is flawed. The problem with this endpoint is that PTH is a poor predictor of underlying bone histomorphometry [29] and significant numbers of patients with this level of PTH will have evidence of adynamic bone disease. Therefore, bringing PTH down to this range will simply result in exchanging high turnover bone disease for adynamic bone disease. Indeed, it is questionable whether any of the subjects needed "additional" control of PTH given that a key inclusion criterion of the study was a PTH of 300–800 pg/ml, which is broadly in line with the KDIGO targets for PTH. Furthermore, the use of cinacalcet in the paricalci-

tol arm potentially mitigates the calcemic effects of paricalcitol, while fixing the dose of alfacalcidol in the cinacalcet arm will simply accentuate the number of patients at risk of hypocalcemia. Moreover, there is little evidence to suggest that paricalcitol provides better biochemical control of SHPT than either alfacalcidol [30] or cinacalcet and the cost-effectiveness of paricalcitol is unclear.

There are observational data to suggest that paricalcitol use is associated with improved survival among hemodialysis patients [31], and there is increasing interest in the fact that vitamin D analogues such as paricalcitol may have cardioprotective and renoprotective effects by negative regulation of renin, thereby inhibiting the renin–angiotensin system. However, there are no positive interventional data with paricalcitol on meaningful patient-centered outcomes such as mortality or hospitalization, and the recently published PRIMO study showed no effect of paricalcitol on left ventricular mass index in patients with CKD [32]. Similarly, there are conflicting data on whether paricalcitol can reduce albuminuria [33], and this is further confounded by the fact that vitamin D therapy may increase urinary creatinine excretion, thereby "artificially" reducing albuminuria when measured using urinary albumin–creatinine ratio.

Evaluation of Cinacalcet Hydrochloride to Lower Cardiovascular Disease (EVOLVE)

Publication: *Effect of cinacalcet on cardiovascular disease in patients undergoing dialysis*

Authors: EVOLVE Trial Investigators, Chertow GM, Block GA, Correa-Rotter R, Drüeke TB, Floege J, Goodman WG, Herzog CA, Kubo Y, London GM, Mahaffey KW, Mix TC, Moe SM, Trotman ML, Wheeler DC, Parfrey PS

Reference: *N Engl J Med*. 2012. 27;367(26):2482–94

Abstract

Background: Disorders of mineral metabolism, including secondary hyperparathyroidism, are thought to contribute to extraskeletal (including vascular) calcification among patients with chronic kidney disease. It has been hypothesized that treatment with the calcimimetic agent cinacalcet might reduce the risk of death or nonfatal cardiovascular events in such patients.

Methods: In this clinical trial, we randomly assigned 3,883 patients with moderate-to-severe secondary hyperparathyroidism (median level of intact parathyroid hormone, 693 pg/ml [10th–90th percentile, 363–1,694]), who were undergoing hemodialysis, to receive either cinacalcet or placebo. All patients were eligible to receive conventional therapy, including phosphate binders, vitamin D sterols, or both. The patients were followed up for up to 64 months. The primary composite endpoint was the time until death, myocardial infarction, hospitalization for unstable angina, heart failure, or a peripheral vascular event. The primary analysis was performed on the basis of the intention-to-treat principle.

Results: The median duration of study–drug exposure was 21.2 months in the cinacalcet group versus 17.5 months in the placebo group. The primary composite endpoint was reached in 938 of 1,948 patients (48.2 %) in the cinacalcet group and 952 of 1,935 patients (49.2 %) in the placebo group (relative hazard in the cinacalcet group vs. the placebo group, 0.93; 95 % confidence interval, 0.85–1.02; $P = 0.11$). Hypocalcemia and gastrointestinal adverse events were significantly more frequent in patients receiving cinacalcet.

Conclusions: In an unadjusted intention-to-treat analysis, cinacalcet did not significantly reduce the risk of death or major cardiovascular events in patients with moderate-to-severe secondary hyperparathyroidism who were undergoing dialysis.

Critical Appraisal

Parameters	Yes	No	Comment
Validity			
Is the **randomization** procedure well described?	+1		Well described with well-balanced baseline variables. There was slight difference in age but was not statistically significant
Double **blinded**?	+2		Yes
Is the **sample size** calculation described/adequate?	+3		They also took into account the expected dropout and drop-in rate. The power level was 90 % with higher projected event rate compared to the actual one, which resulted in extension for 16 months more than planned
Does it have a hard primary **endpoint**?	+1		All-cause mortality, nonfatal MI, hospitalization for unstable angina, heart failure, and arterial revascularization
Is the endpoint surrogate?		0	No
Is the follow-up appropriate?	+1		Yes with minimum of 4 years and as long as 64 months
Was there a **bias**?		+2	No other than slight difference in baseline age between the two groups. There was an analysis that accounted for study–drug exposure that appeared to show a benefit of cinacalcet. However, the authors rightly state that the prespecified intention-to-treat analysis showed no benefit of cinacalcet

Parameters	Yes	No	Comment
Is the dropout >25 %?	−1		Yes with high dropout and drop-in rate in both arms
Is the analysis **ITT**?	+3		Yes
Utility/usefulness			
Can the findings be generalized?	+1		Yes, it is a negative study of hemodialysis patients aged more than 18 years old with serum intact PTH >300 pg/ml. It was a global study involving 500 hospitals in 22 countries
Are the findings easily translatable?	+1		Yes
Is the NNT <100			Not applicable as a negative outcome study
Score	87.5 %		

Comments and Discussion

Cinacalcet is a calcimimetic agent that activates the calcium-sensing receptor on the parathyroid gland, increasing its sensitivity to calcium and thereby reducing PTH secretion. When the FDA approved cinacalcet for clinical use, it relied mainly on its biochemical efficacy and safety with a phase 3, double-blind, placebo-controlled study demonstrating its efficacy in significantly reducing PTH levels in dialysis patients with associated reductions in both serum calcium and phosphorus [34]. At the time of licensing, there was no evidence that cinacalcet had any effect on hard clinical outcomes. Prior to the publication of the EVOLVE study [35], there were only limited data that cinacalcet may have a beneficial effect on fractures [36] and surrogates such as VC. For example, the ADVANCE study [24] was an open-label RCT with a relatively short follow-up of 52 weeks, which demonstrated that the progression of coronary artery and valvular calcification was less in those randomized to cinacalcet as compared to those on flexible vitamin D dosing. However, whether an impact on a surrogate outcome such as VC has any meaningful impact of patient-centered outcomes is far from clear.

EVOLVE, therefore, is a landmark study in nephrology that moves beyond surrogates such as VC and PTH levels with a composite primary endpoint of death, myocardial infarction, or hospitalization of a cardiovascular or peripheral vascular event. A particular strength of the study is not only its large size but also the flexibility in phosphate binder and phosphate binder dosing, which means that the study protocol reflects "real world" clinical use of cinacalcet. A problem with the study was that subjects in the placebo arm were slightly younger at baseline and there also appeared to be considerable crossover between the two arms of the study – a high dropout rate in the placebo arm and a high drop-in rate into the active arm. A per protocol analysis with adjustment of baseline variables suggested a statistical benefit for cinacalcet. However, the reality is that this is another negative outcome study with the intention-to-treat analysis highlighting not only the lack of effect of cinacalcet on cardiovascular outcomes, but also a significantly higher risk of significant side effects such as nausea and hypocalcemia. Indeed, the latter can be fatal, and it is worth noting that the FDA has now withdrawn the license for cinacalcet in the pediatric population. Cinacalcet did, however, reduce the risk of parathyroidectomy by half, and the study confirms that this is its main clinical benefit. However, cinacalcet is expensive, and there has been little pharmacoeconomic analysis using quality-adjusted life years (QALYS) incorporating the hard clinical data from EVOLVE. Therefore, for clinicians who practice in an environment where cost is an issue, the UK National Institute of Health and Clinical Excellence guidelines on the use of cinacalcet seem eminently sensible, namely, that it should only be used in patients with refractory, uncontrolled levels of PTH (defined as greater than 800 pg/ml), with normal/high adjusted calcium levels, in whom the risks of parathyroidectomy outweigh its benefits.

General Discussion and Conclusions

In this chapter, we have reviewed some of the key RCTs that have informed clinical practice in the field of CKD-MBD. What is striking is how poorly most trials score when subject to critical appraisal. This reflects the difficulty in conducting clinical trials with meaningful hard clinical endpoints in such a heterogeneous population with fast changing clinical variables. Furthermore, while registry data indicate that good biochemical control of calcium, phosphorus, and PTH associates with improved survival, it is far from clear whether specific interventions per se improve patient-centered outcomes. In fact, what the large RCTs such as DCOR and EVOLVE suggest is that improved control of biochemical surrogates does not translate into better patient outcomes.

As regards phosphorus control, there is simply no RCT data to inform what the optimal phosphorus level is in dialysis patients nor is there an RCT to show whether phosphate binders improve outcomes in the dialysis population. Much of the research has focused on the potential benefit of expensive, non-calcium binders (particularly sevelamer) over cheaper calcium-based binders. Again, while there are potential benefits on surrogate outcomes such as VC, the benefit of sevelamer in mortality is much harder to prove. A recent meta-analysis by Jamal suggests that non-calcium binders were associated with reduced mortality in the CKD population [37]. However, as already discussed, there are significant flaws in many of the positive outcome studies, such as the INDEPENDENT studies that make the interpretation of such meta-analyses difficult. Furthermore, given the cost of non-calcium binders such as lanthanum and sevelamer, there has been very little, robust pharmacoeconomic analysis of the use of such drugs.

Similarly, the cost-benefit of either VDRAs such as paricalcitol or calcimimetics such as cinacalcet is far from clear. While there has been huge interest in the cardio- and nephroprotective effects of VDRAs, there is little hard outcome data from interventional studies. Similarly, while cinacalcet clearly reduces the risk of parathyroidectomy [38] and is a useful therapeutic in the management of SHPT, it is not clear whether it is a cost-effective intervention for patients on dialysis. There is also increasing interest in replacement of native vitamin D, and a recent study suggests that cholecalciferol replacement is both safe and may reduce PTH levels [39]. Again there are no data to show whether this impacts on harder endpoints such as fractures or mortality.

The salutary lesson from these studies in CKD-MBD is that it is unlikely that there is a single "magic bullet" targeting a single biochemical parameter which will translate into clinically meaningful impact on patient mortality, morbidity, and quality of life. Future studies are likely to need to look at "bundle of care" interventions that take a multifaceted approach at targeting multiple risk factors.

References

1. Evenepoel P, Rodriguez M, Ketteler M. Laboratory abnormalities in CKD-MBD: markers, predictors, or mediators of disease? Semin Nephrol. 2014;34(2):151–63.
2. Kuro-o M. Klotho, phosphate and FGF-23 in ageing and disturbed mineral metabolism. Nat Rev Nephrol. 2013;9(11):650–60.
3. KDIGO clinical practice guideline for the diagnosis, evaluation, prevention, and treatment of Chronic Kidney Disease-Mineral and Bone Disorder (CKD-MBD). Kidney Disease: Improving Global Outcomes (KDIGO) CKD-MBD Work Group. Kidney Int Suppl. 2009;(113):S1–130.
4. Alexopoulos N, Raggi P. Calcification in atherosclerosis. Nat Rev Cardiol. 2009;6:681–8.
5. Blacher J, Guerin AP, Pannier B, et al. Arterial calcifications, arterial stiffness, and cardiovascular risk in end-stage renal disease. Hypertension. 2001;38:938–42.
6. Goodman WG, Goldin J, Kuizon BD, et al. Coronary-artery calcification in young adults with end-stage renal disease who are undergoing dialysis. N Engl J Med. 2000;342:1478–83.
7. Cleveland M. Calcium on trial: beyond a reasonable doubt? Kidney Int. 2003;63(1):383; author reply 383–4.
8. Canavese C, Bergamo D, Dib H, Bermond F, Burdese M. Calcium on trial: beyond a reasonable doubt? Kidney Int. 2003;63(1):381–2; author reply 383–4.
9. Goudas PC. Renal disease medications and evidence-biased medicine. Kidney Int. 2003;64(4):1533–4.
10. Block GA, Spiegel DM, Ehrlich J, Mehta R, Lindbergh J, Dreisbach A, Raggi P. Effects of sevelamer and calcium on coronary artery calcification in patients new to hemodialysis. Kidney Int. 2005;68(4):1815–24.
11. Chertow GM, Burke SK, Raggi P, Treat to Goal Working Group. Sevelamer attenuates the progression of coronary and aortic calcification in hemodialysis patients. Kidney Int. 2002;62(1):245–52.
12. Block GA, Raggi P, Bellasi A, Kooienga L, Spiegel DM. Mortality effect of coronary calcification and phosphate binder choice in incident hemodialysis patients. Kidney Int. 2007;71(5):438–41.

13. Qunibi WY, Hootkins RE, McDowell LL, Meyer MS, Simon M, Garza RO, Pelham RW, Cleveland MV, Muenz LR, He DY, Nolan CR. Treatment of hyperphosphatemia in hemodialysis patients: The Calcium Acetate Renagel Evaluation (CARE Study). Kidney Int. 2004;65(5):1914–26.

14. Qunibi W, Moustafa M, Muenz LR, He DY, Kessler PD, Diaz-Buxo JA, Budoff M. A 1-year randomized trial of calcium acetate versus sevelamer on progression of coronary artery calcification in hemodialysis patients with comparable lipid control: the Calcium Acetate Renagel Evaluation-2 (CARE-2) study. Am J Kidney Dis. 2008; 51(6):952–65.

15. Shanahan CM, Crouthamel MH, Kapustin A, Giachelli CM. Arterial calcification in chronic kidney disease: key roles for calcium and phosphate. Circ Res. 2011;109(6):697–711.

16. Suki WN, Zabaneh R, Cangiano JL, Reed J, Fischer D, Garrett L, Ling BN, Chasan-Taber S, Dillon MA, Blair AT, Burke SK. Effects of sevelamer and calcium-based phosphate binders on mortality in hemodialysis patients. Kidney Int. 2007;72(9):1130–7.

17. St Peter WL, Liu J, Weinhandl E, Fan Q. A comparison of sevelamer and calcium-based phosphate binders on mortality, hospitalization, and morbidity in hemodialysis: a secondary analysis of the Dialysis Clinical Outcomes Revisited (DCOR) randomized trial using claims data. Am J Kidney Dis. 2008;51(3):445–54.

18. Palmer SC, Hayen A, Macaskill P, Pellegrini F, Craig JC, Elder GJ, Strippoli GF. Serum levels of phosphorus, parathyroid hormone, and calcium and risks of death and cardiovascular disease in individuals with chronic kidney disease. A systematic review and meta-analysis. JAMA. 2011;305:1119–27.

19. Russo D, Corrao S, Battaglia Y, Andreucci M, Caiazza A, Carlomagno A, Lamberti M, Pezone N, Pota A, Russo L, Sacco M, Scognamiglio B. Progression of coronary artery calcification and cardiac events in patients with chronic renal disease not receiving dialysis. Kidney Int. 2011;80(1):112–8.

20. Di Iorio B, Bellasi A, Russo D. Mortality in kidney disease patients treated with phosphate binders: a randomized study. Clin J Am Soc Nephrol. 2012;7:487–93.

21. Di Iorio B, Molony D, Bell C, Cucciniello E, Bellizzi V, Russo D, Bellasi A. Sevelamer versus calcium carbonate in incident hemodialysis patients: results of an open-label 24-month randomized clinical trial. Am J Kidney Dis. 2013;62(4):771–8.

22. Gutiérrez OM, Mannstadt M, Isakova T, Rauh-Hain JA, Tamez H, Shah A, Smith K, Lee H, Thadhani R, Jüppner H, Wolf M. Fibroblast growth factor 23 and mortality among patients undergoing hemodialysis. N Engl J Med. 2008;359(6):584–92.

23. Block GA, Wheeler DC, Persky MS, Kestenbaum B, Ketteler M, Spiegel DM, Allison MA, Asplin J, Smits G, Hoofnagle AN, Kooienga L, Thadhani R, Mannstadt M, Wolf M, Chertow GM. Effects of phosphate binders in moderate CKD. J Am Soc Nephrol. 2012;23(8):1407–15.

24. Raggi P, Chertow GM, Torres PU, Csiky B, Naso A, Nossuli K, Moustafa M, Goodman WG, Lopez N, Downey G, Dehmel B, Floege J, ADVANCE Study Group. The ADVANCE study: a randomized study to evaluate the effects of cinacalcet plus low-dose vitamin D on vascular calcification in patients on hemodialysis. Nephrol Dial Transplant. 2011;26(4):1327–39.

25. Jean G, Chazot C. Questions about the ADVANCE study. Nephrol Ther. 2012;8(3):131–4.

26. Ketteler M, Martin KJ, Wolf M, Amdahl M, Cozzolino M, Goldsmith D, Sharma A, Marx S, Khan S. Paricalcitol versus cinacalcet plus low-dose vitamin D therapy for the treatment of secondary hyperparathyroidism in patients receiving hemodialysis: results of the IMPACT SHPT study. Nephrol Dial Transplant. 2012;27(8):3270–8.

27. Ketteler M, Martin KJ, Cozzolino M, Goldsmith D, Sharma A, Khan S, Dumas E, Amdahl M, Marx S, Audhya P. Paricalcitol versus cinacalcet plus low-dose vitamin D for the treatment of secondary hyperparathyroidism in patients receiving hemodialysis: study design and baseline characteristics of the IMPACT SHPT study. Nephrol Dial Transplant. 2012;27(5):1942–9.

28. Dyer CA. Safety and tolerability of paricalcitol in patients with chronic kidney disease. Expert Opin Drug Saf. 2013;12(5): 717–28.

29. Barreto FC, Barreto DV, Moysés RMA, Neves KR, Canziani ME, Draibe SA, Jorgetti V, Carvalho AB. K/DOQI-recommended intact PTH levels do not prevent low-turnover bone disease in hemodialysis patients. Kidney Int. 2008;73:771–7.

30. Hansen D, Rasmussen K, Danielsen H, Meyer-Hofmann H, Bacevicius E, Lauridsen TG, Madsen JK, Tougaard BG, Marckmann P, Thye-Roenn P, Nielsen JE, Kreiner S, Brandi L. No difference between alfacalcidol and paricalcitol in the treatment of secondary hyperparathyroidism in hemodialysis patients: a randomized cross-over trial. Kidney Int. 2011;80(8):841–50.

31. Teng M, Wolf M, Lowrie E, Ofsthun N, Lazarus JM, Thadhani R. Survival of patients undergoing hemodialysis with paricalcitol or calcitriol therapy. N Engl J Med. 2003;349(5):446–56.

32. Thadhani R, Appelbaum E, Pritchett Y, Chang Y, Wenger J, Tamez H, Bhan I, Agarwal R, Zoccali C, Wanner C, Lloyd-Jones D, Cannata J, Thompson BT, Andress D, Zhang W, Packham D, Singh B, Zehnder D, Shah A, Pachika A, Manning WJ, Solomon SD. Vitamin D therapy and cardiac structure and function in patients with chronic kidney disease: the PRIMO randomized controlled trial. JAMA. 2012;307(7):674–84.

33. Agarwal R, Hynson JE, Hecht TJ, Light RP, Sinha AD. Short-term vitamin D receptor activation increases serum creatinine due to increased production with no effect on the glomerular filtration rate. Kidney Int. 2011;80(10):1073–9.

34. Lindberg JS, Culleton B, Wong G, Borah MF, Clark RV, Shapiro WB, Roger SD, Husserl FE, Klassen PS, Guo MD, Albizem MB, Coburn JW. Cinacalcet HCl, an oral calcimimetic agent for the treatment of secondary hyperparathyroidism in hemodialysis and peritoneal dialysis: a randomized, double-blind, multicenter study. J Am Soc Nephrol. 2005;16(3):800–7.

35. EVOLVE Trial Investigators, Chertow GM, Block GA, Correa-Rotter R, Drüeke TB, Floege J, Goodman WG, Herzog CA, Kubo Y, London GM, Mahaffey KW, Mix TC, Moe SM, Trotman ML, Wheeler DC, Parfrey PS. Effect of cinacalcet on cardiovascular disease in patients undergoing dialysis. N Engl J Med. 2012; 367(26):2482–94.

36. Cunningham J, Danese M, Olson K, Klassen P, Chertow GM. Effects of the calcimimetic cinacalcet HCl on cardiovascular disease, fracture, and health-related quality of life in secondary hyperparathyroidism. Kidney Int. 2005;68(4):1793–800.

37. Jamal SA, Vandermeer B, Raggi P, Mendelssohn DC, Chatterley T, Dorgan M, Lok CE, Fitchett D, Tsuyuki RT. Effect of calcium-based versus non-calcium-based phosphate binders on mortality in patients with chronic kidney disease: an updated systematic review and meta-analysis. Lancet. 2013;382(9900):1268–77.

38. Palmer SC, Nistor I, Craig JC, Pellegrini F, Messa P, Tonelli M, Covic A, Strippoli GF. Cinacalcet in patients with chronic kidney disease: a cumulative meta-analysis of randomized controlled trials. PLoS Med. 2013;10(4):e1001436.

39. Delanaye P, Weekers L, Warling X, Moonen M, Smelten N, Médart L, Krzesinski JM, Cavalier E. Cholecalciferol in hemodialysis patients: a randomized, double-blind, proof-of-concept and safety study. Nephrol Dial Transplant. 2013;28(7):1779–86.

Diabetic Nephropathy Clinical Trials: A Critical Appraisal

Meguid El Nahas and Bo Feldt-Rasmussen

Over the last quarter of a century, diabetic nephropathy has steadily increased in incidence and prevalence to become one of the most common causes of ESRD. Worldwide, obesity and the associated type 2 diabetes mellitus (T2DM) have reached epidemic proportions leading to a significant rise in those suffering from diabetic kidney disease (DKD) [1]. This has coincided with considerable preclinical research aimed at a better understanding of the pathophysiology of diabetic nephropathy (DN) and its progression [2].

Clearly, one of the main targets of intervention to slow the progression of DM and its complications has always focused on the optimization of glycemia control. A number of studies have explored whether intensive glycemia control offers advantages in terms of the progression of diabetic nephropathy and other vascular complications [3].

Another key focus has been the control of hypertension and the choice of anti-hypertensive agents [4]. In the 1980s, the Brenner hypothesis focused attention on the role of changes in glomerular hemodynamics, glomerular hyperperfusion-hyperfiltration, and hypertension, in the pathogenesis of diabetic nephropathy. A major role emerged for the RAAS implicating it in the initiation and progression of experimental diabetic nephropathy [5]. This has led to the clinical translation of these studies to humans with the pioneer work of Lewis and collaborators who showed for the first time in 1993 the beneficial effect of ACE inhibition of the progression of DN [6]. Since then, thousands of publications confirmed the importance of the RAAS system in the progression of DN and the beneficial impact of its inhibition [4]. Inhibition of RAAS has become the cornerstone of the management of diabetic nephropathy.

Over the last decade, other approaches based on the inhibition of putative mediators of DN and related scarring have been tested including endothelin antagonists, inhibitors of oxidative stress, as well as interventions based on vitamin D supplementation [2, 7–9].

Major RCTs that impacted our practice and the management of patients with DKD will be reviewed in this chapter with emphasis on a critical appraisal of their value, strengths, and shortcomings. We hope that such analysis will give a balanced view of the background for current clinical practice and draw attention to potential new interventions.

RCTs Based on Glycemia Control

The optimization of glycemia control has been the cornerstone of the management of people with diabetes mellitus. A large number of studies have examined, over the last 30 years, the impact of glycemia control on DM complications including macro- and micro-vascular complications. They have also included analyses of the effect of intensive glycemia control on the development and progression of diabetic nephropathy. Discussed below are the UKPDS study in T2DM and the DCCT study in T1DM.

UKPDS Trial

Lancet. 1998 Sep 12;352(9131):837–53.

Intensive blood-glucose control with sulphonylureas or insulin compared with conventional treatment and risk of complications in patients with type 2 diabetes (UKPDS 33).

UK Prospective Diabetes Study (UKPDS) Group.
[No authors listed]

M. El Nahas, MD, PhD, FRCP
Sheffield Kidney Institute, Global Kidney Academy, Sheffield, UK
e-mail: m.el-nahas@sheffield.ac.uk

B. Feldt-Rasmussen, MD, DMSc
Department of Nephrology, Rigshospitalet, University of Copenhagen, Blegdamsvej 9, Copenhagen 2100, Denmark
e-mail: bo.feldt-rasmussen@regionh.dk

Abstract

Background: Improved blood-glucose control decreases the progression of diabetic microvascular disease, but the effect on macrovascular complications is unknown. There is concern that sulphonylureas may increase cardiovascular mortality in patients with type 2 diabetes and that high insulin concentrations may enhance atheroma formation. We compared the effects of intensive blood-glucose control with either sulphonylurea or insulin and conventional treatment on the risk of microvascular and macrovascular complications in patients with type 2 diabetes in a randomized controlled trial.

Methods: Three thousand eight hundred and sixty-seven newly diagnosed patients with type 2 diabetes, median age 54 years (IQR 48–60 years), who after 3 months' diet treatment had a mean of two fasting plasma glucose (FPG) concentrations of 6.1–15.0 mmol/L were randomly assigned intensive policy with a sulphonylurea (chlorpropamide, glibenclamide, or glipizide) or with insulin, or conventional policy with diet. The aim in the intensive group was FPG less than 6 mmol/L. In the conventional group, the aim was the best achievable FPG with diet alone; drugs were added only if there were hyperglycemic symptoms or FPG greater than 15 mmol/L. Three aggregate endpoints were used to assess differences between conventional and intensive treatment: any diabetes-related endpoint (sudden death, death from hyperglycemia or hypoglycemia, fatal or non-fatal myocardial infarction, angina, heart failure, stroke, renal failure, amputation [of at least one digit], vitreous hemorrhage, retinopathy requiring photocoagulation, blindness in one eye, or cataract extraction); diabetes-related death (death from myocardial infarction, stroke, peripheral vascular disease, renal disease, hyperglycemia or hypoglycemia, and sudden death); and all-cause mortality. Single clinical endpoints and surrogate subclinical endpoints were also assessed. All analyses were by intention to treat and frequency of hypoglycemia was also analyzed by actual therapy.

Findings: Over 10 years, hemoglobin A1c (HbA1c) was 7.0 % (6.2–8.2) in the intensive group compared with 7.9 % (6.9–8.8) in the conventional group – an 11 % reduction. There was no difference in HbA1c among agents in the intensive group. Compared with the conventional group, the risk in the intensive group was 12 % lower (95 % CI 1–21, $p = 0.029$) for any diabetes-related endpoint; 10 % lower (−11 to 27, $p = 0.34$) for any diabetes-related death; and 6 % lower (−10 to 20, $p = 0.44$) for all-cause mortality. Most of the risk reduction in the any diabetes-related aggregate endpoint was due to a 25 % risk reduction (7–40, $p = 0.0099$) in microvascular endpoints, including the need for retinal photocoagulation. There was no difference for any of the three aggregate endpoints between the three intensive agents (chlorpropamide, glibenclamide, or insulin). Patients in the intensive group had more hypoglycemic episodes than those in the conventional group on both types of analysis (both $p < 0.0001$). The rates of major hypoglycemic episodes per year were 0.7 % with conventional treatment, 1.0 % with

chlorpropamide, 1.4 % with glibenclamide, and 1.8 % with insulin. Weight gain was significantly higher in the intensive group (mean 2.9 kg) than in the conventional group ($p < 0.001$), and patients assigned insulin had a greater gain in weight (4.0 kg) than those assigned chlorpropamide (2.6 kg) or glibenclamide (1.7 kg).

Interpretation: Intensive blood-glucose control by either sulphonylureas or insulin substantially decreases the risk of microvascular complications, but not macrovascular disease, in patients with type 2 diabetes.

Critical Appraisal

Parameters	Yes	No	Comment
Validity			
Is the **Randomization** Procedure well described?	+1		Randomization was by means of centrally produced, computer-generated therapy allocations in sealed, opaque envelopes which were opened in sequence
Double **blinded**?		−2	Open study
Is the **sample size** calculation described/adequate?	+3		Sample size and power calculation modified as the study went on, with changes implemented in 1987. The study was extended to include randomization of 3,867 patients with a median time from randomization of 11 years to the end of the study in 1997. In 1992, at the 1 % level of significance, the power for any diabetes-related endpoint and for diabetes-related death was calculated as 81 and 23 %, respectively 1138: Conventional DM control 2729: Intensive DM control
Does it have a hard primary **endpoint**?		−1	21 endpoints including: ESRD or serum creatinine reaching 250 umol/l
Is the endpoint surrogate?	−2		
Is the follow-up appropriate?	+1		Median follow-up was 10 year Parameters checked every 1–3 years
Was there a **Bias**?		+2	
Is the dropout >25 %?		+1	
Is the analysis **ITT**?	+3		
Utility/usefulness			
Can the findings be generalized?	+1		T2DM aged 25–65, normal serum creatinine, normoalbuminuric
Was the NNT <100?	+1		The number needed to treat to prevent one patient developing any of the single endpoints over 10 years was 19.6 patients (95 % CI 10–500)
Score	**50 %**		

Comments and Discussion

This is one of the most quoted studies in DM relating to the quality of glycemia control on outcomes. It also has the merit to be one of the largest and longest follow-up studies. It has the merit to have maintained a difference in glycemia control between the standard (HbA1c ~7 %) and the intensive control (HbA1c ~7.9 %) groups throughout the study duration averaging 10 years. The study showed a 25 % reduction in risk of developing microvascular complications, mostly retinal.

The development of microalbuminuria was reduced on intensive therapy (−34 %) but overt proteinuria did not significantly differ between the groups. There was a 67 % reduction in the number of patients who had a doubling of serum creatinine in the intensive therapy arm. Too few patients developed ESRD.

There was no significant effect on the macrovascular endpoints; major adverse cardiovascular events. This has been confirmed by more recent trials on intensive glycemia control in T2DM, such as ACCORD, ADVANCE, and VADT, that also failed to show benefit of cardiovascular outcomes (reviewed in [10]).

UKPDS has a number of limitations including:

1. Reliance of changes in microalbuminuria as a surrogate marker for kidney disease, when nowadays serious reservations exist regarding the specificity of this surrogate endpoint for renal disease [11]. It is more likely to reflect the potential beneficial effect of more intensive glycemia control on microvascular disease in general.
2. The reduction in the number of patients whose creatinine doubled on intensive therapy was large, but it was not statistically significant over the 10–15 years' observation time.
3. Serum creatinine and its changes can be confounded by numerous factors in T2DM including changes in weight/muscle mass or appetite.
4. The study was not powered to investigate progression of diabetic nephropathy to ESRD, in view of the fact that the cohort started with normal renal function. Consequently, it is impossible to evaluate whether the observed numerical reduction in doubling of serum creatinine translated into a reduction in the incidence of ESRD in this cohort in the long term.
5. The age range of the cohort study 25–65 years raises concern over the heterogeneity of the population studied. A more focused approach on a more homogeneous patients' group may have yielded different outcomes. Age, duration of diabetes, and presence of underlying cardiovascular disease at baseline may influence response to glycemia control [10]. Also, the impact of strict glycemia control on cardiovascular outcomes may be confounded by the impact of hypoglycemia itself as well as that of some oral hypoglycemic agents on cardiovascular events [10].

Conclusion

UKPDS showed some benefit of tighter glycemia control on microvascular complications and more specifically diabetic proliferative retinopathy. It showed little significant impact on other variables and endpoints, including proteinuria, doubling of serum creatinine, or ESRD.

DCCT Trial

Kidney Int. 1995 Jun;47(6):1703–20.

Effect of intensive therapy on the development and progression of diabetic nephropathy in the diabetes control and complications trial. The Diabetes Control and Complications (DCCT) Research Group

Abstract

The Diabetes Control and Complications Trial (DCCT) has demonstrated that intensive diabetes treatment delays the onset and slows the progression of retinopathy, nephropathy, and neuropathy in patients with IDDM. A detailed description of the effects of this treatment on diabetic nephropathy is presented here. In the primary prevention cohort, intensive treatment reduced the mean adjusted risk of the cumulative incidence of microalbuminuria (≥28 μg/min) by 34 % (95 % CI 2, 56 %; $P=0.04$). Furthermore, intensive treatment decreased the albumin excretion rate (AER) by 15 % after the first year of therapy (6.5 vs. 7.7 μg/min, $P<0.001$). Thereafter the rates of change for AER within each treatment group were no different from zero, retaining a constant difference in AER between groups in the trial. In the secondary intervention cohort with baseline AER <28 μg/min, intensive therapy reduced the mean adjusted risk of microalbuminuria (≥28 μg/min) by 43 % (95 % CI 21, 58 %; $P<0.0001$); the risk of a more advanced level of microalbuminuria (≥70 μg/min) by 56 % (95 % CI 26, 74 %; $P=0.002$); and the risk of clinical albuminuria (≥208 μg/min) by 56 % (95 % CI 18, 76 %; $P<0.01$). In the secondary intervention cohort, values for AER at year 1 were identical at 9 μg/min, but the 6.5 % change per year in the conventional group greatly exceeded the rate of change of −0.3 % in the intensive group ($P<0.001$). Among the 73 secondary cohort subjects with AER levels ≥28 μg/min but ≤139 μg/min at baseline, the reduction of progression to clinical albuminuria with intensive therapy was not statistically significant. The longitudinal treatment effect of conventional versus intensive therapy (11.0 % vs. 2.5 % per year, respectively, $P=0.087$) was similar in magnitude to that among patients with AER <28 μg/min at baseline. For the primary, secondary, and combined cohorts, there were no significant differences in the rates of change in creatinine clearance (CCr) between treatment groups during the study. Only seven subjects in the entire study (2 intensive, 5 conventional) developed urinary AER ≥208 μg/min coupled with a CCr< 70 ml/min/1.73 m². Neither the rate of change of blood pressure nor the appearance of hypertension (BP> 140/90 mmHg) differed significantly between treatment groups in the primary, secondary, or combined cohorts.

Critical Appraisal

Parameters	Yes	No	Comment
Validity			
Is the **Randomization** Procedure well described?	+1		Primary prevention cohort Secondary prevention cohort with microalbuminuria
Double **blinded**?		−2	
Is the **sample size** calculation described/ adequate?	+3		1441 T1DM randomized
Does it have a hard primary **endpoint**?		−1	Albuminuria changes
Is the endpoint surrogate?	−2		Albuminuria
Is the follow-up appropriate?	+1		6.5 years
Was there a **Bias**?		+2	
Is the dropout >25 %?		+1	
Is the analysis **ITT**?	+3		
Utility/usefulness			
Can the findings be generalized?	+1		T1DM with normal renal function and normoalbuminuria
Was the NNT <100?	+1		
Score	**50 %**		

Comments and Discussion

The DCCT trial had previously demonstrated a beneficial effect of intensive glycemia control on diabetic complications including retinopathy and neuropathy [12]. In this study, it focused on renal outcomes, both prevention and development/progression of albuminuria.

It showed that intensive and sustained glycemia control, with an HbA1c around 7 % compared to 9 % in standard therapy group, reduced the incidence of microalbuminuria and its progression by 34 and 43 %, respectively.

Limitations of the DCCT study:
1. It was not powered to study changes in renal function with age and thus failed to detect any difference between the groups in the renal functional parameters including the measurement of GFR (iothalamate clearance).
2. It assumed that low-level albuminuria (microalbuminuria) was a valid surrogate for diabetic nephropathy; a commonly held view then that has been challenged since [13].
3. It also assumed that changes in albuminuria would imply subsequent changes in renal function, an assumption since challenged by a number of observations including the RASS study showing a dissociation between changes in microalbuminuria and renal function or histology [14]. However, the subsequent DCCT EDIC 22-year follow-up study in terms of renal functional decline supported the association of better functional (eGFR) outcomes in those

initially on intensive glycemia control and lower levels of albuminuria as well as putting forward the notion of metabolic memory [15].

Conclusion

The DCCT study has been the key study underlying the importance of tight glycemia control in minimizing the complications of T1DM. It was supported by the long-term DCCT EDIC follow-up (22 years) observations of persistent benefit [15]. It was also supported by the STENO multi-intervention study that showed a protective effect on T2DM vascular and renal complications with intensive multi-targeted therapy [15]. The primary endpoint of the STENO study was a composite of death from cardiovascular causes, nonfatal myocardial infarction, nonfatal stroke, revascularization, and amputation.

However, other studies in T2DM such as ACCORD, ADVANCE, and VADT failed to show an impact of strict glycemia control on cardiovascular outcomes (reviewed in [16]). It has been argued that the potential beneficial effect of strict glycemia control may largely depend on patients' characteristics, including age, diabetes duration, previous glucose control, presence of cardiovascular disease, and risk of hypoglycemia. Other confounders include the extent and frequency of hypoglycemic events and the impact of glucose-lowering medication itself on the cardiovascular system [16].

RCTs Based on RAAS Inhibition

Since Brenner and colleagues put forward their hypothesis related to the role of glomerular hyperperfusion-hyperfiltration, glomerular hypertension, and the related role of angiotensin II on the pathogenesis of diabetic nephropathy (DN), a very large number of clinical trials addressed the question of whether ACE inhibition slowed the development and progression of DN. More specifically, these trials aimed to show whether ACE inhibition or angiotensin receptor blockade (ARB) slowed DN progression independently of their anti-hypertensive effect. This started with the publication in 1993 of the seminal study of the collaborative study group in patients with T1DM. More recently, studies also examined the impact of renin blockade (AVOID and ALTITUDE studies) and dual ACE inhibition and ARB therapy on renal and cardiovascular outcomes (ONTARGET and VA-NEPHRON D).

The Collaborative Study Group (Lewis) Trial

N Engl J Med. 1993 Nov 11;329(20):1456–62.

The effect of angiotensin-converting-enzyme inhibition on diabetic nephropathy. The Collaborative Study Group

Lewis EJ, Hunsicker LG, Bain RP, Rohde RD.

Abstract

Background: Renal function declines progressively in patients who have diabetic nephropathy, and the decline may be slowed by antihypertensive drugs. The purpose of this study was to determine whether captopril has kidney-protecting properties independent of its effect on blood pressure in diabetic nephropathy.

Methods: We performed a randomized, controlled trial comparing captopril with placebo in patients with insulin-dependent diabetes mellitus in whom urinary protein excretion was ≥500 mg/day and the serum creatinine concentration was ≤2.5 mg/dl (221 μmol/l). Blood-pressure goals were defined to achieve control during a median follow-up of 3 years. The primary endpoint was a doubling of the baseline serum creatinine concentration.

Results: Two hundred and seven patients received captopril and 202 placebo. Serum creatinine concentrations doubled in 25 patients in the captopril group, as compared with 43 patients in the placebo group ($P=0.007$). The associated reductions in risk of a doubling of the serum creatinine concentration were 48 % in the captopril group as a whole, 76 % in the subgroup with a baseline serum creatinine concentration of 2.0 mg/dl (177 μmol/l), 55 % in the subgroup with a concentration of 1.5 mg/dl (133 μmol/l), and 17 % in the subgroup with a concentration of 1.0 mg/dl (88.4 μmol/l). The mean (±SD) rate of decline in creatinine clearance was 11 ± 21 % per year in the captopril group and 17 ± 20 % per year in the placebo group ($P=0.03$). Among the patients whose baseline serum creatinine concentration was ≥1.5 mg/dl, creatinine clearance declined at a rate of 23 ± 25 % per year in the captopril group and at a rate of 37 ± 25 % per year in the placebo group ($P=0.01$). Captopril treatment was associated with a 50 % reduction in the risk of the combined endpoints of death, dialysis, and transplantation that was independent of the small disparity in blood pressure between the groups.

Conclusions: Captopril protects against deterioration in renal function in insulin-dependent diabetic nephropathy and is significantly more effective than blood-pressure control alone.

Comments and Discussion

There is little doubt that this clinical trial changed the practice of nephrologists in terms of management of progressive diabetic nephropathy. It pioneered the universal use of RAAS inhibitors to slow the progression of DN. While the authors concluded that Captopril reduced the rate of doubling of serum creatinine by 48 %, they emphasized that the beneficial effect was predominantly due to a slowing of DN progression in patients with a baseline serum creatinine >1.5 mg/dl. Proteinuria was reduced significantly in the Captopril group.

The Lewis study has a number of shortcomings:

1. There was a patients' selection bias as baseline proteinuria was significantly higher in the placebo group (3 g/24 h versus 2.5 g/24 h). Also the percentage of those with heavy proteinuria was higher in the placebo group. In view of the known association of higher proteinuria and worse outcomes in CKD and DN, such a bias could have impacted the subsequent outcome of the two groups.
2. Reliance on doubling of serum creatinine as a primary endpoint has been challenged as it does not always translate into progression to ESRD [17].
3. Reliance of changes in serum creatinine, without measuring GFR and its changes, raises concern about confounders such as the impact of ACE inhibitors on tubular secretion of creatinine [18].
4. Secondary endpoints such as ESRD or transplantation were not protocolized in terms of prespecified cutoffs for interventions.
5. Blood pressure (diastolic) was lower in the captopril group (MAP=96 mmHg) compared to placebo (MAP=100 mmHg); however, the difference did not exceed 5 mmHg and adjustments were made in relation to its impact on the rate of doubling of serum creatinine. Of note, blood pressure was measured casually at the office at given intervals and did not rely on a more accurate recording such as day- and nighttime measurements or 24 h ABPM recording. Those may have shown a bigger difference in BP between the groups. They are also more relevant to DN complications than office BP readings [19, 20].

Critical Appraisal

Parameters	Yes	No	Comment
Validity			
Is the **Randomization** Procedure well described?	+1		Standard urn design
Double **blinded**?	+2		
Is the **sample size** calculation described/adequate?		−3	Sample size calculation assumption not given: Captopril group: 207 patients Placebo: 202 patients
Does it have a hard primary **endpoint**?		−1	Doubling of serum creatinine
Is the endpoint surrogate?	−2		GFR was not measured
Is the follow-up appropriate?	+1		36 months
Was there a **Bias**?	−2		The placebo group had more severe DN at baseline based on a higher urine albumin excretion rate
Is the dropout >25 %?	−1		301/409 completed the study
Is the analysis **ITT**?	+3		
Utility/usefulness			
Can the findings be generalized?	+1		T1DM with proteinuria and serum creatinine <2.5 mg/dl
Was the NNT <100?	+1		Risk reduction of 48 % for doubling of serum creatinine in the captopril group
Score	**0 %**		

Conclusion

The Lewis trial remains a reference RCT in diabetic nephropathy and the impact of ACE inhibition. Its results are primarily confounded by the patients' selection bias of those with worse prognosis being allocated to the placebo group.

The RENAAL Trial

N Engl J Med. 2001;345(12):861–9.

Effects of losartan on renal and cardiovascular outcomes in patients with type 2 diabetes and nephropathy

Brenner BM, Cooper ME, de Zeeuw D, Keane WF, Mitch WE, Parving HH, Remuzzi G, Snapinn SM, Zhang Z, Shahinfar S; RENAAL Study Investigators.

Abstract

Background: Diabetic nephropathy is the leading cause of end-stage renal disease. Interruption of the renin-angiotensin system slows the progression of renal disease in patients with type 1 diabetes, but similar data are not available for patients with type 2, the most common form of diabetes. We assessed the role of the angiotensin-II-receptor antagonist losartan in patients with type 2 diabetes and nephropathy.

Methods: A total of 1,513 patients were enrolled in this randomized, double-blind study comparing losartan (50–100 mg once daily) with placebo, both taken in addition to conventional antihypertensive treatment (calcium-channel antagonists, diuretics, alpha-blockers, beta-blockers, and centrally acting agents), for a mean of 3.4 years. The primary outcome was the composite of a doubling of the baseline serum creatinine concentration, end-stage renal disease, or death. Secondary endpoints included a composite of morbidity and mortality from cardiovascular causes, proteinuria, and the rate of progression of renal disease.

Results: A total of 327 patients in the losartan group reached the primary endpoint, as compared with 359 in the placebo group (risk reduction, 16 %; $P=0.02$). Losartan reduced the incidence of a doubling of the serum creatinine concentration (risk reduction, 25 %; $P=0.006$) and end-stage renal disease (risk reduction, 28 %; $P=0.002$) but had no effect on the rate of death. The benefit exceeded that attributable to changes in blood pressure. The composite of morbidity and mortality from cardiovascular causes was similar in the two groups, although the rate of first hospitalization for heart failure was significantly lower with losartan (risk reduction, 32 %; $P=0.005$). The level of proteinuria declined by 35 % with losartan ($P<0.001$ for the comparison with placebo).

Conclusions: Losartan conferred significant renal benefits in patients with type 2 diabetes and nephropathy, and it was generally well tolerated.

Critical Appraisal

Parameters	Yes	No	Comment
Validity			
Is the **Randomization** Procedure well described?	+1		Previously described [21]
Double **blinded**?	+2		
Is the **sample size** calculation described/adequate?	+3		751 T2DM patients in Losartan group
			762 in placebo
Does it have a hard primary **endpoint**?		+1	The first event of the composite endpoint of a doubling of the serum creatinine concentration, end-stage renal disease, or death
Is the endpoint surrogate?	−2		GFR was not measured
Is the follow-up appropriate?		−1	Mean follow-up time = 3.4 years. Discontinued early by unanimous decision of the steering committee in view of reported benefits of cardiovascular outcomes by ACE inhibitors (HOPE study) [22]
Was there a **Bias**?	+2		
Is the dropout >25 %?	+1		
Is the analysis **ITT**?	+3		Study terminated prematurely
Utility/usefulness			
Can the findings be generalized?	+1		T2DM and nephropathy; serum creatinine between 1.3 and 3 mg/dl with overt proteinuria
Was the NNT <100?	+1		Treatment with Losartan led to a 16 % reduction in primary composite endpoints
Score	75 %		

Comments and Discussion

The RENAAL study is the pivotal study on angiotensin receptor blockade (ARB) efficacy in slowing the progression of T2DM-associated nephropathy. It showed a significant (16 %) reduction in the rate of reaching the composite endpoints of doubling of serum creatinine, ESRD or death. It also showed a significant reduction in proteinuria. Of interest, there was no significant difference between the groups in secondary CVD outcomes, as anticipated by the premature termination of the study based on the reported data from HOPE [22].

Limitations of the RENAAL study:

1. The study was powered for a mean follow-up duration of 4.5 years and was prematurely terminated thus having a much shorter mean follow-up period of 3.4 years. This could have impacted the power of the study and the appropriateness of the sample size.

2. Reliance on serum creatinine-based co-primary endpoint (doubling of serum creatinine and ESRD) without measuring GFR and its changes, raises concern about confounders such as the impact of ACE inhibitors on tubular secretion of creatinine [23, 24].

3. The co-primary endpoint of ESRD was not protocolized in terms of prespecified cutoffs for intervention; renal replacement therapy.

4. Reliance on composite and interrelated endpoints has its limitations [25].

5. Blood pressure (diastolic) was lower in the Losartan group (MAP = 100 mmHg) compared to placebo (MAP = 103 mmHg); however, adjustments were made in relation to the impact of BP differences on the composite endpoints and hardly affected the study outcome.

6. Blood pressure was measured casually at the office at given intervals and did not rely on a more accurate recording such as day- and nighttime measurements or 24 h ABPM recording. Those may have shown a bigger difference in BP between the groups. They are also more relevant to DN complications than office BP readings [26]. In fact, this was noted in the HOPE study upon which the study premature termination was based, as casual BP recording did not show differences between the Ramipril and placebo groups, while more accurate BP monitoring showed a significant difference and lower BP in those treated with Ramipril [27] possibly explain the better cardioprotection.

Conclusion

RENAAL is a major study that claimed that ARB slows the progression of DN. Its conclusion is confounded by the premature termination of the study thus raising concerns over its power and the use of serum creatinine as a primary endpoint without measuring changes in GFR.

IDNT Trial

N Engl J Med. 2001;345(12):851–60.

Renoprotective effect of the angiotensin-receptor antagonist irbesartan in patients with nephropathy due to type 2 diabetes

Lewis EJ, Hunsicker LG, Clarke WR, Berl T, Pohl MA, Lewis JB, Ritz E, Atkins RC, Rohde R, Raz I; Collaborative Study Group.

Abstract

Background: It is unknown whether either the angiotensin-II-receptor blocker irbesartan or the calcium-channel blocker amlodipine slows the progression of nephropathy in patients with type 2 diabetes independently of its capacity to lower the systemic blood pressure.

Methods: We randomly assigned 1,715 hypertensive patients with nephropathy due to type 2 diabetes to treatment with irbesartan (300 mg daily), amlodipine (10 mg daily), or placebo. The target blood pressure was 135/85 mmHg or less in all groups. We compared the groups with regard to the time to the primary composite endpoint of a doubling of the baseline serum creatinine concentration, the development of end-stage renal disease, or death from any cause. We also compared them with regard to the time to a secondary, cardiovascular composite endpoint.

Results: The mean duration of follow-up was 2.6 years. Treatment with irbesartan was associated with a risk of the

Critical Appraisal

Parameters	Yes	No	Comment
Validity			
Is the **Randomization** Procedure well described?	+1		Protocol previously published [28] Randomization into three groups: Irbesartan, amlodipine, placebo
Double **blinded**?	+2		
Is the **sample size** calculation described/adequate?	+3		On the basis of the results of study in type 1 diabetes, in which the 3-year rate of a doubling of the baseline serum creatinine concentration, end-stage renal disease, or death was 36 %, authors estimated that 550 patients per treatment group were needed for an analysis of the primary outcome. The sample size was selected to achieve 90 % power to detect a 26 % difference in the primary endpoint between the irbesartan group and the placebo group at a 5 % alpha level
Does it have a hard primary **endpoint**?		−1	Composite endpoint of doubling of serum creatinine, ESRD or death
Is the endpoint surrogate?	−2		GFR was not measured
Is the follow-up appropriate?	+1		~mean 3 years
Was there a **Bias**?		+2	
Is the dropout >25 %?		+1	
Is the analysis **ITT**?	+3		
Utility/usefulness			
Can the findings be generalized?	+1		T2DM with hypertension and serum creatinine between 1 and 3 mg/dl and proteinuria >900 mg/24 h
Was the NNT <100?	+1		Risk reduction by Irbesartan 20 % compared to placebo and 23 % compared to amlodipine
Score	**75 %**		

primary composite endpoint that was 20 % lower than that in the placebo group ($P=0.02$) and 23 % lower than that in the amlodipine group ($P=0.006$). The risk of a doubling of the serum creatinine concentration was 33 % lower in the irbesartan group than in the placebo group ($P=0.003$) and 37 % lower in the irbesartan group than in the amlodipine group ($P<0.001$). Treatment with irbesartan was associated with a relative risk of end-stage renal disease that was 23 % lower than that in both other groups ($P=0.07$ for both comparisons). These differences were not explained by differences in the blood pressures that were achieved. The serum creatinine concentration increased 24 % more slowly in the irbesartan group than in the placebo group ($P=0.008$) and 21 % more slowly than in the amlodipine group ($P=0.02$). There were no significant differences in the rates of death from any cause or in the cardiovascular composite endpoint.

Conclusions: The angiotensin-II-receptor blocker irbesartan is effective in protecting against the progression of nephropathy due to type 2 diabetes. This protection is independent of the reduction in blood pressure it causes.

Comments and Discussion

The IDNT study results are similar to those of RENAAL in that an ARB slowed the rate of changes in serum creatinine over a reasonably long observation period.

It has the same limitations as RENAAL:
1. Reliance of changes in serum creatinine to ascertain DN progression; Inhibition of RAS has been associated with increased tubular secretion of creatinine [29, 30], thus confounding the interpretation of this parameter in terms of changes in GFR.
2. GFR was not measured. This has to be considered the gold standard for RCTs evaluating the rate of progression of CKD or DKD.
3. The use of interrelated composite endpoints subject to limitations and criticism [31].
4. Blood pressure measured casually/office readings rather than the more accurate 24 h ABPM recording can give the misleading impression that BP was comparable between the Irbesartan and Amlodipine groups.
5. Sample size estimation was made on the assumption that the rate of progression of T2DM-associated nephropathy was similar to that of T1DM. This is unlikely to be the case as most would argue that T2DM-associated DKD progressed more slowly than DKD in younger patients with T1DM [32, 33].

Conclusion

IDNT along with RENAAL are often cited as the ultimate proof that ARBs are protective against the decline in kidney function in DN. While this may be the case, these studies have their limitations highlighted above that confound irrefutable evidence.

VA-Nephron D Trial

N Engl J Med. 2013 Nov 14;369(20):1892–903. doi: 10.1056/NEJMoa1303154. Epub 2013 Nov 9.

Combined angiotensin inhibition for the treatment of diabetic nephropathy

Fried LF, Emanuele N, Zhang JH, Brophy M, Conner TA, Duckworth W, Leehey DJ, McCullough PA, O'Connor T, Palevsky PM, Reilly RF, Seliger SL, Warren SR, Watnick S, Peduzzi P, Guarino P; VA NEPHRON-D Investigators. Collaborators (248)

Abstract

Background: Combination therapy with angiotensin-converting-enzyme (ACE) inhibitors and angiotensin-receptor blockers (ARBs) decreases proteinuria; however, its safety and effect on the progression of kidney disease are uncertain.

Methods: We provided losartan (at a dose of 100 mg/day) to patients with type 2 diabetes, a urinary albumin-to-creatinine ratio (with albumin measured in milligrams and creatinine measured in grams) of at least 300, and an estimated glomerular filtration rate (GFR) of 30.0–89.9 ml/min/1.73 m^2 of body-surface area and then randomly assigned them to receive lisinopril (at a dose of 10–40 mg/day) or placebo. The primary endpoint was the first occurrence of a change in the estimated GFR (a decline of ≥ 30 ml/min/1.73 m^2 if the initial estimated GFR was ≥ 60 ml/min/1.73 m^2 or a decline of ≥ 50 % if the initial estimated GFR was <60 ml/min/1.73 m^2), end-stage renal disease (ESRD), or death. The secondary renal endpoint was the first occurrence of a decline in the estimated GFR or ESRD. Safety outcomes included mortality, hyperkalemia, and acute kidney injury.

Results: The study was stopped early owing to safety concerns. Among 1,448 randomly assigned patients with a median follow-up of 2.2 years, there were 152 primary end-point events in the monotherapy group and 132 in the combination-therapy group (hazard ratio with combination therapy, 0.88; 95 % confidence interval [CI], 0.70–1.12; $P=0.30$). A trend toward a benefit from combination therapy with respect to the secondary endpoint (hazard ratio, 0.78; 95 % CI, 0.58–1.05; $P=0.10$) decreased with time ($P=0.02$ for nonproportionality). There was no benefit with respect to mortality (hazard ratio for death, 1.04; 95 % CI, 0.73–1.49; $P=0.75$) or cardiovascular events. Combination therapy increased the risk of hyperkalemia (6.3 events per 100 person-years vs. 2.6 events per 100 person-years with monotherapy; $P<0.001$) and acute kidney injury (12.2 vs. 6.7 events per 100 person-years, $P<0.001$).

Conclusions: Combination therapy with an ACE inhibitor and an ARB was associated with an increased risk of adverse events among patients with diabetic nephropathy. (Funded by the Cooperative Studies Program of the Department of Veterans Affairs Office of Research and Development; VA NEPHRON-D ClinicalTrials.gov number, NCT00555217.).

Critical Appraisal

Parameters	Yes	No	Comment
Validity			
Is the **Randomization** Procedure well described?	+1		Protocol previously described Randomization into Losartan alone versus Losartan+Lisinopril on outcomes in T2DM with eGFR from 30 to 89 ml/min and overt proteinuria (ACR >300 mg/g)
Double **blinded**?	+2		
Is the **sample size** calculation described/adequate?	+3		Assuming a 45 % cumulative event rate and a 10 % loss to follow-up, authors initially calculated that they would need to enroll 1,850 patients over a period of 3 years, with a minimum follow-up of 2 years, for the study to have 85 % power to detect an 18 % relative reduction in the primary endpoint at a two-sided alpha level of 0.05. 1448 underwent randomization
Does it have a hard primary **endpoint**?		−1	Decrease in eGFR
Is the endpoint surrogate?		−2	GFR not measured
Is the follow-up appropriate?		−1	Terminated prematurely (~2 years) due to high rate of side effects; hyperkalemia and AKI in the combination arm of the study
Was there a **Bias**?		+2	
Is the dropout >25 %?	−1		Terminated prematurely
Is the analysis **ITT**?	+3		
Utility/usefulness			
Can the findings be generalized?	+1		T2DM with eGFR from 30 to 89 ml/min
Was the NNT <100?			Negative study
Score	**50 %**		

Comments and Discussion

The VA NEPHRON-D study confirmed the observations made in previous studies on the negative impact of dual RAS blockade; ONTARGET in high cardiovascular risk patients including people with high risk diabetes mellitus [34] as well as the ALTITUDE study that investigated the combination of a renin antagonist with ACE inhibition in patients with diabetic nephropathy [35]. These studies had to be discontinued due to a high rate of side effects and morbidity. VA NEPHRON-D was also stopped prematurely due to the

increased rate of side effects, hyperkalemia, and AKI. During the observation time, the study failed to show benefit on the primary endpoint of decline in eGFR or in other endpoints of cardiovascular complications or mortality. Of note the highest rate of albuminuria decline took place in the combination group.

Limitations of the VA NEPHRON-D trial:

1. Clearly the main limitation of the VA NEPHRON-D trial is its early termination that impacts the power of the study and the interpretation of its final results.
2. Like most studies, if not all studies, of DKD progression reliance on serum creatinine changes and the derived eGFR can be misleading.
3. GFR was not measured.
4. BP was casually assessed at office visits.

Conclusion

The VA NEPHRON-D study was the third major RCT that showed the risks associated with dual blockade of the RAS. Like previous studies such focus has been on older patients with DM (mean age 64 years) compared to 66 years in ONTARGET and 60 years in ALTITUDE. Whether dual RAS blockade is equally harmful in younger patients with lower cardiovascular risk is unknown.

AVOID Trial

N Engl J Med. 2008 Jun 5;358(23):2433–46. doi: 10.1056/NEJMoa0708379.

Aliskiren combined with losartan in type 2 diabetes and nephropathy

Parving HH, Persson F, Lewis JB, Lewis EJ, Hollenberg NK; AVOID Study Investigators.

Collaborators (351)

Abstract

Background: Diabetic nephropathy is the leading cause of end-stage renal disease in developed countries. We evaluated the renoprotective effects of dual blockade of the renin-angiotensin-aldosterone system by adding treatment with aliskiren, an oral direct renin inhibitor, to treatment with the maximal recommended dose of losartan (100 mg daily) and optimal antihypertensive therapy in patients who had hypertension and type 2 diabetes with nephropathy.

Methods: We enrolled 599 patients in this multinational, randomized, double-blind study. After a 3-month, open-label, run-in period during which patients received 100 mg of losartan daily, patients were randomly assigned to receive 6 months of treatment with aliskiren (150 mg daily for 3 months, followed by an increase in dosage to 300 mg daily for another 3 months) or placebo, in addition to losartan. The primary outcome was a reduction in the ratio of albumin to creatinine, as measured in an early-morning urine sample, at 6 months.

Results: The baseline characteristics of the two groups were similar. Treatment with 300 mg of aliskiren daily, as compared with placebo, reduced the mean urinary albumin-to-creatinine ratio by 20 % (95 % confidence interval, 9–30; $P<0.001$), with a reduction of 50 % or more in 24.7 % of the patients who received aliskiren as compared with 12.5 % of those who received placebo ($P<0.001$). A small difference in blood pressure was seen between the treatment groups by the end of the study period (systolic, 2 mmHg lower [$P=0.07$] and diastolic, 1 mmHg lower [$P=0.08$] in the aliskiren group). The total numbers of adverse and serious adverse events were similar in the groups.

Conclusions: Aliskiren may have renoprotective effects that are independent of its blood-pressure-lowering effect in patients with hypertension, type 2 diabetes, and nephropathy who are receiving the recommended renoprotective treatment. (ClinicalTrials.gov number, NCT00097955 [ClinicalTrials.gov].).

Critical Appraisal

Parameters	Yes	No	Comment
Validity			
Is the **Randomization** Procedure well described?	+1		599 patients enrolled Losartan versus Losartan + Aliskiren (301 patients) (298 patients)
Double **blinded**?	+2		
Is the **sample size** calculation described/adequate?	+3		Assuming a dropout rate of 20 %, authors planned to randomly assign 496 patients. This sample size would have provided 90 % power to detect, at a two-sided level of significance of 0.05, a treatment difference of 18 % in the primary endpoint
Does it have a hard primary **endpoint**?		−1	Changes in urine ACE from baseline to 24 weeks
Is the endpoint surrogate?	−2		Albuminuria
Is the follow-up appropriate?		−1	6 months
Was there a **Bias**?	−2		Aliskiren group younger and shorter duration of T2DM
Is the dropout >25 %?	−1		
Is the analysis **ITT**?	+3		
Utility/usefulness			
Can the findings be generalized?	+1		T2DM with nephropathy and ACR >300 mg/g. GFR >30 ml/min
Was the NNT <100?	+1		18 % reduction in ACR by Aliskiren compared to control
Score	**25 %**		

Comments and Discussion

The AVOID study opened the way to dual blockade of RAS combining an ARB with a renin inhibitor (Aliskiren). It showed a significant reduction in albuminuria over and above that achieved with an ARB (Losartan) alone. This effect was obtained independently of changes in eGFR or blood pressure control.

The AVOID trial limitations are:

1. The reliance of albuminuria as a surrogate endpoint for DN progression. Studies such as ACCOMPLISH (in nondiabetic kidney disease) [36] and ONTARGET (in high-risk people with diabetes) [37] showed that a reduction in albuminuria may take place regardless of a faster decline in eGFR, thus dissociating the reduction in albuminuria from a protective long-term effect of CKD and DKD progression. Albuminuria is a very soft and unpredictable endpoint.

Conclusion

It is imperative that studies relying on changes in albuminuria as the primary endpoint are conducted long enough to ascertain the impact of the intervention on renal function (measured GFR) as well as blood pressure control and side effects. The assumption that a reduction of albuminuria by a given intervention will inevitably lead to a slowing of CKD progression is no longer tenable in view of the results of ALTITUDE [38] but also ONTARGET [37] and ACCOMPLISH [36].

ALTITUDE Trial

N Engl J Med. 2012 Dec 6;367(23):2204–13. doi: 10.1056/NEJMoa1208799. Epub 2012 Nov 3.

Cardiorenal endpoints in a trial of aliskiren for type 2 diabetes

Parving HH, Brenner BM, McMurray JJ, de Zeeuw D, Haffner SM, Solomon SD, Chaturvedi N, Persson F, Desai AS, Nicolaides M, Richard A, Xiang Z, Brunel P, Pfeffer MA; ALTITUDE Investigators.

Collaborators (817)

Abstract

Background: This study was undertaken to determine whether use of the direct renin inhibitor aliskiren would reduce cardiovascular and renal events in patients with type 2 diabetes and chronic kidney disease, cardiovascular disease, or both.

Methods: In a double-blind fashion, we randomly assigned 8,561 patients to aliskiren (300 mg daily) or placebo as an adjunct to an angiotensin-converting-enzyme inhibitor or an angiotensin-receptor blocker. The primary endpoint was a composite of the time to cardiovascular death or a first occurrence of cardiac arrest with resuscitation; nonfatal myocardial infarction; nonfatal stroke; unplanned hospitalization for heart failure; end-stage renal disease, death attributable to kidney failure, or the need for renal-replacement therapy with no dialysis or transplantation available or initiated; or doubling of the baseline serum creatinine level.

Results: The trial was stopped prematurely after the second interim efficacy analysis. After a median follow-up of 32.9 months, the primary endpoint had occurred in 783 patients (18.3 %) assigned to aliskiren as compared with 732 (17.1 %) assigned to placebo (hazard ratio, 1.08; 95 % confidence interval [CI], 0.98–1.20; $P=0.12$). Effects on secondary renal endpoints were similar. Systolic and diastolic blood pressures were lower with aliskiren (between-group differences, 1.3 and 0.6 mmHg, respectively) and the mean reduction in the urinary albumin-to-creatinine ratio was greater (between-group difference, 14 percentage points; 95 % CI, 11–17). The proportion of patients with hyperkalemia (serum potassium level, ≥6 mmol/l) was significantly higher in the aliskiren group than in the placebo group (11.2 % vs. 7.2 %), as was the proportion with reported hypotension (12.1 % vs. 8.3 %) ($P<0.001$ for both comparisons).

Conclusions: The addition of aliskiren to standard therapy with renin-angiotensin system blockade in patients with type 2 diabetes who are at high risk for cardiovascular and renal events is not supported by these data and may even be harmful (Funded by Novartis; ALTITUDE ClinicalTrials.gov number, NCT00549757.).

Critical Appraisal

Parameters	Yes	No	Comment
Validity			
Is the **Randomization** Procedure well described?	+1		Protocol previously published [39]
			Standard care including RAS inhibitor versus standard care + Aliskiren
			>4,200 in each group
Double **blinded**?	+2		
Is the **sample size** calculation described/adequate?	+3		The trial was designed to enroll 8,600 patients and to continue until 1,620 patients reached the primary composite endpoint, with the assumption of an annual event rate of 8 % in the placebo group, in order to provide 90 % power to detect a reduction in risk of 15 % or more at a significance level of 5 %

Parameters	Yes	No	Comment
Does it have a hard primary **endpoint**?		−1	The primary outcome was a composite of death from cardiovascular causes or the first occurrence of cardiac arrest with resuscitation; nonfatal myocardial infarction; nonfatal stroke; unplanned hospitalization for heart failure; end-stage renal disease, death attributable to kidney failure, or the need for renal-replacement therapy with no dialysis or transplantation available or initiated; or a serum creatinine value that was at least double the baseline value and that exceeded the upper limit of the normal range (>80 μmol/l [0.9 mg/dl] in women and >106 μmol/l [1.2 mg/dl] in men), sustained for at least a month
Is the endpoint surrogate?		0	GFR not measured but MACE well defined
Is the follow-up appropriate?		−1	Early termination of the study due to adverse events
			Mean follow-up 32 months
Was there a **Bias**?	−2		Early termination
Is the dropout >25 %?		+1	
Is the analysis **ITT**?	+3		
Utility/usefulness			
Can the findings be generalized?	+1		T2DM with CKD and proteinuria
Was the NNT <100?			Negative study
Score	**43 %**		

Comments and Discussion

ALTITUDE showed that dual RAS blockade including a renin inhibitor (Aliskiren) was potentially harmful and poorly tolerated in older patients with T2DM and CKD (mean GFR=57 ml/min). In spite of a more significant reduction in blood pressure and albuminuria, the dual blockade led to a faster rate of decline of eGFR and a higher rate of complications including hyperkalemia and hypotension. This has led to the premature termination of the study on safety grounds.

ALTITUDE's limitations included:
1. Early termination for adverse events, thus somewhat compromising the power of the study
2. Reliance on eGFR and not measured GFR to ascertain the rate of CKD progression
3. Casual/office BP recording, when using hypotensive agents to control CKD progression; these may underestimate the overall, 24 h, extent of BP reduction

Conclusion

Dual RAS blockade is potentially harmful in older patients at high cardiovascular risk, this in spite of a significant reduction in albuminuria. Such harmful effect may be due to excessive blood pressure lowering in older age groups with cardiovascular complications and potential renal underperfusion exacerbated by dual blockade-induced hypotension. The reduction of albuminuria may be the reflection of a marked reduction in intraglomerular pressure seriously compromising renal function. This was also noted in the ONTARGET study [39].

RASS Trial

N Engl J Med. 2009 Jul 2;361(1):40–51. doi: 10.1056/NEJMoa0808400.

Renal and retinal effects of enalapril and losartan in type 1 diabetes

Mauer M, Zinman B, Gardiner R, Suissa S, Sinaiko A, Strand T, Drummond K, Donnelly S, Goodyer P, Gubler MC, Klein R.

Abstract

Background: Nephropathy and retinopathy remain important complications of type 1 diabetes. It is unclear whether their progression is slowed by early administration of drugs that block the renin-angiotensin system.

Methods: We conducted a multicenter, controlled trial involving 285 normotensive patients with type 1 diabetes and normoalbuminuria and who were randomly assigned to receive losartan (100 mg daily), enalapril (20 mg daily), or placebo and followed for 5 years. The primary endpoint was a change in the fraction of glomerular volume occupied by mesangium in kidney-biopsy specimens. The retinopathy endpoint was a progression on a retinopathy severity scale of two steps or more. Intention-to-treat analysis was performed with the use of linear regression and logistic-regression models.

Results: A total of 90 and 82 % of patients had complete renal-biopsy and retinopathy data, respectively. Change in mesangial fractional volume per glomerulus over the 5-year period did not differ significantly between the placebo group (0.016 units) and the enalapril group (0.005, $P=0.38$) or the losartan group (0.026, $P=0.26$), nor were there significant treatment benefits for other biopsy-assessed renal structural variables. The 5-year cumulative incidence of microalbuminuria was 6 % in the placebo group; the incidence was higher with losartan (17 %, $P=0.01$ by the log-rank test) but not with enalapril (4 %, $P=0.96$ by the log-rank test). As compared with placebo, the odds of retinopathy progression by two steps or more was reduced by 65 % with enalapril (odds ratio, 0.35; 95 % confidence interval [CI], 0.14–0.85) and by 70 % with losartan (odds ratio, 0.30; 95 % CI, 0.12–0.73), independently of changes in blood pressure. There were three biopsy-related serious adverse events that completely resolved. Chronic cough occurred in 12 patients receiving enalapril, 6 receiving losartan, and 4 receiving placebo.

Conclusions: Early blockade of the renin-angiotensin system in patients with type 1 diabetes did not slow nephropathy progression but slowed the progression of retinopathy. (ClinicalTrials.gov number, NCT00143949.)

Critical Appraisal

Parameters	Yes	No	Comment
Validity			
Is the **Randomization** Procedure well described?	+1		Protocol described elsewhere [40]
			Enalapril v Losartan v Placebo
Double **blinded**?	+2		
Is the **sample size** calculation described/adequate?	+3		Investigators calculated that a sample size of 86 patients per group would be required for the study to have a statistical power of 80 % to detect a 50 % reduction in the change in mesangial fractional volume over the 5-year period, with a significance level of 5 % that was reduced to 2.5 % to allow for the two contrasts of the primary analysis (losartan vs. placebo and enalapril vs. placebo)
			256 in renal biopsy study
			223 in retinopathy study
Does it have a hard primary **endpoint**?		−1	Renal Histology; Mesangial volume expansion
			Secondary endpoints included measured GFR (Iohexol clearance)
			Also progression of diabetic retinopathy
Is the endpoint surrogate?	0		
Is the follow-up appropriate?	+1		5 years
Was there a **Bias**?		+2	
Is the dropout >25 %?		+1	
Is the analysis **ITT**?	+3		
Utility/usefulness			
Can the findings be generalized?	+1		T1DM with normal renal function (GFR >90 ml/min) and normoalbuminuric
Was the NNT <100?			Negative renal outcome
Score	**93 %**		

Comments and Discussion

The RASS study comparing an ACE inhibitor, an ARN, and placebo in patients with T1DM, normal function, and normoalbuminuria is worth including in this chapter for a number of reasons:

1. It shows that ACE inhibition did not differ from placebo in the prevention of microalbuminuria development. This is in contrast with a previous and less well-designed study in T2DM (BENEDICT) [40].
2. It showed that ARB increased the incidence of microalbuminuria, also in disagreement with ROADMAP that showed a protective effect in T2DM [41]. Of note in ROADMAP, Olmesartan had a detrimental effect on cardiovascular events rate.
3. The rate of decline of measured GFR was not different between the groups and generally fairly slow; around 6–8 ml/min/5 years; 1–1.5 ml/min/year, an unexpectedly slow rate of GFR decline in diabetic nephropathy, specially T1DM.
4. Neither ACE inhibition nor ARB changed the rate of progression of mesangial expansion over 5 years.
5. Blood pressure levels and the incidence of hypertension were favorably affected by RAS inhibitors.
6. Both ACE inhibition and ARB reduced the rate of progression of diabetic retinopathy.
7. Glycemia control was comparable between the groups.

Strength and limitations of RASS:

1. The strength of this study is that it shows that serial measurement of GFR is achievable in patients with DM.
2. It also showed that serial renal biopsy is achievable.
3. The limitation is the assumption that changes in mesangial volume fraction would inevitably translate in the long term to parallel changes in glomerulosclerosis and kidney function.

ABCD Trial

Kidney Int. 2002;61(3):1086–97.

Effects of aggressive blood pressure control in normotensive type 2 diabetic patients on albuminuria, retinopathy, and strokes

Schrier RW, Estacio RO, Esler A, Mehler P.

Abstract

Background: Although several important studies have been performed in hypertensive type 2 diabetic patients, it is not known whether lowering blood pressure in normotensive (BP <140/90 mmHg) patients offers any beneficial results on vascular complications. The current study evaluated the effect of intensive versus moderate diastolic blood pressure (DBP) control on diabetic vascular complications in 480 normotensive type 2 diabetic patients.

Methods: The current study was a prospective, randomized controlled trial in normotensive type 2 diabetic subjects. The subjects were randomized to intensive (10 mmHg below the baseline DBP) versus moderate (80–89 mmHg) DBP control. Patients in the moderate therapy group were given placebo, while the patients randomized to intensive therapy received either nisoldipine or enalapril in a blinded manner as the initial antihypertensive medication. The primary endpoint evaluated was the change in creatinine clearance with the secondary endpoints consisting of change in urinary albumin excretion, progression of retinopathy and neuropathy, and the incidence of cardiovascular disease.

Critical Appraisal

Parameters	Yes	No	Comment
Validity			
Is the **Randomization** Procedure well described?	+1		Protocol previously described [42]. Premuted block randomization with strata
			Patients were randomized into two treatment arms consisting of an intensive treatment with a diastolic blood pressure goal of 10 mmHg below the randomization diastolic blood pressure and moderate (placebo) treatment with a diastolic blood pressure goal between 80 and 89 mmHg. Intensive arms nisoldipine or enalapril
Double **blinded**?	+2		
Is the **sample size** calculation described/adequate?	+3		Moderate BP control: $n = 243$ Intensive BP therapy: $n = 237$
Does it have a hard primary **endpoint**?		−1	Changes in serum creatinine clearance
Is the endpoint surrogate?		−2	GFR was not measured
Is the follow-up appropriate?	+1		5 years
Was there a **Bias**?		+2	
Is the dropout >25 %?	−1		
Is the analysis **ITT**?		−3	
Utility/usefulness			
Can the findings be generalized?	+1		T2DM, normotensive, normal renal function. Results may not be applicable to patients with diabetic nephropathy
Was the NNT <100?			Negative study
Score	**20 %**		

Results: The mean follow-up was 5.3 years. Mean BP in the intensive group was $128\pm0.8/75\pm0.3$ mmHg versus $137\pm0.7/81\pm0.3$ mmHg in the moderate group, $P<0.0001$. Although no difference was demonstrated in creatinine clearance ($P=0.43$), a lower percentage of patients in the intensive group progressed from normoalbuminuria to microalbuminuria ($P=0.012$) and microalbuminuria to overt albuminuria ($P=0.028$). The intensive BP control group also demonstrated less progression of diabetic retinopathy ($P=0.019$) and a lower incidence of strokes ($P=0.03$). The results were the same whether enalapril or nisoldipine was used as the initial antihypertensive agent.

Conclusion: Over a 5-year follow-up period, intensive (approximately 128/75 mmHg) BP control in normotensive type 2 diabetic patients: (1) slowed the progression to incipient and overt diabetic nephropathy; (2) decreased the progression of diabetic retinopathy; and (3) diminished the incidence of stroke.

Comments and Discussion

The ABCD study was one of the first to explore the impact on intensive BP control compared to standard control on the progression of diabetic complications in patients with T2DM. Its primary endpoint was the changes in creatinine clearance over the 5 year observation time.

Intensive BP control had no impact on renal function decline. Subgroup analysis suggested a benefit for intensive BP control in patients with over proteinuria.

On the other hand, intensive BP control reduced the progression of normoalbuminuria to microalbuminuria and that of microalbuminuria to macroalbuminuria.

In the intensive BP control, there was no difference on renal function or albuminuria between those treated with nisoldipine and enalapril. Blood pressure control was comparable in both arms. Also no difference between nisoldipine and enalapril was noted in relation to albuminuria.

Strength and limitations of ABCD:

This was a well-conducted study in patients with T2DM, mostly normoalbuminuria, normotensive and with normal renal function.

Blood pressure difference between the standard and intensive BP control groups was maintained throughout the study. Also an effort was made to measure BP at peak drug action rather than a randomly defined time.

A preliminary study established the agreement between creatinine clearance and iothalamate clearance measured GFR in this patients' group [43]. The authors rightly attributed that agreement to that limited contribution of tubular secretion of creatinine at that level of GFR.

Secondary endpoints showed a beneficial effect of intensive BP control on the progression of diabetic retinopathy but not neuropathy or cardiovascular complications.

Limitations include:

1. Absence of measured GFR, although, as outlined above, this may be less important at this early stage of T2DM complications.
2. Blood pressure not recorded over 24 h; this is all the more relevant in a study whose focal point is BP control.
3. The study is also limited to patients with T2DM who are normotensive and with essentially normal renal function, thus limited its applicability to those with overt diabetic nephropathy. The beneficial effect observed in those with overt nephropathy of intensive BP control is limited by the lack of power of this sub-study and the small sample size of those with overt nephropathy, precluding any meaningful conclusions.

Conclusions

The ABCD study showed that more intensive BP control in normoalbuminuric T2DM individuals had little impact on CKD progression. It suggested a dissociation between the impact of lower BP on the progression of albuminuria from that of renal dysfunction. It also suggested a dissociation between the progression of diabetic nephropathy and retinopathy; the latter being affected by lower blood pressure levels. Finally, ABCD showed no superiority of enalapril over nisoldipine in any aspect of the progression of early diabetic complications.

Endothelin Antagonists

A role has been put forward for endothelin 1 in the pathogenesis of hypertension, albuminuria, as well as the progression of CKD including DKD. It made therefore good sense to follow promising preclinical data, showing a protective effect on the progression of renal scarring by endothelin antagonists, with clinical trials. Emphasis has been, to a large extent, on the selective blockade of endothelin type A (ETA) receptor thought to activate potentially inflammatory and fibrogenic intracellular signaling pathways and mediators.

ASCEND Trial

J Am Soc Nephrol. 2010 Mar;21(3):527–35. doi: 10.1681/ ASN.2009060593. Epub 2010 Feb 18.

Avosentan for overt diabetic nephropathy

Mann JF, Green D, Jamerson K, Ruilope LM, Kuranoff SJ, Littke T, Viberti G; ASCEND Study Group.

Abstract

In the short term, the endothelin antagonist avosentan reduces proteinuria, but whether this translates to protection from progressive loss of renal function is unknown. We examined the effects of avosentan on progression of overt diabetic nephropathy in a multicenter, multinational, double-blind, placebo-controlled trial. We randomly assigned 1,392 participants with type 2 diabetes to oral avosentan (25 or 50 mg) or placebo in addition to continued angiotensin-converting-enzyme inhibition and/or angiotensin receptor blockade. The composite primary outcome was the time to doubling of serum creatinine, ESRD, or death. Secondary outcomes included changes in albumin-to-creatinine ratio (ACR) and cardiovascular outcomes. We terminated the trial prematurely after a median follow-up of 4 months (maximum 16 months) because of an excess of cardiovascular events with avosentan. We did not detect a difference in the frequency of the primary outcome between groups. Avosentan significantly reduced ACR: In patients who were treated with avosentan 25 mg/day, 50 mg/day, and placebo, the median reduction in ACR was 44.3, 49.3, and 9.7 %, respectively. Adverse events led to discontinuation of trial medication significantly more often for avosentan than for placebo (19.6 and 18.2 versus 11.5 % for placebo), dominated by fluid overload and congestive heart failure; death occurred in 21 (4.6 %; P=0.225), 17 (3.6 %; P=0.194), and 12 (2.6 %), respectively. In conclusion, avosentan reduces albuminuria when added to standard treatment in people with type 2 diabetes and overt nephropathy but induces significant fluid overload and congestive heart failure.

Critical Appraisal

Parameters	Yes	No	Comment
Validity			
Is the **Randomization** Procedure well described?	+1		Randomization 1:1:1 Avosentan 25 mg: 50 mg: placebo On a background of standard therapy including RAS inhibitors
Double **blinded**?	+2		
Is the **sample size** calculation described/adequate?	+3		A sample size of 2,364 patients and 747 primary outcomes were calculated to provide a 90 % power at the 5 % level (two-sided) to detect a 7 % (25-mg dose) and 10 % (50-mg dose) absolute reduction of the primary outcome compared with the placebo group, assuming a placebo cumulative incidence of 40 % at 36 months for the primary outcome

Parameters	Yes	No	Comment
Does it have a hard primary **endpoint**?		−1	The primary outcome was defined as the composite of time to doubling of serum creatinine, ESRD, or death ESRD prespecified in protocol
Is the endpoint surrogate?	−2		GFR was not measured
Is the follow-up appropriate?		−1	Study terminated prematurely after 4 months
Was there a **Bias**?		+2	
Is the dropout >25 %?			Not applicable in view of early termination of the study due to serious adverse events
Is the analysis **ITT**?			Same as above
Utility/usefulness			
Can the findings be generalized?	−1		Inconclusive study
Was the NNT <100?			Inconclusive study
Score	**20 %**		Inconclusive trial due to premature termination

Comments and Discussion

ASCEND was the first major study investigating the impact of an endothelin type A (ETA) receptor on the progression of diabetic nephropathy. It had to be terminated early on safety grounds.

Avosentan reduced blood pressure, accelerated the decline in eGFR, and reduced albuminuria (ACR). The reduction in albuminuria was not entirely attributable to the decline in GFR most notable at 6 months on Avosentan 50 mg/daily.

While Avosentan significantly reduced albuminuria, the study had to be prematurely terminated due to serious adverse events related to fluid retention, congestive heart failure, and related death. Consequently, any meaningful conclusions cannot be drawn from this study on the value of endothelin ETAR antagonists on the progression of diabetic nephropathy.

Fluid retention may have been attributable to the dose of Avosentan used but also the study design and inappropriate usage of diuretics in patients with advanced renal insufficiency.

The results of the ASCEND study were reproduced with another ETA receptor antagonist, Atrasentan, that also reduced albuminuria and blood pressure along with an increased rate of side effects including weight gain, fluid retention, and heart failure [44]. Anemia was also noted with Atrasentan and attributed to the fluid retention and hemodilution effect of this class of compounds.

Conclusions

The addition of ETA receptor antagonists to RAS inhibitors for the management of progressive and proteinuric diabetic nephropathy further reduce blood pressure and proteinuria but appears to be unsafe.

Antioxidant Therapy

A role has been postulated for chronic inflammation and reactive oxygen species (ROS) in the pathogenesis of the complications of DM. ROS have the capacity to cause direct tissue and renal injury as well as activate a range of intracellular inflammatory as well as fibrogenic mediators implicated in renal scarring and the progression of CKD. It makes therefore good sense to attempt to inhibit some of the ROS-mediated signaling pathways in order to minimize renal injury and the progression of CKD.

BEACON Trial

N Engl J Med. 2013 Dec 26;369(26):2492–503. doi: 10.1056/NEJMoa1306033. Epub 2013 Nov 9.

Bardoxolone methyl in type 2 diabetes and stage 4 chronic kidney disease

de Zeeuw D, Akizawa T, Audhya P, Bakris GL, Chin M, Christ-Schmidt H, Goldsberry A, Houser M, Krauth M, Lambers Heerspink HJ, McMurray JJ, Meyer CJ, Parving HH, Remuzzi G, Toto RD, Vaziri ND, Wanner C, Wittes J, Wrolstad D, Chertow GM; BEACON Trial Investigators.

Collaborators (347)

Abstract

Background: Although inhibitors of the renin-angiotensin-aldosterone system can slow the progression of diabetic kidney disease, the residual risk is high. Whether nuclear 1 factor (erythroid-derived 2)-related factor 2 activators further reduce this risk is unknown.

Methods: We randomly assigned 2,185 patients with type 2 diabetes mellitus and stage 4 chronic kidney disease (estimated glomerular filtration rate [GFR], 15 to <30 ml/min/1.73 m^2 of body-surface area) to bardoxolone methyl, at a daily dose of 20 mg, or placebo. The primary composite outcome was end-stage renal disease (ESRD) or death from cardiovascular causes.

Results: The sponsor and the steering committee terminated the trial on the recommendation of the independent data and safety monitoring committee; the median follow-up was 9 months. A total of 69 of 1,088 patients (6 %) randomly assigned to bardoxolone methyl and 69 of 1,097 (6 %) randomly assigned to placebo had a primary composite outcome (hazard ratio in the bardoxolone methyl group vs. the placebo group, 0.98; 95 % confidence interval [CI], 0.70–1.37; $P=0.92$). In the bardoxolone methyl group, ESRD developed in 43 patients, and 27 patients died from cardiovascular causes; in the placebo group, ESRD developed in 51 patients, and 19 patients died from cardiovascular causes. A total of 96 patients in the bardoxolone methyl group were hospitalized for heart failure or died from heart failure, as compared with 55 in the placebo group (hazard ratio, 1.83; 95 % CI, 1.32–2.55; $P<0.001$). Estimated GFR, blood pressure, and the urinary albumin-to-creatinine ratio increased significantly and body weight decreased significantly in the bardoxolone methyl group, as compared with the placebo group.

Conclusions: Among patients with type 2 diabetes mellitus and stage 4 chronic kidney disease, bardoxolone methyl did not reduce the risk of ESRD or death from cardiovascular causes. A higher rate of cardiovascular events with bardoxolone methyl than with placebo prompted termination of the trial. (Funded by Reata Pharmaceuticals; BEACON ClinicalTrials.gov number, NCT01351675.).

Critical Appraisal

Parameters	Yes	No	Comment
Validity			
Is the **Randomization** Procedure well described?	+1		Bardoxolone methyl on a background of RAS inhibition Placebo = 1,097 Bardoxolone = 1,088
Double **blinded**?	+2		
Is the **sample size** calculation described/adequate?	+3		It was calculated that we needed to enroll 2,000 patients on the basis of the following assumptions: a two-sided type I error rate of 5 %, an event rate of 24 % for the primary composite outcome in the placebo group during the first 2 years of the study
Does it have a hard primary **endpoint**?	+1		ESRD or death from cardiovascular causes
Is the endpoint surrogate?	−2		
Is the follow-up appropriate?		−1	Median follow-up = 9 months due to the premature termination of the study due to serious adverse events
Was there a **Bias**?	−2		Control group was not progressive
Is the dropout >25 %?			
Is the analysis **ITT**?	+3		
Utility/usefulness			
Can the findings be generalized?		−1	Inconclusive study prematurely terminated
Was the NNT <100?			Inconclusive study prematurely terminated
Score	**27 %**		Inconclusive trial due to premature termination

Comments and Discussion

It has long been assumed that oxidant stress plays an important role in the initiation and progression of diabetic nephropathy. A number of interventions aimed at reducing oxidant-induced renal injury have been tested in RCTs aimed at reducing renal injury and slowing the progression of diabetic kidney disease

[45, 46]. This has included Bardoxolone methyl, a nuclear 1 factor (erythroid-derived 2)–related factor 2 activator, that showed promise in experimental models [47].

Following the BEAM proof of concept study of the efficacy of Bardoxolone methyl, a nuclear 1 factor (erythroid-derived 2)–related factor 2 activator, on renal function in T2DM nephropathy that showed an acute and sustained increase in eGFR [48], BEACON was designed to confirm such potential benefit and its impact on the incidence of ESRD and cardiovascular events in T2DM.

BEACON, like BEAM [48] before it, showed that Bardoxolone methyl reduced serum creatinine and increased eGFR over the observation period. But the two studies also showed that patients suffered significant weight loss.

Of note, BEACON also showed a significant increase in blood pressure and albuminuria on Bardoxolone.

BEACON was terminated prematurely due to increased morbidity and mortality attributed to Bardoxolone.

Limitations and lessons from the BEAM/BEACON trials:

1. Changes in eGFR do not equate to measured GFR.
2. Changes in serum creatinine and eGFR are confounded by variables such as weight and muscle loss as observed with a toxic compound such as Bardoxolone.
3. Changes in serum creatinine and eGFR can also be affected by tubular effects of drugs such as Bardoxolone that may also have affected the urinary excretion of magnesium, uric acid, and phosphate with consequent lower blood levels compared to placebo.
4. GFR has to be measured to evaluate CKD and DKD progression.
5. ESRD incidence based on changes in serum creatinine and eGFR has the same limitations outlined above.
6. In the BEAM study, the nature of progressive DKD was not established prior to randomization, hence the non-progressive nature of eGFR in the placebo group.

Conclusions

The BEAM/BEACON tragedy highlights the serious and potentially dangerous practice of relying on changes in serum creatinine and its derived eGFR to measure renal function decline in RCTs [48–50]. This reflects that dangerous oversight that serum creatinine changes can be confounded by a number of factors including diet, metabolism, and muscle mass as well as tubular secretion.

The BEAM-BEACON "improved GFR" myth was also noted in a study of another potential antioxidant pirfenidone that showed an increase in eGFR in diabetic nephropathy along with serious gastrointestinal side effects that would have undoubtedly impacted protein intake, weight and serum creatinine levels, without necessarily affecting measured GFR [49].

It is high time nephrologists realize that eGFR does not always reflect measured GFR and that RCTs have to rely on the latter to avoid confounders affecting the former.

Miscellaneous Interventions

Pirfenidone

Pirfenidone has been at the forefront of anti-fibrotic agents for more than a decade. It has proved effective in minimizing a number of experimental fibrosis models. While the precise anti-fibrotic effect of pirfenidone is not fully understood, it has shown great promise for the management of patients with lung fibrosis. Translational studies based on the treatment of patients with CKD and DKD with Pirfenidone have tested whether such agent is capable of slowing the progression of the underlying nephropathy.

J Am Soc Nephrol. 2011;22(6):1144–51. doi: 10.1681/ASN.2010101049. Epub 2011 Apr 21.
Pirfenidone for diabetic nephropathy

Sharma K, Ix JH, Mathew AV, Cho M, Pflueger A, Dunn SR, Francos B, Sharma S, Falkner B, McGowan TA, Donohue M, Ramachandrarao S, Xu R, Fervenza FC, Kopp JB.

Abstract

Pirfenidone is an oral antifibrotic agent that benefits diabetic nephropathy in animal models, but whether it is effective for human diabetic nephropathy is unknown. We conducted a randomized, double-blind, placebo-controlled study in 77 subjects with diabetic nephropathy who had elevated albuminuria and reduced estimated GFR (eGFR) (20–75 ml/min/1.73 m^2). The prespecified primary outcome was a change in eGFR after 1 year of therapy. We randomly assigned 26 subjects to placebo, 26 to pirfenidone at 1,200 mg/day, and 25 to pirfenidone at 2,400 mg/day. Among the 52 subjects who completed the study, the mean eGFR increased in the pirfenidone 1,200-mg/day group (+3.3±8.5 ml/min/1.73 m^2) whereas the mean eGFR decreased in the placebo group (−2.2±4.8 ml/min/1.73 m^2; $P=0.026$ versus pirfenidone at 1,200 mg/day). The dropout rate was high (11 of 25) in the pirfenidone 2,400-mg/day group, and the change in eGFR was not significantly different from placebo (−1.9±6.7 ml/min/1.73 m^2). Of the 77 subjects, 4 initiated hemodialysis in the placebo group, 1 in the pirfenidone 2,400-mg/day group, and none in the pirfenidone 1,200-mg/day group during the study ($P=0.25$). Baseline levels of plasma biomarkers of inflammation and fibrosis significantly correlated with baseline eGFR but did not predict response to therapy. In conclusion, these results suggest that pirfenidone is a promising agent for individuals with overt diabetic nephropathy.

Critical Appraisal

Parameters	Yes	No	Comment
Validity			
Is the **Randomization** Procedure well described?	+1		Randomly assigned 26 subjects to placebo, 26 to pirfenidone at 1,200 mg/day, and 25 to pirfenidone at 2,400 mg/day
Double **blinded**?	+2		
Is the **sample size** calculation described/adequate?		−3	
Does it have a hard primary **endpoint**?		−1	Changes in eGFR after 1 year follow-up
Is the endpoint surrogate?	−2		
Is the follow-up appropriate?		−1	1 year
Was there a **Bias**?	+2		
Is the dropout >25 %?		−1	52 of 77 completed the study and were analyzed. Biggest dropout in the 2,400 mg/day pirfenidone group due to gastrointestinal side effects
Is the analysis **ITT**?		−3	52 of 77 analyzed
Utility/usefulness			
Can the findings be generalized?		−1	T2DM with eGFR 20–75 ml/min and albuminuria
Was the NNT <100?			Negative study
Score	**0 %**		

Comments and Discussion

The Pirfenidone in diabetic nephropathy study is another example of a badly conducted and interpreted study [51]. In view of large dropout rate and missing data for the final analysis, it required statistical assistance, permutation tests, and ANCOVA with iterated re-weighted least squares, controlling for baseline values and their inter- action with treatment, to conclude that there was an improvement in eGFR between the Pirfenidone 1,200 mg/day group and placebo. This conclusion is confounded by the serious study limitations, mostly the likely misinterpretation of changes in serum creatinine (and eGFR) levels due to the side effects of the compound. It bears similarities to the BEAM/BEACON studies [52] where claims of improved eGFR sadly reflected the investigators' choice of wrong primary endpoint (serum creatinine/eGFR) when using a compound/pirfenidone that affects gastric emptying and may therefore impact food/protein intake [53].

Limitations:

1. This is not an intention to treat analysis and in view of the large dropout rate (>30 %), the study is clearly underpowered and therefore inconclusive.
2. Pirfinedone at 2,400 mg/day had so many gastrointestinal side effects that few patients completed the study in this arm, thus excluding it from any meaningful analysis.
3. The known gastrointestinal side effects of Pirfenidone, abdominal discomfort, nausea, vomiting, and decreased appetite make the use of serum creatinine unacceptable at best and misleading at worst. Changes reported in serum creatinine (fall) and in eGFR(rise +3 ml/min) in the Pirfenidone 1,200 mg/day group are most likely related to decreased food intake and consequent fall in serum creatinine; little to do with renal function and/or its improvement.
4. GFR was not measured.

Conclusions

The Pirfenidone study is fraught by its numerous limitations including its inadequate power and inappropriate use of serum creatinine as the primary endpoint and, therefore, is inconclusive. Pirfenidone may be a compound with too many side effects to be safely administered to patients with CKD, never mind those with diabetes mellitus who are often already suffering from underlying autonomic neuropathy and impaired gastric emptying [53].

AGE Inhibition

Advanced glycation end products (AGE) have been implicated in the pathogenesis of a number of degenerative diseases including diabetes mellitus. In diabetes, sustained glycation of endogenous proteins through the Amadori nonenzymatic reaction has been linked to all the micro- and macro- vascular complications of the disease including DN. Inhibitors of AGE formation have shown promise in experimental models of diabetic nephropathy in rodents, hence their translation into the treatment of patients with DKD.

J Am Soc Nephrol. 2012 Jan;23(1):131–6. doi: 10.1681/ASN.2011030272. Epub 2011 Oct 27.

Pyridorin in type 2 diabetic nephropathy

Lewis EJ, Greene T, Spitalewiz S, Blumenthal S, Berl T, Hunsicker LG, Pohl MA, Rohde RD, Raz I, Yerushalmy Y, Yagil Y, Herskovits T, Atkins RC, Reutens AT, Packham DK, Lewis JB; Collaborative Study Group.

Abstract

Pyridoxamine dihydrochloride (Pyridorin, NephroGenex) inhibits formation of advanced glycation end products and scavenges reactive oxygen species and toxic carbonyls, but whether these actions translate into renoprotective effects is unknown. In this double-blind, randomized, placebo-controlled trial, we randomly assigned 317 patients with proteinuric type 2 diabetic nephropathy to twice-daily placebo; Pyridorin, 150 mg twice daily; or Pyridorin, 300 mg twice daily, for 52 weeks. At baseline, the mean age ± SD was 63.9 ± 9.5 years, and the mean duration of diabetes was 17.6 ± 8.5 years; the mean serum creatinine level was 2.2 ± 0.6 mg/dl, and the mean protein-to-creatinine ratio was

$2,973 \pm 1,932$ mg/g. Regarding the primary endpoint, a statistically significant change in serum creatinine from baseline to 52 weeks was not evident in either Pyridorin group compared with placebo. However, analysis of covariance suggested that the magnitude of the treatment effect differed by baseline renal function. Among patients in the lowest tertile of baseline serum creatinine concentration, treatment with Pyridorin associated with a lower average change in serum creatinine concentration at 52 weeks (0.28, 0.07, and 0.14 mg/dl for placebo, Pyridorin 150 mg, and Pyridorin 300 mg, respectively; $P=0.05$ for either Pyridorin dose versus placebo); there was no evidence of a significant treatment effect in the middle or upper tertiles. In conclusion, this trial failed to detect an effect of Pyridorin on the progression of serum creatinine at 1 year, although it suggests that patients with less renal impairment might benefit.

Critical Appraisal

Parameters	Yes	No	Comment
Validity			
Is the **Randomization** Procedure well described?		−1	
Double **blinded**?	+2		
Is the **sample size** calculation described/adequate?	+3		The sample size estimate for this study was determined using data from previous Pyridorin studies (PYR 206, PYR 205/207) and the IDNT. The study was powered to detect a 40 % difference between the Pyridorin groups and placebo
			Placebo: 106, Pyridorin 150 mg/bid=105, pyridorin 300 mg/bid=106
Does it have a hard primary **endpoint**?		−1	Changes in serum creatinine over 12 months
Is the endpoint surrogate?		−2	GFR not measured, prespecified ESRD not considered
Is the follow-up appropriate?		−1	12 months too short for progression study
Was there a **Bias**?		+2	
Is the dropout >25 %?		+1	
Is the analysis **ITT**?	+3		
Utility/usefulness			
Can the findings be generalized?	+1		T2DM with serum creatinine between 1.3 and 3 mg/dl and overt albuminuria >1,200 mg/g
Was the NNT <100?			Negative study
Score	**47 %**		

Comments and Discussion

One of the main hypotheses related to the pathogenesis of the complications of DM focuses on the role of advanced glycation endproducts (AGE) and their deposition in tissues [54]. The kidney is no exception as it has been argued that the glomerular as well as tubular accumulation of AGE initiate and contribute to the progression of glomerulosclerosis and tubulointerstitial fibrosis, respectively [55]. Consequently, experimental and clinical attempts at the prevention of AGE formation and deposition have become one of the main therapeutic targets and strategy for the management of DM and its complications [55].

Earlier experimental [56] and clinical [57] studies suggested that an inhibitor of advanced glycation endproducts (pyridoxine/pyridorin) may slow the rate of increase in serum creatinine. However, the proof of concept (POC) study under discussion above failed to confirm such findings as serum creatinine changes were not affected by treatment with pyridorin. Pyridorin had no effect on albuminuria. Diabetes control was comparable between groups.

This study has a number of limitations:

1. Relatively small sample size.
2. Short duration of follow-up; 12 months' follow-up period does not allow for a comprehensive evaluation of an intervention aimed to inhibit the ongoing deposition of AGE on the progression of DN.
3. The study relied on the soft endpoint of changes in serum creatinine rather than the hard endpoint of measured GFR.
4. Changes in Cystatin C were measured, although these may be affected in obesity and inflammation associated with T2DM.
5. Proof of compound efficacy was not ascertained by measurement of AGE in circulation.

Conclusions

A study with a flawed design and short follow-up period that does not allow the drawing of any meaningful conclusions.

Suledoxide

Suledoxide and other naturally occurring glycosaminoglycans as well as heparinoids have shown in a number of experimental renal models a capacity to reduce albuminuria and decrease renal fibrosis. Pilot studies have also shown an anti-proteinuric effect in patients with diabetic nephropathy.

The Sun-MACRO Trial

J Am Soc Nephrol. 2012;23(1):123–30. doi: 10.1681/ASN.2011040378. Epub 2011 Oct 27.

Sulodexide fails to demonstrate renoprotection in overt type 2 diabetic nephropathy

Packham DK, Wolfe R, Reutens AT, Berl T, Heerspink HL, Rohde R, Ivory S, Lewis J, Raz I, Wiegmann TB, Chan JC, de Zeeuw D, Lewis EJ, Atkins RC; Collaborative Study Group.

Abstract

Sulodexide, a mixture of naturally occurring glycosaminoglycan polysaccharide components, has been reported to reduce albuminuria in patients with diabetes, but it is unknown whether it is renoprotective. This study reports the results from the randomized, double-blind, placebo-controlled sulodexide macroalbuminuria (Sun-MACRO) trial, which evaluated the renoprotective effects of sulodexide in patients with type 2 diabetes, renal impairment, and significant proteinuria (>900 mg/day) already receiving maximal therapy with angiotensin II receptor blockers. The primary endpoint was a composite of a doubling of baseline serum creatinine, development of ESRD, or serum creatinine ≥ 6.0 mg/dl. We planned to enroll 2,240 patients over approximately 24 months but terminated the study after enrolling 1,248 patients. After 1,029 person-years of follow-up, we did not detect any significant differences between sulodexide and placebo; the primary composite endpoint occurred in 26 and 30 patients in the sulodexide and placebo groups, respectively. Side effect profiles were similar for both groups. In conclusion, these data do not suggest a renoprotective benefit of sulodexide in patients with type 2 diabetes, renal impairment, and macroalbuminuria.

Critical Appraisal

Parameters	Yes	No	Comment
Validity			
Is the **Randomization** Procedure well described?	+1		1,248 studied instead of the anticipated 2,240: sulodexide=619 patients
Double **blinded**?	+2		
Is the **sample size** calculation described/adequate?		−3	
Does it have a hard primary **endpoint**?		−1	The primary endpoint was a composite of a doubling of baseline serum creatinine, development of ESRD, or serum creatinine >6.0 mg/dl
Is the endpoint surrogate?	−2		GFR not measured
Is the follow-up appropriate?		−1	Premature termination of the study for futility; follow-up <12 months
Was there a **Bias**?		+2	
Is the dropout >25 %?			Premature termination
Is the analysis **ITT**?		−3	Premature termination
Utility/usefulness			
Can the findings be generalized?	+1		T2DM, with renal impairment (serum creatinine: 1.5–3 mg/dl) and significant proteinuria (>900 mg/day)
Was the NNT <100?			Inconclusive study
Score	**0 %**		Inconclusive study

Comments and Discussion

Sulodexide is a mixture of naturally occurring glycosaminoglycan polysaccharide. It has heparin-like effects. It has shown anti-proteinuric properties in preclinical studies [58]. Early experimental [59] and clinical [60, 61] evidence confirmed such impression in patients with early and advanced diabetic nephropathy.

The Sun-MACRO study aimed to test this hypothesis in T2DM patients with a median GFR of 30 ml/min and macro-proteinuria (>900 mg/day). While the study was meant to run for 3 years and recruit >2,200 patients, it was terminated early (<12 months) with <1,500 patients recruited.

Limitations of the Sun-MACRO trial

The study has many of the limitations of other RCTs in patients with DN.

1. GFR was not measured and it relied on the soft endpoint of changes in serum creatinine.
2. A decision to terminate prematurely is difficult to explain as the study neither reached its power or had a long enough follow-up to determine renal functional outcome. To some extent the lack of the early and anticipated (within 4 months) effect on the secondary endpoint of proteinuria, for which the authors claim that the study was powered to detect, seems to have been the decisive factor in the study termination.
3. The advanced stage of DN (CKD3b-4) may have confounded the likelihood of response to a compound that may have otherwise altered early changes in glomerular basement membrane structure and charge.
4. As with many experimental compounds, investigators have failed to show that the oral administration of sulodexide effected some anticipated actions, for instance, Factor Xa inhibition.

Conclusions

The premature termination of this study precludes any meaningful conclusions regarding the efficacy of sulodexide in diabetic nephropathy. As only one tenth of endpoints were reached during the short follow-up of a small number of patients, a type 2 statistical error cannot be excluded.

Vitamin D

Increasingly, vitamin D deficiency has been implicated in the pathogenesis of a range of chronic diseases including CKD. Vitamin D deficiency has also been associated with increased cardiovascular morbidity and all-cause mortality. Patients with CKD and ESRD with vitamin D deficiency are at increased risk of mortality. While initially thought to act primarily on calcium absorption and bone mineralization, it is becoming apparent that vitamin D is a pleomorphic hormone that modulates the physiology of a number of organs as well as the immune system. This has prompted the administration of vitamin D and its analogues to patients with DN in an attempt to improve outcomes.

VITAL Trial

Lancet. 2010 Nov 6;376(9752):1543–51. doi: 10.1016/S0140-6736(10)61032-X.

Selective vitamin D receptor activation with paricalcitol for reduction of albuminuria in patients with type 2 diabetes (VITAL study): A Randomized Controlled Trial

de Zeeuw D, Agarwal R, Amdahl M, Audhya P, Coyne D, Garimella T, Parving HH, Pritchett Y, Remuzzi G, Ritz E, Andress D.

Abstract

Background: Despite treatment with renin–angiotensin–aldosterone system (RAAS) inhibitors, patients with diabetes have increased risk of progressive renal failure that correlates with albuminuria. We aimed to assess whether paricalcitol could be used to reduce albuminuria in patients with diabetic nephropathy.

Methods: In this multinational, placebo-controlled, double-blind trial, we enrolled patients with type 2 diabetes and albuminuria who were receiving angiotensin-converting-enzyme inhibitors or angiotensin receptor blockers. Patients were assigned (1:1:1) by computer-generated randomization sequence to receive 24 weeks' treatment with placebo, 1 μg/day paricalcitol, or 2 μg/day paricalcitol. The primary endpoint was the percentage change in geometric mean urinary albumin-to-creatinine ratio (UACR) from baseline to last measurement during treatment for the combined paricalcitol groups versus the placebo group. Analysis was by intention to treat. This trial is registered with ClinicalTrials.gov, number NCT00421733.

Findings: Between February 2007 and October 2008, 281 patients were enrolled and assigned to receive placebo ($n=93$), 1 μg paricalcitol ($n=93$), or 2 μg paricalcitol ($n=95$); 88 patients on placebo, 92 on 1 μg paricalcitol, and 92 on 2 μg paricalcitol received at least one dose of study drug, and had UACR data at baseline and at least one time-point during treatment, and so were included in the primary analysis. Change in UACR was: −3 % (from 61 to 60 mg/mmol; 95 % CI −16 to 13) in the placebo group; −16 % (from 62 to 51 mg/mmol; −24 to −9) in the combined paricalcitol groups, with a between-group difference versus placebo of −15 % (95 % CI −28 to 1; $p=0.071$); −14 % (from 63 to 54 mg/mmol; −24 to −1) in the 1 μg paricalcitol group, with a between-group difference versus placebo of −11 % (95 % CI −27 to 8; $p=0.23$); and −20 % (from 61 to 49 mg/mmol; −30 to −8) in the 2 μg paricalcitol group, with a between-group difference versus placebo of −18 % (95 % CI −32 to 0; $p=0.053$). Patients on 2 μg paricalcitol showed a nearly, sustained reduction in UACR, ranging from −18 to −28 % ($p=0.014$ vs placebo). Incidence of hypercalcemia, adverse events, and serious adverse events was similar between groups receiving paricalcitol versus placebo.

Interpretation: Addition of 2 μg/day paricalcitol to RAAS inhibition safely lowers residual albuminuria in patients with diabetic nephropathy and could be a novel approach to lower residual renal risk in diabetes.

Funding: Abbott.

Critical Appraisal

Parameters	Yes	No	Comment
Validity			
Is the **Randomization** Procedure well described?	+1		1:1:1 Paricalcitol 1 ug/day: 2 ug/day: Placebo Patients continued on standard therapy including RAAS inhibition
Double **blinded**?	+2		
Is the **sample size** calculation described/adequate?	+3		We calculated that a total sample size of 258 patients was needed for at least 82 % power to detect an absolute difference in log-transformed UACR of 0.034 mg/mmol (SD 0.088) from baseline to last measurement during treatment between the combined paricalcitol group and placebo at a two-sided significance level of 0.05. Paricalcitol 1: 93 patients, Paricalcitol 2: 95 patients and Placebo: 93 patients
Does it have a hard primary **endpoint**?	+1		Percentage change in geometric mean of urinary ACR (UACR)
Is the endpoint surrogate?	−2	0	
Is the follow-up appropriate?	+1		24 weeks
Was there a **Bias**?		+2	
Is the dropout >25 %?		+1	
Is the analysis **ITT**?	+3		
Utility/usefulness			
Can the findings be generalized?	+1		T2DM (eGFR 15–90 ml/min) and albuminuria (11–339 mg/mmol)
Was the NNT <100?			Negative study
Score	**73 %**		

Comments and Discussion

The interest in the potential benefit of vitamin D and its analogues in CKD has stemmed from a number of observations including the correlations between low circulating calcitriol levels and raised albuminuria [62], as well as observations made in preclinical studies, showing that the selective vitamin D receptor activator, paricalcitol, reduced albuminuria and reduced the renal scarring process [63].

The VITAL study tested the hypothesis that activation of the Vitamin D receptor reduces albuminuria in T2DM. The study was negative overall as no statistically significant difference was detected between placebo and those treated with paricalcitol. Subgroup analysis suggested that the higher dose (2 ug/day) of paricalcitol reduced albuminuria compared to placebo.

Paricalcitol was also associated with a reduction in blood pressure that considerably attenuated the putative beneficial effect on albuminuria reduction.

Of note, paricalcitol (2 ug/day) also reduced eGFR.

Limitations of the VITAL study:

1. This is at best a proof-of-concept (POC) study of a small number of patients with T2DM followed up for 24 weeks.
2. The population studied was quite heterogeneous with eGFR from 15 to 90 ml/min and UACR from 11 to 339 mg/mmol. Such heterogeneity would affect the expected response to a given intervention.
3. As with many studies pertaining to the effect of vitamin D on UACR, it somewhat underestimated the known effect of vitamin D supplementation on serum creatinine and its excretion [64]. Increased urinary excretion of creatinine may explain to some extent the fall in UACR. However, there was also a fall in the geometric mean of 24 h urine albumin excretion.
4. Changes in serum creatinine due to vitamin D administration may also explain the "fall" in GFR; eGFR is entirely a reflection of serum creatinine levels and its changes that could be confounded in this study by the impact of vitamin D on creatinine metabolism.
5. Subgroup analysis showing differences compared to placebo is at best hypothesis generating and should not be considered conclusive evidence.
6. Finally, studies based on changes in albuminuria assume a surrogate value for that parameter for progression of DN; a number of studies have now shown that this is not the case; ONTARGET [65] and VA NEPHRON-D [66] as well as ASCEND [67] show the two parameters to be dissociated.

Conclusions

Hypothesis-generating study on the potential of vitamin D and its analogues at reducing albuminuria.

General Discussion

The history and critical appraisal of RCTs on the progression of DN are most informative.

Studies focusing on strict and intensive glycemia control on diabetes micro- and macro-vascular outcomes, including progression of DKD, have shown conflicting results. This is most likely due to a large number of confounders including the heterogeneity of the populations studied as well as the complexity of DM and its complications as well as treatment modalities [68].

Regarding hypertension control, there remains little evidence to support recommendations that patients with DM and DKD warrant tighter blood pressure control; <130/80 mmHg [69], although blood pressure levels <140/90 mmHg seem protective and therapeutic inertia unjustifiable [70].

As to the choice of anti-hypertensive agents, while a stream of RCTs supports the suggestion that RAAS inhibition slows the progression of type 1 and 2 DN, most of these studies have their limitations. Meta-analyses have been conflicting with some being unable to separate the anti-hypertensive advantage of RAAS inhibition from its impact on DN progression [71], while others suggesting an undeniable benefit on DN progression [72]. This is also the case of meta-analyses analyzing the impact of RAAS inhibition of cardiovascular events [73, 74]. The critical appraisal of RAAS inhibition studies in DN reveals that not a single study (other than RASS that investigated people with DM and normal renal function) on progressive DN evaluated progression by measuring GFR. They invariably rely on serum creatinine and eGFR that have proved unreliable measures of renal function in intervention studies where the intervention may impact appetite and protein intake, muscle metabolism (BEAM-BEACON as well as Pirfenidone), as well as the potential confounder of changes in tubular secretion of creatinine that seems underestimated and seldom considered in RCTs of RAAS inhibition [75, 76].

Many studies have relied on the short-term surrogate endpoint of changes in albuminuria as a surrogate for the longer term outcome of decline in renal function. Such assumption is no longer tenable in view of the increasing number of studies showing a dissociation between albuminuria and renal function decline; ACCOMPLISH [77] and in people with diabetes ASCEND (Endothelin receptor blockade), ONTARGET (dual RAS blockade), and VA NEPHRON-D (dual RAS blockade), among others, are all discussed above.

A large number of interventions have not been reviewed in this chapter as they had no impact on clinical practice and are unlikely to do so in the future. They have been outlined in a number of recent publications [78, 79]. They are mostly proof-of-concept studies that have no advanced to large Phase 3 RCTs to date.

Recommendations for RCTs on DKD

1. GFR has to be measured if the aim of the RCT is the evaluation of the impact on an intervention of DKD progression. Too many compounds with gastrointestinal side

effects and/or inducing weight loss (low protein diets, Pirfenidone, Bardoxolone) have been inappropriately tested by using serum creatinine/eGFR as primary endpoint to claim improved renal function when in reality these changes in these parameters reflected serious adverse effects and harm to patients.

2. Serum creatinine /eGFR are soft and unpredictable surrogate endpoints that should not be used as primary endpoint in RCTs testing new therapeutic compounds.

3. Microalbuminuria/albuminuria is no longer acceptable as a surrogate marker for DKD progression in view of the numerous disconnect between changes in its excretion rate and the harder endpoint/outcome of disease progression [80].

4. Interventions impacting blood pressure levels should be supported by accurate BP recordings and not occasional office BP measurements. 24 h ABPM would be recommended in studies focusing on the impact of BP control or using agents that affect blood pressure.

5. A well-defined and mostly homogeneous and progressive population would increase the likelihood of positive outcomes with smaller sample size. To include patients with type 1 and 2 DM and GFR ranging from 90 to 15 ml/min or albuminuria from normal to macroalbuminuria reflect poor RCT design that seriously compromises the likelihood of a meaningful outcome.

6. RCTs should also focus on progressive DN, as studies where the control/placebo group is not progressive (as in BEAM) raise questions regarding the whole premise of the clinical trial.

7. Focus on DM patients with detectable renal/cardiovascular disease (secondary prevention) may yield more results than those aimed at primary prevention warranting much larger sample size and longer follow-up.

8. A better understanding of the changing nature of DM [81] and DKD with slower CKD progression and less albuminuria in older T2DM [82] has to be taken into consideration. Many have primarily a hypertensive and ischemic nephropathy rather than the putative hyperperfused and hyperfiltering kidneys upon which many interventions have been based over the recent decades.

References

1. Hossain P, Kawar B, El Nahas M. Obesity and diabetes in the developing world – a growing challenge. N Engl J Med. 2007;356(3):213–5.
2. Harjutsalo V, Groop PH. Epidemiology and risk factors for diabetic kidney disease. Adv Chronic Kidney Dis. 2014;21(3):260–6.
3. Giorgino F, Leonardini A, Laviola L. Cardiovascular disease and glycemic control in type 2 diabetes: now that the dust is settling from large clinical trials. Ann N Y Acad Sci. 2013;1281:36–50.
4. Yamout H, Lazich I, Bakris GL. Blood pressure, hypertension, RAAS blockade, and drug therapy in diabetic kidney disease. Adv Chronic Kidney Dis. 2014;21(3):281–6.
5. Anderson S, Brenner BM. Influence of antihypertensive therapy on development and progression of diabetic glomerulopathy. Diabetes Care. 1988;11(10):846–9.
6. Lewis EJ, Hunsicker LG, Bain RP, Rohde RD. The effect of angiotensin-converting-enzyme inhibition on diabetic nephropathy. The Collaborative Study Group. N Engl J Med. 1993;329(20): 1456–62.
7. Stanton RC. Clinical challenges in diagnosis and management of diabetic kidney disease. Am J Kidney Dis. 2014;63(2 Suppl 2):S3–21.
8. Khwaja A, El Kossi M, Floege J, El Nahas M. The management of CKD: a look into the future. Kidney Int. 2007;72(11):1316–23.
9. Fernandez-Fernandez B, Ortiz A, Gomez-Guerrero C, Egido J. Therapeutic approaches to diabetic nephropathy-beyond the RAS. Nat Rev Nephrol. 2014;10:325–46. doi:10.1038/nrneph.2014.74.
10. Giorgino F, Leonardini A, Laviola L. Cardiovascular disease and glycemic control in type 2 diabetes: now that the dust is settling from large clinical trials. Ann N Y Acad Sci. 2013;1281:36–50.
11. Macisaac RJ, Ekinci EI, Jerums G. Progressive diabetic nephropathy. How useful is microalbuminuria?: contra. Kidney Int. 2014;86:50–7. doi:10.1038/ki.2014.98.
12. The Diabetes Control and Complications Trial Research Group. The effect of intensive treatment of diabetes on the development and progression of long-term complications in insulin-dependent diabetes mellitus. N Engl J Med. 1993;329(14):977–86.
13. Bakris GL, Molitch M. Microalbuminuria as a risk predictor in diabetes: the continuing saga. Diabetes Care. 2014;37(3):867–75.
14. Mauer M, Zinman B, Gardiner R, Suissa S, Sinaiko A, Strand T, Drummond K, Donnelly S, Goodyer P, Gubler MC, Klein R. Renal and retinal effects of enalapril and losartan in type 1 diabetes. N Engl J Med. 2009;361(1):40–51.
15. DCCT/EDIC Research Group, de Boer IH, Sun W, Cleary PA, Lachin JM, Molitch ME, Steffes MW, Zinman B. Intensive diabetes therapy and glomerular filtration rate in type 1 diabetes. N Engl J Med. 2011;365(25):2366–76.
16. Giorgino F, Leonardini A, Laviola L. Cardiovascular disease and glycemic control in type 2 diabetes: now that the dust is settling from large clinical trials. Ann N Y Acad Sci. 2013;1281:36–50.
17. Rosansky SJ, Glassock RJ. Is a decline in estimated GFR an appropriate surrogate end point for renoprotection drug trials? Kidney Int. 2014;85(4):723–7.
18. Thomas MC, Jerums G, Tsalamandris C, Macisaac R, Panagiotopoulos S, Cooper ME, MDNSG Study Group. Increased tubular organic ion clearance following chronic ACE inhibition in patients with type 1 diabetes. Kidney Int. 2005;67(6):2494–9.
19. Mancia G, et al. 2013 ESH/ESC guidelines for the management of arterial hypertension: the Task Force for the Management of Arterial Hypertension of the European Society of Hypertension (ESH) and of the European Society of Cardiology (ESC). Eur Heart J. 2013;34(28):2159–219.
20. Niiranen TJ, Mäki J, Puukka P, Karanko H, Jula AM. Office, home, and ambulatory blood pressures as predictors of cardiovascular risk. Hypertension. 2014. pii: HYPERTENSIONAHA.114.03292. [Epub ahead of print].
21. Brenner BM, Cooper ME, de Zeeuw D, et al. The Losartan Renal Protection Study: rationale, study design and baseline characteristics of RENAAL (Reduction of Endpoints in NIDDM with the Angiotensin II Antagonist Losartan). J Renin Angiotensin Aldosterone Syst. 2000;1(4):328–35.
22. Heart Outcomes Prevention Evaluation Study Investigators. Effects of ramipril on cardiovascular and microvascular outcomes in people with diabetes mellitus: results of the HOPE study and MICRO-HOPE substudy. Lancet. 2000;355(9200):253–9.
23. Thomas MC, Tikellis C, Burns WC, Thallas V, Forbes JM, Cao Z, Osicka TM, Russo LM, Jerums G, Ghabrial H, Cooper ME,

Kantharidis P. Reduced tubular cation transport in diabetes: prevented by ACE inhibition. Kidney Int. 2003;63(6):2152–61.

24. Thomas MC, Jerums G, Tsalamandris C, Macisaac R, Panagiotopoulos S, Cooper ME, MDNSG Study Group. Increased tubular organic ion clearance following chronic ACE inhibition in patients with type 1 diabetes. Kidney Int. 2005;67(6):2494–9.

25. Montori VM, Permanyer-Miralda G, Ferreira-González I, Busse JW, Pacheco-Huergo V, Bryant D, Alonso J, Akl EA, Domingo-Salvany A, Mills E, Wu P, Schünemann HJ, Jaeschke R, Guyatt GH. Validity of composite end points in clinical trials. BMJ. 2005;330:594.

26. Niiranen TJ, Mäki J, Puukka P, Karanko H, Jula AM. Office, home, and ambulatory blood pressures as predictors of cardiovascular risk. Hypertension. 2014. pii: HYPERTENSIONAHA.114.03292. [Epub ahead of print].

27. Svensson P, de Faire U, Sleight P, Yusuf S, Ostergren J. Comparative effects of ramipril on ambulatory and office blood pressures: a HOPE Substudy. Hypertension. 2001;38(6):E28–32.

28. Rodby RA, Rohde RD, Clarke WR, et al. The Irbesartan type II diabetic nephropathy trial: study design and baseline patient characteristics. Nephrol Dial Transplant. 2000;15:487–97.

29. Thomas MC, Tikellis C, Burns WC, Thallas V, Forbes JM, Cao Z, Osicka TM, Russo LM, Jerums G, Ghabrial H, Cooper ME, Kantharidis P. Reduced tubular cation transport in diabetes: prevented by ACE inhibition. Kidney Int. 2003;63(6):2152–61.

30. Thomas MC, Jerums G, Tsalamandris C, Macisaac R, Panagiotopoulos S, Cooper ME, MDNSG Study Group. Increased tubular organic ion clearance following chronic ACE inhibition in patients with type 1 diabetes. Kidney Int. 2005;67(6):2494–9.

31. Montori VM, Permanyer-Miralda G, Ferreira-González I, Busse JW, Pacheco-Huergo V, Bryant D, Alonso J, Akl EA, Domingo-Salvany A, Mills E, Wu P, Schünemann HJ, Jaeschke R, Guyatt GH. Validity of composite end points in clinical trials. BMJ. 2005;330:594.

32. Packham DK, Ivory SE, Reutens AT, Wolfe R, Rohde R, Lambers Heerspink H, Dwyer JP, Atkins RC, Lewis J, Collaborative Study Group. Proteinuria in type 2 diabetic patients with renal impairment: the changing face of diabetic nephropathy. Nephron Clin Pract. 2011;118(4):c331–8.

33. Tuomi T, Santoro N, Caprio S, Cai M, Weng J, Groop L. The many faces of diabetes: a disease with increasing heterogeneity. Lancet. 2014;383(9922):1084–94.

34. ONTARGET Investigators, Yusuf S, Teo KK, Pogue J, Dyal L, Copland I, Schumacher H, Dagenais G, Sleight P, Anderson C. Telmisartan, ramipril, or both in patients at high risk for vascular events. N Engl J Med. 2008;358(15):1547–59.

35. Parving HH, Brenner BM, McMurray JJ, de Zeeuw D, Haffner SM, Solomon SD, Chaturvedi N, Persson F, Desai AS, Nicolaides M, Richard A, Xiang Z, Brunel P, Pfeffer MA, ALTITUDE Investigators. Cardiorenal end points in a trial of aliskiren for type 2 diabetes. N Engl J Med. 2012;367(23):2204–13.

36. Bakris GL, Sarafidis PA, Weir MR, Dahlöf B, Pitt B, Jamerson K, Velazquez EJ, Staikos-Byrne L, Kelly RY, Shi V, Chiang YT, Weber MA, ACCOMPLISH Trial Investigators. Renal outcomes with different fixed-dose combination therapies in patients with hypertension at high risk for cardiovascular events (ACCOMPLISH): a prespecified secondary analysis of a randomised controlled trial. Lancet. 2010;375(9721):1173–81.

37. ONTARGET Investigators, Yusuf S, Teo KK, Pogue J, Dyal L, Copland I, Schumacher H, Dagenais G, Sleight P, Anderson C. Telmisartan, ramipril, or both in patients at high risk for vascular events. N Engl J Med. 2008;358(15):1547–59.

38. Parving HH, Brenner BM, McMurray JJ, de Zeeuw D, Haffner SM, Solomon SD, Chaturvedi N, Persson F, Desai AS, Nicolaides M, Richard A, Xiang Z, Brunel P, Pfeffer MA, ALTITUDE Investigators. Cardiorenal end points in a trial of aliskiren for type 2 diabetes. N Engl J Med. 2012;367(23):2204–13.

39. ONTARGET Investigators, Yusuf S, Teo KK, Pogue J, Dyal L, Copland I, Schumacher H, Dagenais G, Sleight P, Anderson C. Telmisartan, ramipril, or both in patients at high risk for vascular events. N Engl J Med. 2008;358(15):1547–59.

40. Ruggenenti P, Fassi A, Ilieva AP, Bruno S, Iliev IP, Brusegan V, Rubis N, Gherardi G, Arnoldi F, Ganeva M, Ene-Iordache B, Gaspari F, Perna A, Bossi A, Trevisan R, Dodesini AR, Remuzzi G Bergamo Nephrologic Diabetes Complications Trial (BENEDICT) Investigators. Preventing microalbuminuria in type 2 diabetes. N Engl J Med. 2004;351(19):1941–51.

41. Haller H, Ito S, Izzo Jr JL, Januszewicz A, Katayama S, Menne J, Mimran A, Rabelink TJ, Ritz E, Ruilope LM, Rump LC, Viberti G. ROADMAP Trial Investigators. Olmesartan for the delay or prevention of microalbuminuria in type 2 diabetes. N Engl J Med. 2011;364(10):907–17.

42. Estacio RO, Savage S, Nagel NJ, Schrier RW. Baseline characteristics of participants in the Appropriate Blood Pressure Control in Diabetes trial. Control Clin Trials. 1996;17:242–57.

43. Abstract; Savage et al. American Society of Nephrology Meeting. 1993.

44. Kohan DE, Pritchett Y, Molitch M, Wen S, Garimella T, Audhya P, Andress DL. Addition of atrasentan to renin-angiotensin system blockade reduces albuminuria in diabetic nephropathy. J Am Soc Nephrol. 2011;22(4):763–72.

45. Stanton RC. Clinical challenges in diagnosis and management of diabetic kidney disease. Am J Kidney Dis. 2014;63(2 Suppl 2):S3–21.

46. Miyata T, Suzuki N, van Ypersele de Strihou C. Diabetic nephropathy: are there new and potentially promising therapies targeting oxygen biology? Kidney Int. 2013;84(4):693–702.

47. Arora MK, Singh UK. Oxidative stress: meeting multiple targets in pathogenesis of diabetic nephropathy. Curr Drug Targets. 2014;15(5):531–8.

48. Rojas-Rivera J, Ortiz A, Egido J. Antioxidants in kidney diseases: the impact of bardoxolone methyl. Int J Nephrol. 2012;2012:321714.

49. Pergola PE, Raskin P, Toto RD, Meyer CJ, Huff JW, Grossman EB, Krauth M, Ruiz S, Audhya P, Christ-Schmidt H, Wittes J, Warnock DG, BEAM Study Investigators. Bardoxolone methyl and kidney function in CKD with type 2 diabetes. N Engl J Med. 2011;365(4):327–36.

50. Tayek JA, Kalantar-Zadeh K. The extinguished BEACON of bardoxolone: not a Monday morning quarterback story. Am J Nephrol. 2013;37(3):208–11.

51. Sharma K, Ix JH, Mathew AV, Cho M, Pflueger A, Dunn SR, Francos B, Sharma S, Falkner B, McGowan TA, Donohue M, Ramachandrarao S, Xu R, Fervenza FC, Kopp JB. Pirfenidone for diabetic nephropathy. J Am Soc Nephrol. 2011;22(6):1144–51.

52. Tayek JA, Kalantar-Zadeh K. The extinguished BEACON of bardoxolone: not a Monday morning quarterback story. Am J Nephrol. 2013;37(3):208–11.

53. Pirfenidone. First, do no harm. Prescrire Int. 2013;22(138):117–9.

54. Stanton RC. Clinical challenges in diagnosis and management of diabetic kidney disease. Am J Kidney Dis. 2014;63(2 Suppl 2):S3–21.

55. D'Agati V, Yan SF, Ramasamy R, Schmidt AM. RAGE, glomerulosclerosis and proteinuria: roles in podocytes and endothelial cells. Trends Endocrinol Metab. 2010;21(1):50–6.

56. Degenhardt TP, Alderson NL, Arrington DD, Beattie RJ, Basgen JM, Steffes MW, Thorpe SR, Baynes JW. Pyridoxamine inhibits early renal disease and dyslipidemia in the streptozotocin-diabetic rat. Kidney Int. 2002;61:939–50.

57. Williams ME, Bolton WK, Khalifah RG, Degenhardt TP, Schotzinger RJ, McGill JB. Effects of pyridoxamine in combined phase 2 studies of patients with type 1 and type 2 diabetes and overt nephropathy. Am J Nephrol. 2007;27:605–14.

58. Lauver DA, Lucchesi B. Sulodexide: a renewed interest in this glycos-aminoglycan. Cardiovasc Drug Rev. 2006;24:214–26.

59. Gambaro G, Cavazzana AO, Luzi P, Piccoli A, Borsatti A, Crepaldi G, Marchi E, Venturini AP, Baggio B. Glycosaminoglycans prevent morphological renal alterations and albuminuria in diabetic rats. Kidney Int. 1992;42:285–91.

60. Gambaro G, Kinalska I, Oksa A, Pont'uch P, Hertlová M, Olsovsky J, Manitius J, Fedele D, Czekalski S, Perusicová J, Skrha J, Taton J, Grzeszczak W, Crepaldi G. Oral sulodexide reduces albuminuria in microalbuminuric and macroalbuminuric type 1 and type 2 diabetic patients: the Di.N.A.S. randomized trial. J Am Soc Nephrol. 2002;13:1615–25.

61. Achour A, Kacem M, Dibej K, Skhiri H, Bouraoui S, El May M. One year course of oral sulodexide in the management of diabetic nephropathy. J Nephrol. 2005;18:568–74.

62. Pérez-Gómez MV, Ortiz-Arduán A, Lorenzo-Sellares V. Vitamin D and proteinuria: a critical review of molecular bases and clinical experience. Nefrologia. 2013;33(5):716–26.

63. Wang Y, Deb Dk, Zhang Z, et al. Vitamin D receptor signalling in podocytes protects against diabetic nephropathy. J Am Soc Nephrol, 2012;23:1977–86.

64. Weir MR. Short term effects of vitamin D receptor activation on serum creatinine, creatinine generation and glomerular filtration. Kidney Int. 2011;80:1016–7.

65. ONTARGET Investigators, Yusuf S, Teo KK, Pogue J, Dyal L, Copland I, Schumacher H, Dagenais G, Sleight P, Anderson C. Telmisartan, ramipril, or both in patients at high risk for vascular events. N Engl J Med. 2008;358(15):1547–59.

66. Fried LF, Emanuele N, Zhang JH, Brophy M, Conner TA, Duckworth W, Leehey DJ, McCullough PA, O'Connor T, Palevsky PM, Reilly RF, Seliger SL, Warren SR, Watnick S, Peduzzi P, Guarino P, VA NEPHRON-D Investigators. Combined angiotensin inhibition for the treatment of diabetic nephropathy. N Engl J Med. 2013;369(20):1892–903.

67. Mann JF, Green D, Jamerson K, Ruilope LM, Kuranoff SJ, Littke T, Viberti G, ASCEND Study Group. Avosentan for overt diabetic nephropathy. J Am Soc Nephrol. 2010;21(3):527–35.

68. Giorgino F, Leonardini A, Laviola L. Cardiovascular disease and glycemic control in type 2 diabetes: now that the dust is settling from large clinical trials. Ann N Y Acad Sci. 2013;1281:36–50.

69. Arguedas JA, Leiva V, Wright JM. Blood pressure targets for hypertension in people with diabetes mellitus. Cochrane Database Syst Rev. 2013;10:CD008277. doi:10.1002/14651858.CD008277.pub2.

70. Reboldi G, Gentile G, Manfreda VM, Angeli F, Verdecchia P. Tight blood pressure control in diabetes: evidence-based review of treatment targets in patients with diabetes. Curr Cardiol Rep. 2012;14(1):89–96.

71. Casas JP, Chua W, Loukogeorgakis S, Vallance P, Smeeth L, Hingorani AD, MacAllister RJ. Effect of inhibitors of the renin-angiotensin system and other antihypertensive drugs on renal outcomes: systematic review and meta-analysis. Lancet. 2005;366(9502):2026–33.

72. Wu HY, Huang JW, Lin HJ, Liao WC, Peng YS, Hung KY, Wu KD, Tu YK, Chien KL. Comparative effectiveness of renin-angiotensin system blockers and other antihypertensive drugs in patients with diabetes: systematic review and bayesian network meta-analysis. BMJ. 2013;347:f6008. doi:10.1136/bmj.f6008.

73. Blood Pressure Lowering Treatment Trialists' Collaboration, Ninomiya T, Perkovic V, Turnbull F, Neal B, Barzi F, Cass A, Baigent C, Chalmers J, Li N, Woodward M, MacMahon S. Blood pressure lowering and major cardiovascular events in people with and without chronic kidney disease: meta-analysis of randomised controlled trials. BMJ. 2013;347:f5680. doi:10.1136/bmj.f5680.

74. Savarese G, Costanzo P, Cleland JG, Vassallo E, Ruggiero D, Rosano G, Perrone-Filardi P. A meta-analysis reporting effects of angiotensin-converting enzyme inhibitors and angiotensin receptor blockers in patients without heart failure. J Am Coll Cardiol. 2013;61(2):131–42.

75. Thomas MC, Tikellis C, Burns WC, Thallas V, Forbes JM, Cao Z, Osicka TM, Russo LM, Jerums G, Ghabrial H, Cooper ME, Kantharidis P. Reduced tubular cation transport in diabetes: prevented by ACE inhibition. Kidney Int. 2003;63(6):2152–61.

76. Thomas MC, Jerums G, Tsalamandris C, Macisaac R, Panagiotopoulos S, Cooper ME, MDNSG Study Group. Increased tubular organic ion clearance following chronic ACE inhibition in patients with type 1 diabetes. Kidney Int. 2005;67(6):2494–9.

77. Bakris GL, Sarafidis PA, Weir MR, Dahlöf B, Pitt B, Jamerson K, Velazquez EJ, Staikos-Byrne L, Kelly RY, Shi V, Chiang YT, Weber MA, ACCOMPLISH Trial investigators. Renal outcomes with different fixed-dose combination therapies in patients with hypertension at high risk for cardiovascular events (ACCOMPLISH): a prespecified secondary analysis of a randomised controlled trial. Lancet. 2010;375(9721):1173–81.

78. Fernandez-Fernandez B, Ortiz A, Gomez-Guerrero C, Egido J. Therapeutic approaches to diabetic nephropathy-beyond the RAS. Nat Rev Nephrol. 2014. doi:10.1038/nrneph.2014.74.

79. Khwaja A, El Kossi M, Floege J, El Nahas M. The management of CKD: a look into the future. Kidney Int. 2007;72(11):1316–23.

80. Macisaac RJ, Ekinci EI, Jerums G. Progressive diabetic nephropathy. How useful is microalbuminuria?: contra. Kidney Int. 2014;86:50–7. doi:10.1038/ki.2014.98.

81. Tuomi T, Santoro N, Caprio S, Cai M, Weng J, Groop L. The many faces of diabetes: a disease with increasing heterogeneity. Lancet. 2014;383(9922):1084–94.

82. Packham DK, Ivory SE, Reutens AT, Wolfe R, Rohde R, Lambers Heerspink H, Dwyer JP, Atkins RC, Lewis J, Collaborative Study Group. Proteinuria in type 2 diabetic patients with renal impairment: the changing face of diabetic nephropathy. Nephron Clin Pract. 2011;118(4):c331–8.

Richard J. Glassock

Introduction

The evidence base upon which a rational approach to the management of primary glomerular disease has been building slowly over many decades. Unfortunately, the quality of the studies encompassing this data base has varied widely, in part due to difficulties in study design and subject enrolment. Many studies have been small and underpowered and have used surrogate endpoints, such as a change in proteinuria. Unintentional or unavoidable biases have crept into study execution, and few have been sufficiently long term to evaluate "hard" outcomes such as avoidance of end-stage renal disease (ESRD). The use of estimated rather than measured GFR may have added a further bias in the few studies with renal function endpoints. Due to the limited knowledge of etiology and pathogenesis of primary glomerular disease, most studies have examined the effects of "nonspecific" empirical treatments (such as the use of glucocorticoids or immunosuppressive agents). Nevertheless, there is a "ray of sunshine." Recent trials have employed more rigorous trial design and sample sizes appropriate to minimize the β error (false negatives). Increasingly, the focus has been on more homogeneous group of enrollees with a reasonably well-defined prognosis, in the absence of treatment. Active comparator rather than placebo-controlled trials dominates the landscape, and many trials are not double blinded, leading to the potential for bias.

The studies that have been selected for this review span almost 45 years of history. They have been chosen to illustrate the need for critical appraisal of the individual studies, lest treatments be erroneously accepted as based on high-quality evidence. Not all studies appearing in the literature during this interval have been chosen for critical appraisal, but those discussed are fairly representative of what has transpired over the past four and one half decades. It will be immediately obvious that many gaps in our knowledge still exist and much work still needs to be done in order to provide a rational basis for treatment of these disorders. This analysis will focus on minimal change disease (MCD), focal and segmental glomerulosclerosis (FSGS), membranous nephropathy (MN), IgA nephropathy, and membranoproliferative glomerulonephritis (MPGN). In 2010, the Kidney Disease Improving Global Outcomes (KDIGO) Clinical Practice Guidelines for Glomerulonephritis Work Group undertook a comprehensive study of the quality of evidence base in the treatment of primary (and secondary) glomerular diseases. The reader is referred to this very valuable document for additional information on the quality assessment of published trials [1]. By design, this review will embrace only studies reported as "randomized clinical trials" (RCT) in which the publication included sufficient detail to make its evaluation meaningful and reasonably complete. All trials selected (N=24) have been extensively cited in the literature following their completion and publication in peer-reviewed journals, and many have had a significant impact on clinical practice. Systematic reviews and meta-analyses that "bundle" several RCT have not been included, except by reference citation, as appropriate. Long-term follow-up of the initial trials have been included when available. Early studies did not have the advantage of the CONSORT guideline statement for reporting of RCT, and it is not surprising that they receive much lower ratings than later studies [2].

It is hoped that this analytical review will give the reader some insights on the strengths and weakness of the extant literature on RCTs in treatment of primary glomerular disease.

General Studies

Trial #1

Black DAK, Rose G, Brewer DE. Controlled trial of prednisone in adult patients with the nephrotic syndrome. Brit Med J. 1970;3:421–26.

R.J. Glassock, MD, MACP
Department of Medicine,
Geffen School of Medicine at UCLA,
8 Bethany, Laguna Niguel, CA 92677, USA
e-mail: glassock@cox.net

M. El Kossi, A. Khwaja, and M. El Nahas (eds.), *Informing Clinical Practice in Nephrology: The Role of RCTs*,
DOI 10.1007/978-3-319-10292-4_10, © Springer International Publishing Switzerland 2015

Abstract

A multicenter controlled trial of steroid treatment of the nephrotic syndrome was carried out on 125 patients. Of these, 64 were controls and 61 received prednisone in a recommended dose range of 20–30 mg/24 h. The actual initial dose averaged 29 mg/24 h. Treatment was continued for a variable period, but not less than 6 months. More than 10 mg/24 h was given on average for 12 months to all patients and for longer periods to some. Patients were classified, on the basis of biopsy specimens, into three groups: A, minimal change; B, membranous nephropathy; and C, proliferative glomerulonephritis. In groups B and C, prednisone did not have any strikingly favorable effect on proteinuria or on renal function as compared with the control group. In group A, however, prednisone reduced proteinuria to a striking and statistically significant extent. It had little if any effect on long-term renal function in any group. The death rate was higher in the combined prednisone groups (17/61) than in the control groups (12/64). This difference was not statistically significant, but there was a significantly higher number of deaths from cardiovascular disease in the prednisone group, whereas the numbers of deaths from renal failure were not significantly different in the two groups.

Critical Appraisal

Parameters	Yes	No	Comment
Validity			
Is the **randomization** procedure well described?		−1	
Double **blinded**?		−2	
Is the **sample size** calculation described/adequate?		−3	
Does it have a hard primary **endpoint**?		−1	
Is the endpoint surrogate?	−2		
Is the follow-up appropriate?	+1		
Was there a **bias**?		+2	
Is the dropout >25 %?		+1	
Is the analysis **ITT**?		−3	
Utility/usefulness			
Can the findings be generalized?	+1		
Was the NNT <100?			
Score	**0 %**		

Comments and Discussion

This seminal trial was included mainly for historical purposes as it was the first serious attempt to conduct an RCT in the field of treatment of glomerular diseases. As can be seen from the *Critical Appraisal* above, it had many flaws when judged by a contemporary standard of reference. The power of the study to detect an effect of prednisone in the individual histological groups was low due to the small sample sizes. The dosage of prednisone (about 30 mg/day for about 6 months) would be considered inadequate by current guidelines. Nevertheless, this trial did point to a potential beneficial effect of prednisone in MCD, particularly during the first 2 months of treatment, and a rather high spontaneous remission rate in MCD (about 40 % after 1 year of follow-up). No clear benefits for proteinuria or kidney function could be shown for MN or proliferative glomerulonephritis probably (including cases of IgA N and MPGN), but follow-up was relatively short (2 years). Spontaneous remissions of proteinuria were uncommon in MN (<10 %). Focal and segmental glomerulosclerosis (FSGS) was not separately identified as it had not been widely recognized at the time this study commenced as an important and common lesion underlying nephrotic syndrome in adults and children, although it has been described by Arnold Rich in 1957 [3]. It is noteworthy that adverse events of prednisone treatment were common, including mortality, especially in the early months of treatment and in older individuals – a problem that persists to this day.

Conclusion

Viewed from the prism of history, this seriously flawed study did not have a lasting effect on practice, and its findings were superseded by later (and better) studies to be described below.

Minimal Change Disease

Trial #2

Barratt TM, Soothill JF. Controlled trial of cyclophosphamide in steroid-sensitive relapsing nephrotic syndrome of childhood. Lancet. 1970;2:479–82.

Abstract

A significant reduction in the incidence of relapse of steroid-sensitive nephrotic syndrome has been shown in a controlled trial of cyclophosphamide given during steroid-maintained remission. Toxicity was very minor, and the regimen constitutes a useful advance in management of these patients. The trial had two special features: the use of a semisequential analysis permitting planned repeated access to the trial data and the demonstration of a therapeutic effect of one drug while the manifestations of the disease were completely suppressed by another.

Critical Appraisal

Parameters	Yes	No	Comment
Validity			
Is the **randomization** procedure well described?	+1		Random from sealed envelops
Double **blinded**?		−2	Open label

Parameters	Yes	No	Comment
Is the **sample size** calculation described/ adequate?		−3	No power calculation
Does it have a hard primary **endpoint**?	0		Relapse is the endpoint. Not possible to have a hard endpoint due to infrequency of events
Is the endpoint surrogate?	−2		
Is the follow-up appropriate?	+1		Followed to relapse
Was there a **bias**?		+2	
Is the dropout >25 %?		+1	
Is the analysis **ITT**?	+3		All patients followed to relapse
Utility/usefulness			
Can the findings be generalized?	+1		
Was the NNT <100?	+1		
Score	**25 %**		

Comments and Discussion

While not evaluated as a high-quality study, this trial did have a significant effect on practice as it was the first to show a potential beneficial action of an alkylating agent on relapses in steroid-sensitive, relapsing MCD in children. The trial was well designed, and all patients were followed, making an analysis by intention to treat superfluous. The analysis was sequential, but the P values were not corrected for multiple analyses. All patients (ages 2.9–12.9 years) had steroid-sensitive and frequently relapsing disease (due to MCD, confirmed by renal biopsy) and were in a steroid-induced remission at the time steroids were tapered with or without a pre-taper regimen of oral cyclophosphamide (CYC) (8 weeks at 3 mg/kg/day). Although the duration of steroid treatment was slightly longer in the CYC group, this most likely did not influence the results. After 4 months of observation, 3/15 patients that received CYC and 11/15 that had received steroids only had relapses ($p < 0.02$). After 1 year of observation, 2/10 patients that had received CYC relapsed, while 9/10 patients that tapered steroids without CYC had relapsed. Adverse side effects were minimal (mild alopecia). Leukopenia was seen in only one patient treated with CYC. The duration of CYC treatment (and cumulative dose) proved to be important in subsequent studies [4, 5]. The cumulative dose of CYC in this study was about 168 mg/kg, below the threshold believed to produce gonadal damage and well below the level associated with an increased risk for neoplasia.

Conclusion

This study provided a new way to reduce the harmful effects of repeated courses of glucocorticoids in multiple relapsing MCD. Concerns about the potential for subtle genetic damage from the CYC were well recognized by the authors and

many studies were subsequently performed to try to establish the minimum effective dose and to examine other less toxic regimens [4, 6]. But this study, despite its weaknesses in design and analysis, did have a profound influence practice. Although 40 years later alkylating agents are much less frequently used as steroid-sparing agent in frequently relapsing and steroid-dependent MCD, due to the development of less "toxic" regimens (see below), they still have a role to play in highly selected cases [1]. Less data is available in adults with multiple relapsing MCD, but CYC is also suggested as a steroid-sparing agent in this group as well [7–9].

Trial #3

Coggins CH, and the Collaborative Study. Adult minimal change nephropathy: experience of the collaborative study of glomerular disease. Trans Am Clin Climatol Assoc. 1986;97:18–26.

Abstract

A randomized, double-blind study of the efficacy of oral prednisone (125 mg every other day for 8 weeks) was conducted in 28 adult patients with nephrotic syndrome and a renal biopsy diagnosis of minimal change disease. A complete remission at the end of observation was observed in 13/14 patients assigned to oral prednisone and in 9/14 assigned to placebo. Complete remission occurred more rapidly in the prednisone-treated groups. Steroid-related toxicity was observed in 4/14 patients in the prednisone group, and doubling of serum creatinine was seen in 4/14 patients in the placebo group. Although no important differences between the treated and placebo groups for long-term outcomes were observed, the study is underpowered to demonstrate this with confidence. Short-term administration of steroids in MCD with nephrotic syndrome may be beneficial, but if prolonged repeated courses of steroids are required for relapses or resistant disease, then the hazards may exceed the benefits. Spontaneous remissions do occur, around 25–60 %, but may take 1–2 years to develop, and impaired kidney function can appear will awaiting the development of a spontaneous remission.

Critical Appraisal

Parameters	Yes	No	Comment
Validity			
Is the **randomization** procedure well described?		−1	Randomization not described
Double **blinded**?	+2		

Parameters	Yes	No	Comment
Is the **sample size** calculation described/ adequate?		−3	Underpowered study
Does it have a hard primary **endpoint**?		−1	Incidence of relapse only
Is the endpoint surrogate?		−2	
Is the follow-up appropriate?		+1	50–60 months
Was there a **bias**?		+2	
Is the dropout >25 %?		+1	
Is the analysis **ITT**?		−3	
Utility/usefulness			
Can the findings be generalized?		+1	
Was the NNT <100?		N/A	Low sample size precludes calculation of NNT
Score	**0 %**		

Comments and Discussion

The manner in which this study is reported limits its critical evaluation, as no statistics are provided and the study design is only briefly described. Nevertheless, it's one of a very few RCT of steroid treatment of MCD. The key findings are that oral steroids, given on an alternate-day regimen over 2 months, can rapidly induce a complete remission of proteinuria in many adults (about 65 % at 6 months), whereas spontaneous complete remissions over a comparable period of time are less apparent (about 15 % at 6 months). Impaired renal function can be seen in patients not treated initially with steroids. Due to relapses requiring additional treatment, steroid toxicity was common (about 30 %) in the steroid-treated arm.

Conclusion

Overall, the evidence provided by this study for the efficacy and safety of steroid treatment of MCD in adults is quite weak, and any suggestions for their use in adults with MCD are largely extrapolated from their effects in children [1]. Subsequent observational studies have suggested that the alternate-day regimen is as effective and safe as a daily regimen of steroids [7] and have also supported the viewpoint that remission is delayed in adults compared to children [8]. Acute kidney injury is more common in adults than in children [9].

Trial #4

Ponticelli C, Edefonti A, Ghio L, Rizzoni G, Rinaldi S, Gusmano R, Lama G, Zacchello C, Confalonieri R, Altieri P, Bettinelli A, Maschio G, Cinotti GA, Fuiano G, Schena FP, Castellani A, Della Casa-Alberighi O. Cyclosporin versus cyclophosphamide for patients with steroid dependent and frequently relapsing idiopathic nephrotic syndrome: a multicenter randomized controlled trial. Nephrol Dial Transplant. 1993;8:1326–32.

Abstract

Objective: To compare the efficacy (maintenance of remission), safety, and tolerability of cyclosporin (CsA) with those of cyclophosphamide in patients with steroid-dependent or frequently relapsing nephrotic syndrome (NS).

Design: Open, prospective, randomized, multicenter, controlled study for parallel groups, stratified for adults and children. The setting was in nephrological departments in Italy.

Subjects and Interventions: Seventy-three patients with steroid-sensitive idiopathic NS admitted to the study were randomly assigned to cyclophosphamide (2.5 mg/kg/day) for 8 weeks or CsA (5 mg/kg/day in adults, 6 mg/kg/day in children) for 9 months, tapered off by 25 % every month until complete discontinuation at month 12. Seven patients lost to follow-up were not considered in the analysis. The remaining 66 patients were followed up for 3–24 months after randomization.

Main Outcome Measures: Relapse-free survival, number of N.S. relapses/patient/year, cumulative dose of prednisone/patient, laboratory investigations (kidney and liver functions, hematological parameters), and incidence of adverse events.

Results: At month 9, 26 of 35 CsA-treated patients were still in complete remission, and a further five patients were in partial remission; 18 of 28 cyclophosphamide-treated patients were in complete remission and 1 in partial remission ($P = NS$). No difference between adults and children was seen with either treatment. The risk of relapse was similar between frequent relapsers (19 of 22) and steroid-dependent patients (8 of 14) given CsA and those given cyclophosphamide (5 of 15 and 6 of 15). The mean number of relapses per year and the mean dose of prednisone per year were significantly less ($P < 0.001$) in both groups for the experimental year than for the year before randomization. At 2 years, 25 % of the patients given CsA (50 % adults and 20 % children) and 63 % of those given cyclophosphamide (40 % adults and 68 % children) had not had any relapse of NS. Tolerance to the two drugs was generally good. The CsA-related side effects were mild and disappeared after drug discontinuation.

Conclusions: This study shows that both treatments are effective and well tolerated; more patients given cyclophosphamide had stable remissions.

Critical Appraisal

Parameters	Yes	No	Comment
Validity			
Is the **randomization** procedure well described?		−1	
Double **blinded**?		−2	Open label
Is the **sample size** calculation described/adequate?		−2	Not described
			But likely to be underpowered
Does it have a hard primary **endpoint**?		−1	Relapse-free survival was the main outcome, but relapse frequency, prednisolone dose, laboratories studies, and adverse events examined See Trial #2
Is the endpoint surrogate?		−1	
Is the follow-up appropriate?		−1	3–24 months
Was there a **bias**?		+2	
Is the dropout >25 %?		+1	
Is the analysis **ITT**?	+3		
Utility/usefulness			
Can the findings be generalized?	+1		
Was the NNT <100?	N/A		A comparative study of two regimens
Score	**0 %**		

Comments and Discussion

While the overall appraisal of this study was moderate to low quality, this was primarily the result of its open-label design and inadequate description of sample size calculation. Nevertheless, this seminal study helped to clarify a potential role for calcineurin inhibitor (CNI) agents in the management of frequently relapsing steroid-dependent patients with either MCD ($n=31$) or FSGS ($n=4$). No biopsies were performed in 31 patients. The study included mainly children with MCD (adults, $n=11$; children, $n=55$). At 1 year of follow-up, an 8-week course of oral cyclophosphamide (CYC; 2.5 mg/kg/day) was approximately equal in efficacy to a 12-month tapering dosage schedule of cyclosporin (CsA; initially 5–6 mg/kg/day) when assessed as actuarial probability of relapse-free survival. Furthermore, remissions seemed to be stable after 1 year with CYC, but relapses developed after 1 year when CsA was discontinued. About 25 % of CsA-treated patients and about 60 % of CYC-treated patients entered into long-term remission (maximum follow-up 2 years). Prednisone dosage and relapse frequency were materially decreased in both groups after 1 year. Adverse events included leukopenia in CYC-treated patients ($n=12$) and hyperbilirubinemia or transaminase elevations in

CsA-treated patients ($n=2$). Reversible gingival hyperplasia and/or hypertrichosis was common in CsA-treated patients. There was no evidence of CsA nephrotoxicity over the treatment period.

Conclusion

This study, despite its weaknesses, contributed significantly to the emergence of CsA as an alternate to CYC in the treatment of MCD with a frequently relapsing course. Similar findings were reported by Niaudet et al. [10] in a low-quality RCT comparing CsA (6-month course at 6 mg/kg/day in tapering dosage) to chlorambucil (0.2 mg/kg/day for 40 days). An adjusted dose regimen of CsA designed to maintain a trough level of 60–80 ng/ml was slightly better than a fixed dose of CsA (2.5 mg/kg/day) in a p-ediatric RCT (by Ishikura and colleagues [11]). However, these studies did not settle the issue of what to do with those who continue to relapse or become CsA dependent. This issue is not yet resolved, but the use of mycophenolate mofetil (MMF) [12] or rituximab [13] may have advantages, not yet fully explored in a well-designed, adequately powered RCT (see also Trials #5 and #6 below).

Trial #5

Dorresteijn EM, Kist-vanHolthe JE, Levtchenko EN, Nauta J, Hopp WC, van dedr Heijden AJ. Mycophenolate mofetil versus cyclosporine for remission maintenance in nephrotic syndrome. Pediatr Nephrol. 2008;23:2013–20.

Abstract

We performed a multicenter randomized controlled trial to compare the efficacy of mycophenolate mofetil (MMF) to that of cyclosporine A (CsA) in treating children with frequently relapsing nephrotic syndrome and biopsy-proven minimal change disease. Of the 31 randomized initially selected patients, 7 were excluded. The remaining 24 children received either MMF 1,200 mg/m(2)/day ($n=12$) or CsA 4–5 mg/kg/day ($n=12$) during a 12-month period. Of the 12 patients in the MMF group, 2 discontinued the study medication. Evaluation of the changes from the baseline glomerular filtration rate showed an overall significant difference in favor of MMF over the treatment period ($p=0.03$). Seven of the 12 patients in the MMF group and 11 of the 12 patients in the CsA group remained in complete remission during the entire study period. Relapse rate in the MMF group was 0.83/year compared to 0.08/year in the CsA group ($p=0.08$). None of the patients reported diarrhea. Pharmacokinetic profiles of mycophenolic acid were performed in seven patients.

The patient with the lowest area under the curve had three relapses within 6 months. In children with frequently relapsing minimal change nephrotic syndrome, MMF has a favorable side effect profile compared to CsA; however, there is a tendency towards a higher relapse risk in patients treated with MMF.

Critical Appraisal

Parameters	Yes	No	Comment
Validity			
Is the **randomization** procedure well described?	+1		
Double **blinded**?		−2	
Is the **sample size** calculation described/adequate?		−3	No power calculation
Does it have a hard primary **endpoint**?		−1	Proteinuria remission See Trial #2
Is the endpoint surrogate?		−1	
Is the follow-up appropriate?	+1		12 months
Was there a **bias**?		+2	
Is the dropout >25 %?		+1	
Is the analysis **ITT**?	+3		
Utility/usefulness			
Can the findings be generalized?	+1		Children only
Was the NNT <100?	N/A		Comparative study
Score	**20 %**		

Comment and Discussion

The high frequency of multiple relapse of nephrotic syndrome in 30 % or more of children with steroid-sensitive nephrotic syndrome due to MCD is a challenging problem. As suggested in RCT analyzed above, a short course of CYC (8–12 weeks) or more prolonged treatment with CsA (1–2 years) can reduce exposure to iatrogenic steroid toxicity and prolong the relapse-free interval in such patients. Long-term nephrotoxicity is a concern with prolonged CsA administration, even in modest doses. This underpowered study sought to examine the potential role of MMF as a steroid-sparing agent to prolong remissions in biopsy-proven MCD and frequent relapses. All subjects were children and were in complete steroid-induced remission when randomized to MMF (1.2 g/m^2/day; maximum dose 2 g/day) or CsA (4–5 mg/kg/day for 12 months). Pharmacokinetic assays for MMF were conducted in parallel. During the 12-month study period, 92 % of the CsA-treated patients remained in remission, while 58 % of those treated with MMF remained in complete remission. The relapse rate in MMF-treated patients was nonsignificantly higher than in CsA-treated patients ($p=0.08$). Renal function was better in the MMF-treated group ($p<0.05$). Relapses in MMF-treated patients appeared to be related to low plasma area under the curve levels. Side effects of MMF were mild.

Conclusion

Due to the study design and inadequate sample size, this study is at best hypothesis generating. The better renal function with MMF is offset by the higher relapse rate. MMF was suggested (evidence level 2C) by the KDIGO work group as an alternate to a CNI [1]. Observational studies have now suggested that rituximab may be the preferred agent for difficult-to-treat multiple-relapsing and steroid-dependent MCD in both adults and children, but only one RCT has yet been performed (see Trial # 7).

Trial # 6

Gellermann J, Web er L, Pape L, Tonshoff B, Hoyer P, Querfeld U. Gesellschaft fur Padiatrische Nephrologie. Mycophenolate mofetil versus cyclosporin a in children with frequently relapsing nephrotic syndrome. J Am Soc Nephrol. 2013;245:1689–97.

Abstract

The severe side effects of long-term corticosteroid or cyclosporin A (CsA) therapy complicate the treatment of children with frequently relapsing steroid-sensitive nephrotic syndrome (FR-SSNS). We conducted a randomized, multicenter open-label, crossover study comparing the efficacy and safety of a 1-year treatment with mycophenolate mofetil (MMF; target plasma mycophenolic acid trough level of 1.5–2.5 µg/ml) or CsA (target trough level of 80–100 ng/ml) in 60 pediatric patients with FR-SSNS. We assessed the frequency of relapse as the primary endpoint and evaluated pharmacokinetic profiles (area under the curve [AUC]) after 3 and 6 months of treatment. More relapses per patient per year occurred with MMF than with CsA during the first year ($P=0.03$) but not during the second year ($P=0.14$). No relapses occurred in 85 % of patients during CsA therapy and in 64 % of patients during MMF therapy ($P=0.06$). However, the time without relapse was significantly longer with CsA than with MMF during the first year ($P<0.05$), but not during the second year ($P=0.36$). In post hoc analysis, patients with low mycophenolic acid exposure (AUC <50 µg·h/ml) experienced 1.4 relapses per year compared with 0.27 relapses per year in those with high exposure (AUC > 50 µg·h/ml; $P<0.05$). There were no significant differences between groups with respect to BP, growth, lipid levels, or adverse events. However, cystatin clearance, estimated GFR, and hemoglobin levels increased significantly with MMF compared with CsA. These results indicate that MMF is inferior to CsA in preventing relapses in pediatric patients with FR-SSNS, but may be a less nephrotoxic treatment option.

Critical Appraisal

Parameters	Yes	No	Comment
Validity			
Is the **randomization** procedure well described?	0		Not well described, crossover design
Double **blinded**?		−2	
Is the **sample size** calculation described/adequate?	+3		Non-inferiority design
Does it have a hard primary **endpoint**?	−1		Proteinuria remission. See Trial #2
Is the endpoint surrogate?	−1		
Is the follow-up appropriate?	+1		
Was there a **bias**?		+2	
Is the dropout >25 %?		+1	
Is the analysis **ITT**?	+3		
Utility/usefulness			
Can the findings be generalized?	+1		Children only
Was the NNT <100?	N/A		Comparative study
Score	**47 %**		

Summary and Discussion

This trial supplements and extends the one conducted by Dorresteijn et al. (see Trial #5) in frequently relapsing nephrotic syndrome (presumed to be due to MCD) and is of much higher quality. Although open label, the crossover design is advantageous. The pharmacokinetic (PK) analyses built into the design provide additional strengths to this study. Early relapses were more frequent with MMF than with CsA, but post hoc analysis of the PK data suggested that this might have been due to low MMF exposure. Estimated GFR was improved by MMF but not CsA, suggesting avoidance of nephrotoxicity. Sustained remissions at 1 year were seen in about 80 % of subjects with MMF treatment and an AUC >50 μg·h/ml, and is about 85 % in those treated with CsA. Serious adverse events were uncommon (7 events out of a total of 111 events in 42 patients) and were seen twice with MMF and seven times with CsA.

Conclusion

Thus, MMF (disregarding PK studies) is inferior to CsA in preventing early relapses in this group of subjects, but it may be less nephrotoxic and perhaps safer. This study also generates the hypothesis that dosage adjustment of MMF according to PK studies will improve outcomes, but a well-designed RCT is required to test this hypothesis. This trial, and others like it, has led to the widespread use of MMF, instead of CYC or CsA, as preferred initial treatment for frequently relapsing and/or steroid-dependent MCD in children. Less data on the benefits of MMF in adults is available. The value of PK studies in augmenting benefits of MMF needs further study. Whether MMF (or CsA) is as effective as steroids for treatment of naive subjects with MCD is unknown (not tested).

Trial #7

Iijima K, Sako M, Nozu K, Mori R, Tuchida N, Kamei K, Miura K, Aya K, Nakanishi K, Ohtomo Y, Takahashi S, Tanaka R, Kaito H, Naklam ura H, Ishikura K, Ito S, Ohashi Y; Rituximab for Childhood-Onset Refractory Nephrotic Syndrome (RCRNS) Study Group. Lancet. 2014.

Abstract

Background: Rituximab could be an effective treatment for childhood-onset, complicated, frequently relapsing nephrotic syndrome (FRNS) and steroid-dependent nephrotic syndrome (SDNS). We investigated the efficacy and safety of rituximab in patients with high disease activity.

Methods: We did a multicenter, double-blind, randomized, placebo-controlled trial at nine centers in Japan. We screened patients aged 2 years or older experiencing a relapse of FRNS or SDNS, which had originally been diagnosed as nephrotic syndrome when aged 1–18 years. Patients with complicated FRNS or SDNS who met all other criteria were eligible for inclusion after remission of the relapse at screening. We used a computer-generated sequence to randomly assign patients (1:1) to receive rituximab (375 mg/m^2) or placebo once weekly for 4 weeks, with age, institution, treatment history, and the intervals between the previous three relapses as adjustment factors. Patients, guardians, caregivers, physicians, and individuals assessing outcomes were masked to assignments. All patients received standard steroid treatment for the relapse at screening and stopped taking immunosuppressive agents by 169 days after randomization. Patients were followed up for 1 year. The primary endpoint was the relapse-free period. Safety endpoints were frequency and severity of adverse events. Patients who received their assigned intervention were included in analyses. This trial is registered with the University Hospital Medical Information Network Clinical Trials Registry, number UMIN000001405.

Findings: Patients were centrally registered between November 13, 2008, and May 19, 2010. Of 52 patients who underwent randomization, 48 received the assigned intervention (24 were given rituximab and 24 placebo). The median relapse-free period was significantly longer in the rituximab group (267 days, 95 % CI 223–374) than in the placebo group (101 days, 70–155; hazard ratio: 0.27, 0.14–0.53; $p < 0.0001$). Ten patients (42 %) in the rituximab group and six (25 %) in the placebo group had at least one serious adverse event ($p = 0.36$).

Interpretation: Rituximab is an effective and safe treatment for childhood-onset, complicated FRNS and SDNS.

Critical Appraisal

Parameters	Yes	No	Comment
Validity			
Is the **randomization** procedure well described?	+1		
Double **blinded**?	+2		Rituximab vs placebo
Is the **sample size** calculation described/ adequate?		−1	Sample size calculated for superiority design and a 40 % response rate in active treatment vs 10 % in placebo at 6 months
			Actual randomization was less than anticipated due to an early interim analysis showing "efficacy" of rituximab
Does it have a hard primary **endpoint**?	−1		Relapse-free interval from randomization
Is the endpoint surrogate?	−1		
Is the follow-up appropriate?	+1		
Was there a **bias**?	−2		Possible confounder of other concomitant medication
Is the dropout >25 %?		+1	4/48 nontreatment failure-related dropouts
Is the analysis **ITT**?	+3		Modified to include patients who received assigned treatment
Utility/usefulness			
Can the findings be generalized?	+1		Children only
Was the NNT <100?	+1		
Score	31 %		

Comment and Discussion

This trial adds significant weight to observational studies suggesting a beneficial effect of rituximab in frequently relapsing or steroid-dependent children (and possibly adults) with presumed (but not necessarily biopsy-proven) MCD. But it also raises new questions. Due to limitations in sample size, it needs further confirmation, and the results may not be applicable to adults. Importantly, most patients had been treated with a variety of other agents (but interestingly not including cyclophosphamide) before randomization. Most patients (over 70 %) exhibited steroid toxicity and had MCD confirmed by renal biopsy. A clear reduction in cumulative prednisone dosage, relapse-free interval, frequency of relapses (per person per year), and initial treatment failure (defined as relapse at 85 days from randomization) were all seen in those patients assigned to

receive rituximab compared to the placebo. Serious adverse events were more commonly observed in the rituximab groups, mostly infection related. No deaths were seen in either groups. Depletion of circulating B19+ B cells was complete until about 20–24 weeks after the first dose of rituximab. About 20 % of the patients assigned to rituximab had a relapse in the first 85 days after randomization, at a time when complete B-cell depletion was present. This raises questions about the posited mechanism of action of rituximab that will require further studies to answer (direct effect of rituximab on podocytes; effect of rituximab on T-cell subsets [14, 15]).

Conclusion

This study indicates that rituximab has a meaningful steroid-sparing and remission-prolonging effect in this difficult-to-treat population of children with nephrotic syndrome and MCD. Additional active comparator RCT (especially with MMF combined with PK analysis (see Trial #6)) will be required to assess the proper role of rituximab in this challenging group of patients.

Focal and Segmental Glomerulosclerosis

Trial #8

Ponticelli C, Rizzoni G, Edefonti A, Altieri P, Rivolta E, Rinaldi S, Ghio L, Lusvarghi E, Gusmano R, Locatgelli F, Pasquali S, Castellan I A, Della Casa-Alberighi O. A randomized trial of cyclosporine in steroid-resistant idiopathic nephrotic syndrome. Kidney Int. 1993; 43:1377–84.

Abstract

To compare the efficacy (induction of remission) and safety of cyclosporine (CsA) with those of supportive therapy in patients with steroid-resistant idiopathic nephrotic syndrome (INS), we organized an open, prospective, randomized, multicentric, controlled study for parallel groups, stratified for adults and children. Forty-five patients with steroid-resistant INS were randomly assigned to supportive therapy or CsA (5 mg/kg/day for adults, 6 mg/kg/day for children) for 6 months, then tapered off by 25 % every 2 months until complete discontinuation. Four patients were lost to follow-up. During the first year, 13/22 CsA-treated patients versus 3 of 19 controls attained remission of the nephrotic syndrome ($P < 0.001$). A symptom score was assessed at time 0 and at 6 months. The mean score significantly decreased in the CsA group ($P < 0.001$), but remained unchanged in the controls. At month 6, the mean urinary protein excretion, the mean serum proteins, and the plasma cholesterol had significantly improved in the CsA group but were not changed in the controls. There were no significant differences in serum creatinine and creatinine clearance between treatments (interaction time* treatments, $P=0.089$ and $P=0.935$, respectively) at month 6 versus basal. The CsA-related side effects were mild; no significant difference in blood pressure between the two groups was seen at any time. This study shows that CsA can bring about remission in some 60 % of patients with steroid-resistant INS. In patients with normal renal function and without severe hypertension, CsA at the therapeutic scheme adopted did not produce severe renal or extrarenal toxicity.

Critical Appraisal

Parameters	Yes	No	Comment
Validity			
Is the **randomization** procedure well described?		0	Partial description
Double **blinded**?		−2	Open label
Is the **sample size** calculation described/ adequate?		−1	Small sample size, most likely underpowered study
Does it have a hard primary **endpoint**?		−1	Remission and changes in proteinuria
Is the endpoint surrogate?	−1		
Is the follow-up appropriate?	+1		
Was there a **bias**?		−1	Center-based effect could be confounder. Definition of "steroid resistance" problematic
Is the dropout >25 %?		+1	
Is the analysis **ITT**?	+3		
Utility/usefulness			
Can the findings be generalized?		0	Cannot be generalized to those with reduced renal function
Was the NNT <100?	+1		
Score	**0 %**		

Comments and Discussion

This study was among the first to suggest a short-term beneficial effect of cyclosporin (CsA) on "steroid-resistant" idiopathic nephrotic syndrome in adults ($n=24$) and children ($n=17$). Not surprisingly a lesion of FSGS was found in 28/51 cases (55 %). The number of MCD cases is higher than one might have expected – many of these cases may have been "misdiagnosed" FSGS. "Steroid resistance" was defined as continued nephrotic syndrome after only 6 weeks (adults) or 5 weeks (children) of treatment with high-dose steroids. This may have been too short by contemporary standards, thus adding a potential bias to the observed remission rates post CsA treatment. The control groups received

supportive therapy only, but "rescue treatment" with steroids was permitted, adding another element of potential bias. Treatment with CsA was at 5 mg/kg/day in adults and 6 mg/kg/day in children with trough blood levels of 250–600 ng/ml with dosage adjustments for impairment of renal function. After 6 months, the CsA was stopped in the absence of a remission or continued in reduced levels for an additional 6 months in those who did remit. The cumulative probability of obtaining a complete or partial remission (CR+PR) of nephrotic syndrome at 1 year was 0.65 in the CsA group and only 0.16 in the control group ($p<.0.001$). Thirty-eight percent of the "responders" remained in remission for at least 12 months. No differences in renal function were observed during the treatment interval in either, but in four subjects in the control group and one in the CsA group developed progress in renal impairment or ESRD within 2 years of follow-up. Adverse events were mild and reversible in both groups.

Conclusions

While some potential for bias is present and short follow-up precluded examination of effects on ESRD, overall this trial supports the widely held view that CsA does play a role in management of steroid-resistant nephrotic syndrome, mainly due to FSGS. The high frequency of CR and PR observed would likely predict avoidance of ESRD over the long term unless CsA nephrotoxicity from repeated courses adds an element of iatrogenic kidney injury. The average baseline serum creatinine in the CsA group was only 0.83 ± 0.09 mg/dl, so no inferences can be made regarding the efficacy or safety of CsA treatment when renal function is impaired (serum creatinine >1.5 mg/dl) at the time treatment is begun. KDIGO does suggest that CsA be considered in management of steroid-resistant FSGS [1], in doses not to exceed 5 mg/kg/day, but prolonged therapy may be required, adding to the risk of nephrotoxicity, especially at the higher dosage levels.

Trial #9

Tarshish P, Tobin JN, Bernstein J, Edelmann CM Jr. **Cyclophosphamide does not benefit patients with focal segmental glomerulosclerosis. A report of the international study of kidney disease in children.** Pediatr Nephrol. 1996;10:590–3.

Abstract

Sixty children, with biopsy-diagnosed focal segmental glomerulosclerosis (FSGS) and with unremitting nephrotic syndrome despite intensive therapy with adrenocortical steroids, were randomly allocated into a clinical trial comparing prednisone, 40 mg/m² on alternate days for a period of 12 months (control group), with the same prednisone regimen plus a 90-day course of daily cyclophosphamide, 2.5 mg/kg in a single morning dose (experimental group). One quarter of the children in each group had complete resolution of proteinuria. The proportions of children with increased, unchanged, and decreased proteinuria by the end of the study were the same in the two groups. Treatment failure was defined as an increase in serum creatinine of 30 % or more or greater than 0.4 mg/dl or onset of renal failure. Treatment failure occurred in 36 % of the control group and 57 % of the experimental group ($P>0.1$). Five patients died during the trial, three in the experimental group, and two in the control group. A Kaplan-Meier survival analysis revealed no significant differences between the two groups. Cyclophosphamide therapy for children with steroid-resistant FSGS is not recommended.

Critical Appraisal

81.969 pt	Yes	No	Comment
Validity			
Is the **randomization** procedure well described?	+1		
Double **blinded**?		−2	
Is the **sample size** calculation described/adequate?		−3	No power calculation
Does it have a hard primary **endpoint**?	+1		Changes in serum creatinine
Is the endpoint surrogate?		0	
Is the follow-up appropriate?	+1		
Was there a **bias**?		+2	
Is the dropout >25 %?		+1	
Is the analysis **ITT**?	+3		Not stated but all children followed to death or renal failure
Utility/usefulness			
Can the findings be generalized?		0	To children only
Was the NNT <100?	N/A		Negative study
Score	**27**%		

Comments and Discussion

This otherwise well-done RCT suffers mainly from a possibility of a deficiency of power (β error). Resistance to high-dose steroid therapy (of at least 8-week duration) was an inclusion criterion. That this definition of "steroid resistance" can be inadequate was exemplified by the fact that 28 % of the patients in the control group experienced a complete remission after randomization with continuation of prednisone in doses of 40 mg/m² every morning for 12 months. However, there was no impact on remission rates when cyclophosphamide (CYC) 2.5 mg/kg/day for 90 days

was added to the continued prednisone regimen identical to the control group. Importantly, an increase in serum creatinine of ≥30 % from baseline, or >0.4 mg/dl, or a serum creatinine of >4.0 mg/dl or ESRD occurred with equal frequency in both groups (36 % in the control group and 57 % in the CYC group).

Conclusion

Except for the caveat about the potential for a β error, this study indicates that CYC should *not* be considered effective (or safe) in pediatric patients with persisting nephrotic syndrome due to FSGS unresponsive to high-dose steroids – a statement that has been codified in the KDIGO Clinical Practice guidelines in 2012 [1]. It does not answer questions arising from observational studies regarding the efficacy or safety of CYC in patients with a lesion of FSGS who are steroid responsive, exhibiting a complete or partial remission to steroid therapy.

Trial #10

Cattran DC, Appel GB, Hebert LA, Hunsicker LG, Pohl MA, Hoy WE, Kunis CL. Randomized trial of cyclosporine in patients with steroid-resistant focal segmental glomerulosclerosis. North American Nephrotic Syndrome Study Group. Kidney Int. 1999;56:2220–6.

Abstract

A randomized trial of cyclosporine in patients with steroid-resistant focal segmental glomerulosclerosis.

Background: A clinical trial of cyclosporine in patients with steroid-resistant focal segmental glomerulosclerosis (FSGS) was conducted. Despite the fact that it is the most common primary glomerulonephritis to progress to renal failure, treatment trials have been very limited.

Methods: We conducted a randomized controlled trial in 49 cases of steroid-resistant FSGS comparing 26 weeks of cyclosporine treatment plus low-dose prednisone to placebo plus prednisone. All patients were followed for an average of 200 weeks, and the short- and long-term effects on renal function were assessed.

Results: Seventy percent of the treatment group versus 4 % of the placebo group ($P<0.001$) had a partial or complete remission of their proteinuria by 26 weeks. Relapse occurred in 40 % of the remitters by 52 weeks and 60 % by week 78, but the remainder stayed in remission to the end of the observation period. Renal function was better preserved in the cyclosporine group. There was a decrease of 50 % in baseline creatinine clearance in 25 % of the treated group compared with 52 % of controls ($P < 0.05$). This was a reduction in risk of 70 % (95 % CI, 9–93) independent of other baseline demographic and laboratory variables.

Conclusions: These results suggest that cyclosporine is an effective therapeutic agent in the treatment of steroid-resistant cases of FSGS. Although a high relapse rate does occur, a long-term decrease in proteinuria and preservation of filtration function were observed in a significant proportion of treated patients.

Critical Appraisal

Parameters	Yes	No	Comment
Validity			
Is the **randomization** procedure well described?	+1		
Double **blinded**?		−2	Investigators were not blinded to patients' allocation
Is the **sample size** calculation described/ adequate?		−1	Calculated for remission only
Does it have a hard primary **endpoint**?		−1	Proteinuria remission by 26 weeks. Renal function decline is a secondary endpoint
Is the endpoint surrogate?	−2		
Is the follow-up appropriate?	+1		
Was there a **bias**?		+2	Definition of "steroid resistance" is suspect. Also investigator unblinding raises concern over potential bias
Is the dropout >25 %?		+1	
Is the analysis **ITT**?		−2	Not explicitly stated in the method
Utility/usefulness			
Can the findings be generalized?		0	Very few African-Americans
Was the NNT <100?		N/A	Comparing between two drug regimens
Score	0 %		

Comments and Discussion

This RCT is largely confirmatory of earlier reports of RCTs of CsA in FSGS by Ponticelli et al. (see Trial #8) [26, 53], Lieberman and Tejani [16], and Jha et al. [25]. It does add useful information in that all subjects were adults and all had biopsy-proven FSGS lesion (excluding collapsing FSGS). The definition of "steroid resistance" was a failure to exhibit a remission after a minimum of 8 weeks of high-dose prednisone, but the actual duration of prednisone therapy was

14 weeks in the placebo and 15 weeks in the CsA groups. The dose of CsA averaged 4.2 ± 2.1 mg/kg over the course of the 26-week treatment period. The groups were largely Caucasian, so the results cannot be extrapolated to other ancestral populations. By the end of the treatment period (26 weeks), 69 % of the CsA arm and 4 % of the placebo arm had experienced a remission (12 % complete and 57 % partial). Due to relapses, the fraction of subjects in the CsA arm remaining in remission at 1–2 years was about 30 %. A 50 % reduction in baseline creatinine clearance was seen in 25 % of the CsA patients and 52 % of the placebo patients at 4 years of follow-up ($p < 0.05$). The overall renal survival rate at the end of the study was not different in the CsA and placebo ($p = 0.10$) groups, but the study was not powered to examine this endpoint. It is noteworthy that the baseline creatinine clearance was 86 ml/min in both groups, so this study is not informative concerning the effect (or safety) of CsA in FSGS in the presence of renal impairment. Adverse effects, other than worsening hypertension, requiring more intense anti hypertensive treatment, were mild, but not well described.

Conclusion

A sustained partial remission rate of close to 30 % and a suggestion of a retardation of renal functional progression support the use of CsA as a treatment for steroid-resistant FSGS in adults. Importantly, the study was not powered to test the impact of the intervention on changes in renal function.

Only 11 of the 26 patients in the CsA arm and 10 of 23 patients in the placebo arm were receiving renin-angiotensin system (RAS) inhibitors at the time of randomization, and this frequency increased in both groups post-randomization due to worsening hypertension; so any comments on the interactions of RAS inhibitors and CsA therapy cannot be estimated, but it seems unlikely that the difference in outcomes between the two groups can be attributed to differences in RAS inhibitor usage. However, the unblinding of the investigators always raises concern about potential bias that might influence confounders.

Trial # 11

Plank C, Kalb V, Hinkes B, Hildebrandt F, Gefeller O, Rascher W; Arbeitgemeinschaft fur Padiatrische Nephrologie. Cyclosporin a is superior to cyclophosphamide in children with steroid-resistant nephrotic syndrome: a randomized controlled multicentre trial by the arbeitsgemeinschaft fur padiatrische nephroplogie. Pediatr Nephrol. 2008;23:1483–93.

Abstract

First-line immunosuppressive treatment in steroid-resistant nephrotic syndrome in children is still open to discussion. We conducted a controlled, multicenter, randomized, open-label trial to test the efficacy and safety of cyclosporin A (CSA) versus cyclophosphamide pulses (CPH) in the initial therapy of children with newly diagnosed primary steroid-resistant nephrotic syndrome and histologically proven minimal change disease, focal segmental glomerulosclerosis, or mesangial hypercellularity. Patients in the CSA group ($n=15$) were initially treated with 150 mg/m(2) CSA orally to achieve trough levels of 120–180 ng/ml, while patients in the CPH group ($n=17$) received CPH pulses (500 mg/m(2)/month intravenous). All patients were on alternate prednisone therapy. Patients with proteinuria >40 mg/m(2)/h at 12 weeks of therapy were allocated to a nonresponder protocol with high-dose CSA therapy or methylprednisolone pulses. At week 12, 9 of the 15 (60 %) CSA patients showed at least partial remission, evidenced by a reduction of proteinuria <40 mg/h/m(2). In contrast, 3 of the 17 (17 %) CPH patients responded ($p<0.05$, intention to treat). Given these results, the study was stopped, in accordance with the protocol. After 24 weeks, complete remission was reached by 2 of the 15 (13 %) CSA and 1 of the 17 (5 %) CPH patients ($p=$n.s.). Partial remission was achieved by 7 of the 15 (46 %) CSA and 2 of the 15 (11 %) CPH patients ($p<0.05$). Five patients in the CSA group and 14 patients in the CPH group were withdrawn from the study, most of them during the nonresponder protocol. The number of adverse events was comparable between both groups. We conclude that CSA is more effective than CPH in inducing at least partial remission in steroid-resistant nephrotic syndrome in children.

Critical Appraisal

Parameters	Yes	No	Comment
Validity			
Is the **randomization** procedure well described?	+1		
Double **blinded**?		−2	
Is the **sample size** calculation described/ adequate?		−3	Study was underpowered. Calculated sample size for 80 % power to detect a 38 % difference in remission rate was 28 patients per group. Only 15–17 recruited
Does it have a hard primary **endpoint**?		−1	Remission of proteinuria
Is the endpoint surrogate?	−2		
Is the follow-up appropriate?	+1		
Was there a **bias**?		+2	
Is the dropout >25 %?		+1	
Is the analysis **ITT**?	+3		

Parameters	Yes	No	Comment
Utility/usefulness			
Can the findings be generalized?	+1		But not to African-Americans
Was the NNT <100?		N/A	Comparative study
Score	**0 %**		

Comments and Discussion

This underpowered multicenter study attempted to clarify the utility of oral cyclosporine (150 mg/m²/day over 24 weeks; CsA; $n=15$) versus intravenous pulses of cyclophosphamide (500 mg/m² times 6 doses over 36 weeks-CYC; $n=17$) in children with steroid-resistant nephrotic syndrome, mainly due to FSGS. Steroid resistance was defined as a failure to achieve complete remission within 4 weeks of standard oral high-dose prednisone treatment + three additional pulses of IV methylprednisolone with 2-week follow-up. The protocol allowed for escalation of CsA dosage if treatment failed to induce a remission by 12 weeks or the addition of methyl prednisolone pulses if no response was seen by 12 weeks in the CYC group. Both groups receive oral prednisone in decreasing dosage over 48 weeks. Genetic forms of FSGS were excluded by exon sequencing for *NPHS2 and WT1*. Renal biopsies were required for enrolment. The primary endpoint was complete remission at 24 weeks.

Overall there were 21 cases of FSGS, 10 cases of MCD, and 1 case of mesangial proliferative GN. Renal function was normal in most patients at entry. No African-American was enrolled. RAS inhibitors were used in 20 of 32 patients. A complete or partial remission (CR or PR) of proteinuria developed in 9 of 15 subjects in the CsA arm (60 % with CR in 13 % and PR in 47 %), but a CR or PR developed in only 3 of 17 subjects in the CYC arm (18 % with a CR in 6 % and a PR in 12 %). Adverse events were approximately equal in the two groups. The protocol was terminated early due to apparent superiority of CsA in inducing a CR or PR.

Conclusion

Although this study exhibited several weaknesses, including an inadequate sample size and inadequate power, it supports superiority of CsA over intravenous CYC in treatment of steroid-resistant nephrotic syndrome, mainly due to FSGS. In spite of such shortcomings and therefore the difficulty in interpretation of the study outcome, when considered in the light of other studies, it has seemingly "closed the door" on the use of CYC as a disease-modifying agent in steroid-resistant nephrotic syndrome, at least in European Caucasians (see also KDIGO Clinical Practice Guidelines for Glomerulonephritis [1]).

Trial #12

Gipson DS, Trachtman H, Kaskel FJ, Greene TH, Radeva MK, Gassman JJ, Moxey-Mims MM, Hogg RJ, Watkins SL, Fine RN, Hogan SL, Middleton JP, Vehaskari VM, Flynn PA, Powell LM, Vento SM, McMahan JL, Siegel N, D'Agati VD, Friedman AL. Clinical trial of focal segmental glomerulosclerosis in children and young adults. Kidney Int. 2011;80:868–78.

Abstract

This NIH-funded multicenter randomized study of focal segmental glomerulosclerosis (FSGS) treatment compared the efficacy of a 12-month course of cyclosporine to a combination of oral pulse dexamethasone and mycophenolate mofetil in children and adults with steroid-resistant primary FSGS. Of the 192 patients enrolled, 138 were randomized to cyclosporine (72) or to mycophenolate/dexamethasone (66). The primary analysis compared the levels of an ordinal variable measuring remission during the first year. The odds ratio (0.59) for achieving at least a partial remission with mycophenolate/dexamethasone compared to cyclosporine was not significant. Partial or complete remission was achieved in 22 mycophenolate-/dexamethasone- and 33 cyclosporine-treated patients at 12 months. The main secondary outcome, preservation of remission for 26 weeks following cessation of treatment, was not significantly different between these two therapies. During the entire 78 weeks of the study, 8 patients treated with cyclosporine and 7 with mycophenolate/dexamethasone died or developed kidney failure. Thus, our study did not find a difference in rates of proteinuria remission following 12 months of cyclosporine compared to mycophenolate/dexamethasone in patients with steroid-resistant FSGS. However, the small sample size might have prevented detection of a moderate treatment effect.

Critical Appraisal

Parameters	Yes	No	Comment
Validity			
Is the **randomization** procedure well described?	+1		
Double **blinded**?		−2	Open label. Thus potential observer bias
Is the **sample size** calculation described/ adequate?		−3	Original design aimed to recruit 500 patients to have 80 % chance of detecting 11–12 % an absolute increase in remission rates. Only 138 subjects randomized

Parameters	Yes	No	Comment
Does it have a hard primary **endpoint**?		−1	Remission of proteinuria; 6 level assessment during 12 months. Scores from 1 to 6 for remission and duration
Is the endpoint surrogate?	−2		
Is the follow-up appropriate?	+1		12 months
Was there a **bias**?		+2	Few African-Americans. Few older individuals. Normal renal function. Open label, thus potential observer bias
Is the dropout >25 %?		+1	
Is the analysis **ITT**?	+3		
Utility/usefulness			
Can the findings be generalized?	+1		To children with FSGS with normal renal function
Was the NNT <100?	N/A		Comparative study
Score	**0 %**		

Comments and Discussion

This important study is seriously flawed because of the inadequate sample size, which renders any conclusions regarding comparative efficacy of cyclosporine (CsA) versus mycophenolate mofetil/dexamethasone (MMF/DX) difficult to embrace with enthusiasm. Cyclosporin was given in doses of 4.6 ± 1.7 mg/kg/day for 26–52 weeks depending on the response. MMF was given in doses of 26.2 ± 6.1 mg/kg/day for 26–52 weeks depending on the response. Nearly all patients receive a RAS inhibitor. Steroid resistance was defined as persistent proteinuria following a minimum of only 4 weeks of high-dose steroid therapy. Patients with an eGFR <40 ml/min/1.7 m^2 were excluded. All patients enrolled had eGFR >75 ml/min/1.73 m^2. Subjects could be enrolled with a urine protein to creatinine ratio (UPCR) of as little as 1 g/g. The UPCR was less than 2.0 g/g in 24 % of the randomized subjects, and many had normal serum albumin levels. Not-otherwise-specified FSGS lesions were found in about 70 % of the renal biopsies. Genetic screening was performed but not reported or used in the analysis, and 67 % of the subjects were ≤17 years of age. African-Americans were well represented.

According to a strict endpoint, 46 % of the CsA-treated and 33 % of the MMF/DX-treated subjects achieved a complete or partial remission by 52 weeks. This was a nonsignificant difference, but the study was underpowered to show a difference even if it did exist. However, by all of the endpoint criteria, MMF/DX showed a numerically inferior efficacy compared to CsA.

Conclusion

The inclusion of many non-nephrotic subjects and the inadequate sample size render interpretation of the trends noted in this trial difficult at best [17]. This study also leaves unanswered the question as to whether MMF (with or without DX) offers any benefit to those persistently nephrotic subjects who fail to respond to or become dependent upon CsA, especially in the presence of declining renal function. At present, MMF is only suggested (evidence level 2D) for use in patients with FSGS and nephrotic syndrome who are resistant to both steroids and CNI [1]. Further well-powered RCTs are needed to clarify the relative roles of CsA and MMF in management of steroid-resistant FSGS. In addition claims of efficacy of rituximab, ACTH, and abatacept in such patients need evaluation in RCT [13, 18, 19]. Major gaps continue to exist in our understanding of the optimal treatment of steroid-resistant FSGS [1, 17].

Membranous Nephropathy

Trial #13

Collaborative Study of the Adult Idiopathic Nephrotic Syndrome. A Controlled Study of Short-Term prednisone treatment in adults with membranous nephropathy. N Engl J Med. 1979;301:1301–6.

Critical Appraisal

Parameters	Yes	No	Comment
Validity			
Is the **randomization** procedure well described?		−1	
Double **blinded**?	+2		
Is the **sample size** calculation described/ adequate?		−3	Thus raising questions about study power
Does it have a hard primary **endpoint**?	+1		Remission and renal failure. However, GFR not measured
Is the endpoint surrogate?		0	
Is the follow-up appropriate?	+1		
Was there a **bias**?		−2	Control group having a possibly unusually rapid rate of progression for IMN
Is the dropout >25 %?		+1	
Is the analysis **ITT**?		−3	Not described. Repeated interim analysis without correction of alpha
Utility/usefulness			
Can the findings be generalized?		−1	Questionable due to possible randomization bias
Was the NNT <100?	+1		
Score	**0 %**		

Comments and Discussion

This seriously flawed study (by contemporary standards of study design and execution) is included primarily for historical reasons, as it was the first RCT conducted in MN. Both remissions and progressive loss of kidney function were analyzed as "endpoints," and the double-blind, placebo-controlled nature of the study design is rather unique in RCT involving primary glomerular diseases. The comparison of oral alternate-day steroids versus placebo was an appropriate study design at the time. Repeated interim analysis without correction of alpha error margins would not be acceptable today. The main criticism of this study was the possibility of a bias since the control subjects progressed rapidly (−10 % per year), and 5/38 (13 %) placebo patients developed ESRD after a follow-up of slightly less than 2 years. This was considered to be unusually high relative to data obtained in observational studies of untreated patients with idiopathic MN. Pre-randomization serum creatinine, urine protein excretion, and histological classification of severity were not different between the two groups. On a cumulative basis, 11/38 (28 %) subjects assigned to placebo and 22/34 (64 %) assigned to prednisone developed at least one complete or partial remission of proteinuria by 36 months of observation; however, due to relapses, the number of subjects in remission at the end of the study was no different between the two groups (7/38 [18 %] in placebo and 12/34 [35 %] in prednisone [p=ns]).

Conclusion

Doubts regarding the validity of this study, spawned additional RCT, none of which were ever able to confirm the findings [20, 21]. As a result, the 2012 KDIGO clinical practice guidelines do not recommend that steroid monotherapy be used to treat nephrotic syndrome in idiopathic MN [1]. Nevertheless, these trials may have missed identification of a small subset (? <10 %) of patients who are steroid responsive and relapsing. Also, longer (and more toxic) regimens of steroids may have beneficial effects, but this has never been formally tested, largely due to fears of serious adverse events.

Trial #14

Ponticelli C, Zucchelli P, Imbasciati E, Cagnoli L, Pozzi C, Passerini P, Grassi C, Limido D, Pasquali S, Volpini T, Sasdelli M, Locatelli F. Controlled trial of methylprednisolone and chlorambucil in idiopathic membranous nephropathy. N Engl J Med. 1984;310:946–50.

Abstract

Sixty-seven adults with idiopathic membranous nephropathy and nephrotic syndrome were randomly assigned to symptomatic treatment only or to a 6-month course of methylprednisolone alternated with chlorambucil every other month. Patients were followed for 1–7 years. At the end of follow-up (mean of 31.4 ± 18.2 months for the treated group and 37.0 ± 22.0 for the control group), 23 of 32 treated patients were in complete or partial remission, as compared with 9 of 30 control patients ($P = 0.001$). Twelve of the treated patients were in complete remission, as compared with only two of the controls. In the treated group, there were no changes in renal function during follow-up, whereas in the control group the reciprocal of the plasma creatinine level, which is proportional to the creatinine clearance, decreased significantly ($P = 0.00017$) after 2 years of follow-up. Side effects were minimal in all treated patients except two, who were dropped from the study because of peptic ulcer and gastric intolerance to chlorambucil. We conclude that steroid and chlorambucil treatment for 6 months favors remission of the nephrotic syndrome in adults with idiopathic membranous nephropathy and can preserve renal function for at least some years.

Critical Appraisal

Parameters	Yes	No	Comment
Validity			
Is the **randomization** procedure well described?	+1		
Double **blinded**?		−2	Thus lending itself to observer bias
Is the **sample size** calculation described/adequate?		−2	Sample size calculation not done. Probably underpowered to test ESRD outcomes
Does it have a hard primary **endpoint**?		−1	Proteinuria remission and renal function endpoints. GFR not measured
Is the endpoint surrogate?		0	
Is the follow-up appropriate?	+1		3 years on average
Was there a **bias**?		+1	But only European Caucasians
Is the dropout >25 %?		+1	
Is the analysis **ITT**?		−1	No ITT analysis, but dropout approximately comparable in the two groups
Utility/usefulness			
Can the findings be generalized?	+1		Only to patients with IMN and normal renal function (serum creatinine). Only European Caucasians
Was the NNT <100?	+1		
Score	0 %		

Summary and Discussion

This landmark trial had a marked effect on clinical practice although by contemporary standards it had significant weaknesses. Patients with nephrotic syndrome and normal or near-normal renal function (serum creatinine 1.07 ± 0.27 mg/dl at baseline) presumably due to idiopathic MN (IMN) were included, but none had been followed long enough (8.5–9.4 months) before randomization to exclude those with a spontaneous remission. Nevertheless, complete or partial remission (CR or PR) occurred in 9/30 (30 %) patients in the control (untreated) group compared to 26/32 (81 %) in the treated at the end of the follow-up period (37 and 31 months, respectively, in control and treated groups ($p = 0.001$)). Importantly, in the treated group, complete remissions developed after the end of treatment in 4/16 patients.

Chlorambucil (0.2 mg/kg/day) was chosen as the alkylating agent component of a cyclical regimen that involved alternate-month administration of IV methylprednisolone and oral prednisone over a period of 6 months, now known as the "Ponticelli Regimen" or the "Milan Cocktail." Side effects of active treatment were infrequent and mild. They included leukopenia (reversible with lowering doses of chlorambucil), tremors, gastritis, and transient liver function abnormalities. No patient stopped treatment because of side effects. During the trial, serum creatinine remained unchanged in the actively treated group but increased by 50 % or more in the control group. No bias could be detected in the randomization process. The follow-up was insufficient to determine the effects of treatment on ESRD rates. Also, GFR was not measured to assess IMN progression, and reliance of serum creatinine-based variables may be confounded by the effect of steroid therapy on muscle mass and consequently creatinine levels [22].

The design of the study could not separate the effects of the alkylating agent from the steroid components of the cyclical regimen, but oral prednisolone alone had been shown to be ineffective in IMN (see Trial #11).

A later adequately powered non-inferiority trial showed that oral cyclophosphamide could be substituted for oral chlorambucil in the cyclical regimen without loss of efficacy and some improvements in safety [23].

Subsequent long-term (10 years) follow-up of the original Ponticelli et al. RCT described here confirmed a long-term beneficial effect on the "hard endpoint" of ESRD [24]. Survival free of ESRD was 92 % in the treated arm and 60 % in the control arm ($p = 0.0038$). In addition, the period of time spent free of nephrotic syndrome was increased in the actively treated patients ($p = 0.0001$). The findings initially published by Ponticelli and coworkers were also independently confirmed by Jha et al. in an RCT from India with 10-year follow-up that also indicated a beneficial effect on quality of life [25]. Infectious complications were common (about 30 %) in both actively treated and control groups. At 10 years, malignancies were not seen in the Ponticelli et al. or the Jha et al. trials. A weakness of both trials was that only subjects with relatively normal renal function were randomized, so no definitive statement could be made about the efficacy or safety of the treatment regimen in patients who had progressed to renal impairment (see Trial #14). A subsequent RCT by Ponticelli et al. [26] compared the relative efficacy of the cyclical chlorambucil-prednisone regimen (6 months) to methylprednisolone (MP) alone (6 months). Although at the end of 4 years of follow-up the patients assigned to the two groups did not differ ($p = 0.10$) with respect to remission status, the patients treated with the combination regimen were in remission for longer than those who received MP alone. The study may have been underpowered to show a beneficial effect at 4 years, and the β error was not calculated.

Conclusion

Due to the balance of strengths over weaknesses, the independent confirmation, the long-term follow-up, and the hard endpoints examined, the "Ponticelli Regimen," described here, was recommended by the KDIGO work group as the preferred initial treatment of MN with persisting nephrotic syndrome, providing patients had been observed for long enough to develop a spontaneous remission [1, 27].

Trial #15

Cattran DC, Appel GB, Hebert LA, Hunsicker LG, Pohl MA, Hoy WE, Maxwell DR, Kunis CL; North America Nephrotic Syndrome Study Group. Cyclosporin in patients with steroid-resistant membranous nephropathy: a randomized trial. Kidney Int. 2001;59:1484–90.

Abstract

Background: A clinical trial of cyclosporine in patients with steroid-resistant membranous nephropathy (MGN) was conducted. Although MGN remains the most common cause of adult-onset nephrotic syndrome, its management is still controversial. Cyclosporine has been shown to be effective in cases of progressive MGN, but it has not been used in controlled studies at an early stage of the disease.

Methods: We conducted a randomized trial in 51 biopsy-proven idiopathic MGN patients with nephrotic-range proteinuria comparing 26 weeks of cyclosporine treatment plus low-dose prednisone to placebo plus prednisone. All patients were followed for an average of 78 weeks, and the short- and long-term effects on renal function were assessed.

Results: Seventy-five percent of the treatment group versus 22 % of the control group ($P < 0.001$) had a partial or complete remission of their proteinuria by 26 weeks. Relapse occurred in 43 % ($N = 9$) of the cyclosporine remission group and 40 % ($N = 2$) of the placebo group by week 52. The fraction of the total population in remission then remained almost unchanged and significantly different between the groups until the end of the study (cyclosporine 39 %, placebo 13 %, $P = 0.007$). Renal function was unchanged and equal in the two groups over the test medication period. In the subsequent follow-up, renal insufficiency, defined as doubling of baseline creatinine, was seen in two patients in each group, but remained equal and stable in all of the other patients.

Conclusion: This study suggests that cyclosporine is an effective therapeutic agent in the treatment of steroid-resistant cases of MGN. Although a high relapse does occur, 39 % of the treated patients remained in remission and were subnephrotic for at least 1 year post treatment, with no adverse effect on filtration function.

Critical Appraisal

Parameters	Yes	No	Comment
Validity			
Is the **randomization** procedure well described?	+1		
Double **blinded**?		−2	Thus lending itself to observer bias
Is the **sample size** calculation described/adequate?	+1		Calculated as adequate to avoid a β error for primary endpoint; 25 subjects in each arm required; 23 were randomized in placebo; 28 in active drug arms
Does it have a hard primary **endpoint**?		−1	Proteinuria remission only. Renal function changes were considered secondary endpoints
Is the endpoint surrogate?	−2		
Is the follow-up appropriate?	+1		
Was there a **bias**?	−1		Due to unblinding observer bias cannot be ruled out
Is the dropout >25 %?		+1	
Is the analysis **ITT**?	+3		Not stated but all patients followed
Utility/usefulness			
Can the findings be generalized?	0		Only normal renal function patients
Was the NNT <100?	+1		
Score	**12.5 %**		Yes, for complete remission

Comments and Discussion

Although suffering from some weaknesses in design and execution, this trial had a significant impact on treatment practices for MN.

Since steroid monotherapy had never been proven to be effective in MN (see comments in Trial #11), it is curious that the study required a failure to remit following an 8-week trial of prednisone at 1 mg/kg/day or more for study eligibility. A 6-month pre-randomization observation period may have reduced the likelihood of a spontaneous remission in the control (untreated) group. RAS inhibition therapy was strictly controlled in both groups so as to avoid a bias. The cyclosporine (CsA) dosage was initially 3.5 mg/kg/day, and an identical place was administered to the control group (single blind). Low-dose oral prednisone was given to both groups. The two groups were well balanced for patient characteristics at baseline, and the patients were predominantly Caucasian. Serum creatinine was 1.1 ± 0.3 mg/dl in the placebo and 1.3 ± 0.5 mg/dl in the CsA groups at randomization. At 26 weeks when CsA was stopped, the number of complete remissions (CR) was not different in the two groups (2/28 in the CsA and 1/23 in the placebo groups), but partial remissions (PR) were more frequent in the CsA group (19/28 in CsA and 4/23 in the placebo groups). Due to relapses the number of CR + PR at 78 weeks was 11/28 (39 %) in the CsA group and 4/23 (17 %) in the placebo group ($p = 0.007$). About 50 % of the patients who received CsA and who were in remission at 26 weeks subsequently relapsed. Hypertension worsened in the CsA group (requiring additional antihypertensive treatment), but other side effects were mild and easily manageable. Although not a primary endpoint, a 50 % reduction in creatinine clearance was similar in both groups, 9 % in placebo and 7 % in CsA by 78 weeks; however, the study is underpowered to evaluate renal function outcomes.

Clearly this study shows that a stable CR is not attainable with short-term (26 weeks) treatment with CsA. Longer-term treatment is required, but this can expose patients to the uncertain adverse effect of cumulative nephrotoxicity of CNI, and the risk/benefit ratio of such prolonged regimens has not been rigorously tested in RCT. Finally, this trial applies only to patients with MN, persisting nephrotic syndrome, and reasonably normal and not declining renal function (see Trial # 14).

Conclusion

In spite of its significant shortcomings, this study did add CsA to the treatment armamentarium of MN, but because of the lack of effect on CR and the unproven effects on long-term outcomes, the KDIGO work group only recommended that CsA (or tacrolimus) be used for initial treatment of MN in those patients who chose to receive a calcineurin inhibitor (CNI), who have contraindications to an alkylating agent-based regimen or who fail to achieve a remission with initial treatment using alkylating agent-based regimen [1, 28].

Trial # 16

Howman A, Chapman TL, Langdon MM, Ferguson C, Adu D, Feehally J, Gaskin GJ, Jayne DR, O'Donoghue D, Boutlon-Jones M, Mathieson PW. Immunosuppression for progressive membranous nephropathy. Lancet. 2013; 381:744–51.

Abstract

Background: Membranous nephropathy leads to end-stage renal disease in more than 20 % of patients. Although immunosuppressive therapy benefits some patients, trial evidence for the subset of patients with declining renal function is not available. We aimed to assess whether immunosuppression preserves renal function in patients with idiopathic membranous nephropathy with declining renal function.

Methods: This randomized controlled trial was undertaken in 37 renal units across the UK. We recruited patients (18–75 years) with biopsy-proven idiopathic membranous nephropathy a plasma creatinine concentration of less than 300 μmol/l and at least a 20 % decline in excretory renal function measured in the 2 years before study entry, based on at least three measurements over a period of 3 months or longer. Patients were randomly assigned (1:1:1) by a random number table to receive supportive treatment only, supportive treatment plus 6 months of alternating cycles of prednisolone and chlorambucil or supportive treatment plus 12 months of ciclosporin. The primary outcome was a further 20 % decline in renal function from baseline, analyzed by intention to treat. The trial is registered as an International Standard Randomised Controlled Trial, number 99959692.

Findings: We randomly assigned 108 patients, 33 of whom received prednisolone and chlorambucil, 37 ciclosporin, and 38 supportive therapy alone. Two patients (one who received ciclosporin and one who received supportive therapy) were ineligible and so were not included in the intention-to-treat analysis, and 45 patients deviated from the protocol before study ends, mostly as a result of minor dose adjustments. Follow-up was until primary endpoint or for minimum of 3 years if primary endpoint was not reached. Risk of further 20 % decline in renal function was significantly lower in the prednisolone and chlorambucil group than in the supportive care group (19 [58 %] of 33 patients reached endpoint vs 31 [84 %] of 37, hazard ratio [HR] 0.44 [95 % CI 0.24–0.78];

$p=0.0042$); risk did not differ between the ciclosporin (29 [81 %] of 36) and supportive treatment only groups (HR 1.17 [0.70–1.95]; $p=0.54$), but did differ significantly across all three groups ($p=0.003$). Serious adverse events were frequent in all three groups but were higher in the prednisolone and chlorambucil group than in the supportive care only group (56 events vs 24 events; $p=0.048$).

Interpretation: For the subset of patients with idiopathic membranous nephropathy and deteriorating excretory renal function, 6-month therapy with prednisolone and chlorambucil is the treatment approach best supported by our evidence. Ciclosporin should be avoided in this subset.

Critical Appraisal

Parameters	Yes	No	Comment
Validity			
Is the **randomization** procedure well described?	+1		
Double **blinded**?		−2	Open label. Thus, subject to observer bias
Is the **sample size** calculation described/ adequate?	+3		
Does it have a hard primary **endpoint**?		−1	Changes in creatinine clearance. GFR not measured
Is the endpoint surrogate?	0		
Is the follow-up appropriate?	+1		
Was there a **bias**?	−2		High starting dose of CsA. Also very long recruitment period (>10 years) may have led to confounders in the management of patients
Is the dropout >25 %?		+1	
Is the analysis **ITT**?	+3		
Utility/usefulness			
Can the findings be generalized?		−1	Not to patients receiving CsA 3.5 mg/kg/day or a CYC-based regimen
Was the NNT <100?	N/A		Comparative study
Score	**20 %**		

Comments and Discussion

This trial addresses an important issue: What is the best treatment for a patient with persisting nephrotic syndrome and declining renal function? It was designed in 1997 and conducted between 1998 and 2008, thus explaining, in part, the use of a chlorambucil-based (0.15 mg/kg/day) "Ponticelli

Regimen" and CsA (at 5 mg/kg/day given without steroids as the initial treatment regimens (with appropriate dosing reductions during the trial) for the active drug treatment arms of the trial. Despite these caveats, it does add useful information bearing on the conundrum of what to do for patients with MN and declining renal function.

The power of the study was marginally calculated to detect a 50 % decline in the frequency of a further 20 % loss of kidney function (assumed to be 80 % in the supportive and 40 % in the immunosuppressive groups). Baseline patient characteristics were similar in all groups. Angiotensin-converting enzyme inhibitor treatment was similar in the groups during the trial, but data on angiotensin receptor blockade was not collected. Baseline creatinine clearance was 50, 49, and 50 ml/min in the chlorambucil-steroids, CsA, and supportive groups, respectively.

The risk of a further 20 % decline in renal function was 58 % in the chlorambucil-steroid group, 81 % in the CsA group, and 84 % in the supportive care group ($p=0.003$ for a three-way comparison). Serious adverse events likely to be related to treatment were common (26/56 events [46 %] in the chlorambucil-prednisone group; 13/37 events [35 %] in the CsA-treated groups). Proteinuria declined to a greater extent in the chlorambucil-steroid group.

While the inherent weaknesses of a study that took so long to recruit and complete (10 years) are obvious, the main concern for bias is the higher dose of CsA used for initial treatment. This may have confounded interpretation of the renal function changes (as assessed by endogenous creatinine clearance rather than serum creatinine alone) in the CsA group due to nephrotoxicity, despite the control of trough plasma CsA levels to 100–200 μg/l. The issue whether the lack of concomitant steroid treatment in the CsA group influenced the results is debatable.

Conclusion

It seems that great caution should be employed in ever utilizing a CsA-based regimen, particularly in higher initial dosage, in treatment of IMN and declining renal function. An alkylating agent-based regimen (cyclical cyclophosphamide + prednisone with dosage modification) might be preferred to slow progression, but the risk of adverse events is great. Whether a tacrolimus-based regimen would fare better is unknown [28]. Mycophenolate mofetil plus steroids might have an advantage in such patients, but the relapse rate is very high (>80 %) and the long-term impact on ESRD is unknown [29, 30]. The impact of rituximab [31] or intact ACTH [32] is encouraging, but the effect on hard endpoint is as yet unknown and untested in RCT, and whether impairment of renal function would disallow any posited benefits of these agents is unknown as well.

Trial #17

Ponticelli C, Passerini P, Salvadori M, Manno C, Viola BF, Pasquali S, Mandolofo S, Messa P. Randomized pilot trial comparing methylprednisolone plus a cytotoxic versus synthetic adrenocorticotropic hormone in idiopathic membranous nephropathy. Am J Kidney Dis. 2006;47:233–40.

Abstract

Background: We conducted a pilot trial to compare the effectiveness and safety of two different treatments in patients with membranous nephropathy and nephrotic syndrome.

Methods: To validate the hypothesis that the two treatments were equivalent, patients with biopsy-proven membranous nephropathy and nephrotic syndrome were randomly assigned to methylprednisolone alternated with a cytotoxic drug every other month for 6 months (group A) or to intramuscular synthetic adrenocorticotropic hormone administered twice a week for 1 year (group B).

Results: The primary outcome measure is cumulative number of remissions as a first event. Fifteen of 16 patients in group A and 14 of 16 patients in group B entered complete or partial remission as a first event. After a median follow-up of 24 months (interquartile range, 15–25 months), there were four complete remissions and eight partial remissions in group A versus 8 complete remissions and 6 partial remissions in group B. Median proteinuria decreased from protein of 5.1 g/day (interquartile range, 4.0–7.3 g/day) to 2.1 g/day (interquartile range, 0.4–3.8 g/day; $P=0.004$) in group A and 6.0 g/day (interquartile range, 4.4–8.5 g/day) to 0.3 g/day (interquartile range, 0.2–1.9 g/day; $P=0.049$) in group B. Two patients from each group interrupted treatment because of side effects or inefficacy.

Conclusion: Most nephrotic patients with membranous nephropathy responded to either treatment. Proteinuria was significantly decreased with both methylprednisolone and cytotoxic agents or prolonged administration of synthetic adrenocorticotropic hormone, without significant differences between these two therapies.

Critical Appraisal

Parameters	Yes	No	Comment
Validity			
Is the **randomization** procedure well described?	+1		
Double **blinded**?		0	Difficult in view of routes of drug administration
Is the **sample size** calculation described/adequate?	N/A		Not included/pilot study
Does it have a hard primary **endpoint**?		−1	Remission of proteinuria
Is the endpoint surrogate?	−2		
Is the follow-up appropriate?	+1		
Was there a **bias**?		+2	
Is the dropout >25 %?		+1	
Is the analysis **ITT**?	N/A		Pilot study
Utility/usefulness			
Can the findings be generalized?	N/A		Pilot study
Was the NNT <100?	N/A		Pilot study
Score	**Not scored**		Pilot study

Comments and Discussion

Although this is an exploratory pilot RCT, it is included because of current interest in the use of ACTH-related products (synthetic ACTH and natural [porcine] intact ACTH) in the treatment of primary glomerular disease [32]. The advantage of this pilot study is that it compares synthetic ACTH to a standard-of-care regimen–cyclical cyclophosphamide + steroids. The small sample size, short-term follow-up, and lack of "hard" endpoints preclude any definitive statements on the efficacy of synthetic ACTH (equivalence or superiority to the standard-of-care regimen), but it does generate a testable hypothesis that will need to be examined in additional well-designed RCTs. Prolonged (1 year) administration of synthetic ACTH might be equal in efficacy to a 6-month course of cyclical cyclophosphamide, but this study only provides weak evidence for this suggestion. The mechanism of action of the posited effect of synthetic ACTH (or for that matter natural ACTH) is unknown but might be a direct effect on podocytes [33].

Conclusion

Much more work will be needed to determine the proper role of ACTH in the treatment of MN or other primary glomerular disease, but it is noteworthy that synthetic ACTH is available for this purpose in Europe, but not in the USA, and natural ACTH is approved by the Food and Drug Administration in the USA for induction of remissions of proteinuria in nephrotic syndrome due to primary glomerular disease (without uremia).

IgA Nephropathy

Trial #18

Donadio JV. Jr, Bergstralh EJ, Offord KP, Spencer DC, Holley KE; Mayo Nephrology Collaborative Group. A controlled trial of fish oil in IgA nephropathy. N Engl J Med. 1994;331:1194–99.

Abstract

Background: The n-3 fatty acids in fish oil affect eicosanoid and cytokine production and therefore have the potential to alter renal hemodynamics and inflammation. The effects of fish oil could prevent immunologic renal injury in patients with IgA nephropathy.

Methods: In a multicenter, placebo-controlled, randomized trial, we tested the efficacy of fish oil in patients with IgA nephropathy who had persistent proteinuria. The daily dose of fish oil was 12 g; the placebo was a similar dose of olive oil. Serum creatinine concentrations, elevated in 68 % of the patients at baseline, and creatinine clearance were measured for 2 years. The primary endpoint was an increase of 50 % or more in the serum creatinine concentration at the end of the study.

Results: Fifty-five patients were assigned to receive fish oil and 51 to receive placebo. According to Kaplan-Meier estimation, 3 patients (6 %) in the fish oil group and 14 (33 %) in the placebo group had increases of 50 % or more in their serum creatinine concentrations during treatment (P=0.002). The annual median changes in the serum creatinine concentrations were 0.03 mg/dl (2.7 µmol/l) in the fish oil group and 0.14 mg/dl (12.4 µmol/l) in the placebo group. Proteinuria was slightly reduced and hypertension was controlled to a comparable degree in both groups. The cumulative percentage of patients who died or had end-stage renal disease was 40 % in the placebo group after 4 years and 10 % in the fish oil group (P=0.006). No patient discontinued fish oil treatment because of adverse effects.

Conclusions: In patients with IgA nephropathy, treatment with fish oil for 2 years retards the rate at which renal function is lost.

Critical Appraisal

Parameters	Yes	No	Comment
Validity			
Is the **randomization** procedure well described?		−1	
Double **blinded**?	+2		
Is the **sample size** calculation described/ adequate?		−2	Not described, likely inadequate power and sample size

Parameters	Yes	No	Comment
Does it have a hard primary **endpoint**?		−1	50 % increase in serum creatinine from baseline. GFR not measured
Is the endpoint surrogate?	−2		
Is the follow-up appropriate?	+1		
Was there a **bias**?		+2	ACE inhibition only used in 60 % of patients, but equally in both groups. NaCl intake not evaluated
Is the dropout >25 %?	−1		31 of 106 randomized did not complete the 2 years of the study
Is the analysis **ITT**?		−3	
Utility/usefulness			
Can the findings be generalized?		−1	Uncertain about generalizability due to high rates of progression in placebo
Was the NNT <100?	+1		
Score	**0 %**		

Comments and Discussion

By contemporary standards, this trial only provides only very weak evidence for efficacy of fish oils in IgA nephropathy (IgAN).

Its strengths are that it is placebo controlled, it has a double-blind design, the "hard"-end points are used, and the dosing is with a well-characterized fish oil preparation. Weaknesses were high dropouts and lack of an ITT analysis.

Also GFR was not measured, and a question must be raised about high fish oil intake and its impact on appetite and subsequent protein intake, thus confounding the impact of the intervention on changes in serum creatinine. Fish oil consumption is known to be associated with gastrointestinal side effects including nausea, flatulence, and diarrhea, which may impact overall food and protein intake.

Due to lack of a requirement for uniform RAS inhibition and no control over NaCl intake, a bias may be present. After a follow-up of only 3 years, a total of 18 patients developed ESRD (16 % of the originally randomized subjects), 4 in the fish oil group, and 14 in the placebo groups. Thus, death-censored renal survival in the placebo group was about 75 % at 3 years – higher than is commonly seen in IgA N with >1.0 g proteinuria at baseline (the inclusion criteria) – raising questions about possible bias. Nevertheless, the baseline characteristics of the patients randomized were well balanced in terms of hypertension and its treatment, levels of urinary protein excretion, and impaired renal function. The serum creatinine at baseline was 1.4 ± 0.4 and 1.5 mg ± 0.5 mg/ dl in the active drug and placebo groups, respectively. No patient had a serum creatinine >3.5 mg/dl (exclusion criteria)

Interestingly, there was no evidence for a beneficial effect of fish oils on urinary protein excretion. A longer-term follow-up (6.4 years) supported a continued benefit of fish oils in terms of renal survival but also no benefit on urinary protein excretion [34]. Side effects attributed to fish oils were not serious.

Conclusion

Other smaller studies were unable to confirm the benefits seen in this study, and a meta-analysis of all trials showed only moderate evidence for efficacy [35–37]. Because of the uncertainty surrounding the efficacy of fish oils coupled with a good overall track record of safety, the KDIGO work group suggested (not recommended) that fish oils be used (in doses and duration comparable to this trial) in patients with IgA N if proteinuria persists at >1.0 g/day despite optimal treatment with RAS inhibition. Treatment seems more likely to be effective if started early in the course and used in combination with RAS inhibition, but this has not been formally tested in an RCT. Note that fish oils have no beneficial effect on proteinuria in IgA N.

Trial #19

Pozzi C, Bolasco P, Fogazzi G, Andrulli S, Altieri P, Ponticelli C, Locatelli F. Corticosteroids in IgA nephropathy: a randomized controlled trial. Lancet. 1999; 353:883–7.

Abstract

Background: IgA nephropathy is progressive in most cases and has no established therapy. In this randomized trial, we assessed the efficacy and safety of a 6-month course of steroids in this disorder.

Methods: Between July 1987 and September 1995, we enrolled 86 consecutive patients from seven renal units in Italy. Eligible patients had biopsy-proven IgA nephropathy, urine protein excretion of 1.0–3.5 g daily, and plasma creatinine concentrations of 133 μmol/l (1.5 mg/dl) or less. Patients were randomly assigned either supportive therapy alone or steroid treatment (intravenous methylprednisolone 1 g/day for 3 consecutive days at the beginning of months 1, 3, and 5, plus oral prednisone 0.5 mg/kg on alternate days for 6 months). The primary endpoint was deterioration in renal function defined as a 50 % or 100 % increase in plasma creatinine concentration from baseline. Analyses were by intention to treat.

Findings: Nine of 43 patients in the steroid group and 14 of 43 in the control group reached the primary endpoint (a 50 % increase in plasma creatinine) by year 5 of follow-up ($p < 0.048$). Factors influencing renal survival were vascular sclerosis (relative risk for 1-point increase in score 1.53, $p = 0.0347$), female sex (0.22, $p = 0.0163$), and steroid therapy (0.41, $p = 0.0439$). All 43 patients assigned steroids completed the treatment without experiencing any important side effects.

Interpretation: A 6-month course of steroid treatment protected against deterioration in renal function in IgA nephropathy with no notable adverse effects during follow-up. An increase in urinary protein excretion could be a marker indicating the need for a second course of steroid therapy.

Critical Appraisal

Parameters	Yes	No	Comment
Validity			
Is the **randomization** procedure well described?		−1	Partially described
Double **blinded**?		−2	Open label. Thus subject to observer bias
Is the **sample size** calculation described/ adequate?		−3	Almost certainly underpowered as renal function normal or near-normal at baseline. Prediction of progression on full RAAS inhibition minimal
Does it have a hard primary **endpoint**?		−1	50 % changes in serum creatinine
			GFR not measured. Confounding with muscle wasting due to steroids a problem
			ESRD incidence not evaluated
Is the endpoint surrogate?	−1		See above
Is the follow-up appropriate?	+1		Possible; not all patients treated with optimized RAAS inhibition
Was there a **bias**?	−1		Effects on serum creatinine of steroid-induced muscle wasting
Is the dropout >25 %?		+1	
Is the analysis **ITT**?	+3		
Utility/usefulness			
Can the findings be generalized?	+1		Only to those with IgAN and serum creatinine levels <1.5 mg/dl and proteinuria between 1 and 3.5 g/day
Was the NNT <100?	+1		
Score	**0 %**		

Comments and Discussion

This landmark but potentially biased RCT started a long series of investigations into the benefits and risks of steroid therapy of IgA N – an issue which remains unsettled to this day.

Its strengths of design and execution were outweighed by its weaknesses, primarily the open-label nature of the trial and failing to treat all subjects with optimum RAAS inhibition before enrolment and limitations of the serum creatinine endpoint.

Furthermore, as most patients had normal or near-normal renal function and moderate level proteinuria (not nephrotic range), questions have to be asked about the power of the study and its small sample size. Also, these patients would be expected to have a relatively good prognosis and would be otherwise treated by RAAS inhibition according to current KDIGO guidelines.

Also, concern must be expressed about the fact that progression was not optimally evaluated by measured GFR. Instead changes in serum creatinine-based parameters were used, which raises questions about the impact of prolonged and high-dose steroid therapy on muscle mass and sarcopenia, confounding the value serum creatinine estimation as a specific marker of IgAN progression.

A 10-year follow-up and secondary analysis of this trial provided substantiation of a pronounced effect on renal survival of the steroid regimen used (oral plus IV methyl prednisolone over 6 months), suggesting a "legacy effect" of this treatment [38, 39]. The 10-year actuarial renal survival was 97 % in the steroid-treated group and 53 % in the control group ($p = 0.0003$ log rank test) and was associated with improved urine protein excretion. Other published RCTs of steroids in IgA N will be reviewed below.

Conclusion

An interesting observation that is at best hypothesis generating and worthy of further and more comprehensive testing. A very large multinational RCT of steroid therapy added onto RAAS inhibition in IgA N is currently in progress (TESTING) [40].

Trial #20

Manno C, Torres DD, Rossini M, Pesce F, Schena FP. Randomized controlled clinical trial of corticosteroids plus ACE inhibitors with long-term follow-up in proteinuric IgA nephropathy. Nephrol Dial Transplant. 2009;24:3694–701.

Abstract

Background: Immunoglobulin A nephropathy (IgAN) is the most common cause of chronic renal failure among primary glomerulonephritis patients. The best treatment for IgAN remains poorly defined. We planned a long-term, prospective, open-label, multicenter, centrally randomized controlled trial to assess whether the combination of prednisone and ramipril was more effective than ramipril alone in patients with proteinuric IgAN.

Methods: Ninety-seven biopsy-proven IgAN patients with moderate histologic lesions, 24-h proteinuria > or =1.0 g, and estimated glomerular filtration rate (eGFR) > or =50 ml/min/ 1.73 m^2 were randomly allocated to receive a 6-month course of oral prednisone plus ramipril (combination therapy group) or ramipril alone (monotherapy group) for the total duration of follow-up. The primary outcome was the progression of renal disease defined as the combination of doubling of baseline serum creatinine or end-stage kidney disease (ESKD). The secondary outcomes were the rate of renal function decline defined as the eGFR slope over time and the reduction of 24-h proteinuria.

Results: After a follow-up of up to 96 months, 13/49 (26.5 %) patients in the monotherapy group reached the primary outcome compared with 2/48 (4.2 %) in the combination therapy group. The Kaplan-Meier analysis showed a significantly higher probability of not reaching the combined outcome in the combination therapy group than in the monotherapy group (85.2 % vs 52.1 %; log-rank test $P = 0.003$). In the multivariate analysis, baseline serum creatinine and 24-h proteinuria were independent predictors of the risk of primary outcome; treatment with prednisone plus ramipril significantly reduced the risk of renal disease progression (hazard ratio 0.13; 95 % confidence interval 0.03–0.61; $P = 0.01$). The mean rate of eGFR decline was higher in the monotherapy group than in the combination therapy group (-6.17 ± 13.3 vs -0.56 ± 7.62 ml/min/ 1.73 m(2)/year; $P = 0.013$). Moreover, the combined treatment reduced 24-h proteinuria more than ramipril alone during the first 2 years.

Conclusions: Our results suggest that the combination of corticosteroids and ramipril may provide additional benefits compared with ramipril alone in preventing the progression of renal disease in proteinuric IgAN patients in the long-term follow-up.

Critical Appraisal

Parameters	Yes	No	Comment
Validity			
Is the **randomization** procedure well described?	+1		
Double **blinded**?		−2	

Parameters	Yes	No	Comment
Is the **sample size** calculation described/ adequate?		−2	Premature termination of the study; study stopped after 97 patients enrolled for interim efficacy analysis. 134 were required based on initial power estimation
Does it have a hard primary **endpoint**?		+1	Doubling of serum creatinine or ESRD. GFR not measured. ESRD definition not protocolized in view of open-label nature of study concern about subjectivity of RRT start
Is the endpoint surrogate?	0		See above
Is the follow-up appropriate?	+1		Up to 96 months
Was there a **bias**?	−1		Better study design would be parallel group comparison rather than sequential design
Is the dropout >25 %?		+1	
Is the analysis **ITT**?	+3		
Utility/usefulness			
Can the findings be generalized?	+1		
Was the NNT <100?	+1		
Score	**31** %		

Comments and Discussion

This RCT only suggests that simultaneous treatment with an ACE inhibitor and oral glucocorticoid (using the 6-month oral prednisone regimen described) affords reno-protective benefits that exceed those of ACE inhibitor monotherapy, as the trial was stopped early (for efficacy in a planned interim analysis).

It has a number of limitations including the fact that it was not blinded, probably underpowered (premature termination may also generate a bias), and finally progression of IgAN was not adequately assessed. GFR was not measured, and the reliance on serum creatinine when an agent that could interfere with muscle mass such as corticosteroids is used raises serious reservations.

The study was not powered to examine safety, but most adverse events were mild and reversible. What is not answered is the question about whether sequential treatment with ACEi first and then treating only the unresponsive patients (those with persistent urine protein excretion >1.0 g/ day) with steroids will achieve as good or better long-term outcome and spare the use of steroids in some patients. Other RCTs have demonstrated long-term beneficial effects of RAS inhibition alone on renal function decline and proteinuria in IgA N [41, 42]. Another RCT has also shown

beneficial reno-protective effects of ACEi plus steroids compared to ACEi alone in Chinese subjects with IgA N and proteinuria, but this latter trial suffered from small sample size and imbalances in patient characteristics at baseline (5). This study was also stopped prematurely at 2 years due to an interim analysis showing efficacy.

Conclusion

This is at best a hypothesis-generating study that warrants further testing. For that the testing study is currently underway [40].

In the meantime the KDIGO work group has suggested that steroids be reserved to subjects who fail to achieve a urine protein excretion of <1.0 g/day after an adequate course of treatment with RAS inhibition [1].

Trial #21

Maes BD, Olyen R, Claes K, Evenepoel P, Kuypers D, Vanwalleghem J, Van Damme B, Vanrenterghem YF. Mycophenolate mofetil in IgA nephropathy: results of a 3-year prospective placebo-controlled randomized study. Kidney Int. 2004;65:1842–9.

Abstract

Background: Because humoral immunity is believed to play a pivotal role in the pathogenesis of IgA nephropathy (IgAN), a prospective placebo-controlled randomized study was started in patients with IgAN using mycophenolate mofetil (MMF).

Methods: A total of 34 patients with IgAN were treated with salt intake restriction, angiotensin-converting enzyme (ACE) inhibition, and MMF 2 g/day ($N=21$) or placebo ($N=13$). After 36 months of follow-up, clinical, biochemical, and radiologic data were analyzed using linear mixed models for longitudinal data and Kaplan-Meier survival analysis.

Results: Therapy had to be stopped prematurely in five patients. Two patients (MMF group) evolved to end-stage renal disease (ESRD). There was no difference between groups in the percentage of patients with a decrease of 25 % or more in the inulin clearance or with a serum creatinine increase of 50 % or more over 3 years. There was also no significant difference between groups in an annualized rate of change of serum creatinine, computed by linear regression analysis. No significant difference was noted between groups for inulin clearance, serum creatinine, proteinuria, blood pressure, or other parameters of renal function. Hemoglobin and C-reactive protein were significantly lower in the MMF group compared with the placebo group. As a function of time, a significant decline in both groups was noted of proteinuria, parenchymal thickness of the kidneys, and C3d.

Conclusion: In patients with IgAN at risk for progressive disease, no beneficial effect of 3-year treatment with MMF 2 g/day could be demonstrated on renal function/outcome or proteinuria. However, larger randomized studies are needed to confirm or reject these results.

Critical Appraisal

Parameters	Yes	No	Comment
Validity			
Is the **randomization** procedure well described?		−1	
Double **blinded**?		−2	Observer bias cannot be ruled out
Is the **sample size** calculation described/ adequate?		−3	No sample size calculation. Likely to be underpowered
Does it have a hard primary **endpoint**?	+1		25 % decline in measured GFR (inulin clearance)
Is the endpoint surrogate?	0		
Is the follow-up appropriate?		−1	3 years may be too short
Was there a **bias**?	+2		
Is the dropout >25 %?	+1		
Is the analysis **ITT**?		−3	Not stated
Utility/usefulness			
Can the findings be generalized?	+1		To European Caucasians
Was the NNT <100?	N/A		Comparative study
Score	**0**%		

Comments and Discussion

This is a seriously flawed and underpowered study that cannot exclude an effect on renal functional outcome and/or proteinuria of a 6-month treatment with MMF (combined with RAS inhibition but without steroids) in proteinuric IgAN patients with near-normal or moderately reduced renal function. The only strong point of the study is the effort made by the investigators to measure the progression of IgAN by assessment of GFR through urinary inulin clearance.

A similarly flawed and underpowered study showed benefits on proteinuria from a 6-month course of MMF, without steroids, in Chinese subjects with IgA N and persistent proteinuria after RAS inhibition [43]. Another underpowered study showed no benefit of MMF in patients with IgA N and advanced CKD [44]. In general, most RCT of IgA N using immunosuppression other than steroids or in addition to steroids have been poorly designed, underpowered, or biased

in some way. The addition of azathioprine to steroids in proteinuric IgA N has been shown to be ineffective and possibly more toxic [45].

Conclusion

In spite of the fact that this study is one of the very few where GFR has been measured, a number of serious limitations make it inconclusive. Perhaps ongoing STOP-IgAN will resolve the major uncertainties that exist in this area due to the very weak evidence base [46]. The KDIGO work group suggested that MMF not be used to treat patients with IgAN [1].

Trial #22

Kawamura T, Yoshimura M, Miyazaki Y, Okamoto H, Kimura K, Hirnao K, Matsushima M, Utsunomiya Y, Ogura M, Yokoo T, Okunogi H, Ishii T, Hamaguchi A, Ueda H, Furusu A, Horikoshi S, Suzuki, Shibata T, Yasuda T, Shirai S, Imasawa T, Kanozawa K, Wada A, Yamaji I, Mikura N, Imai H, Kasai K, Soma J, Fujimolto S, Matsduo S, Tomino Y and the Special IgA Nephropathy Study Group. A multicenter randomized controlled trial of tonsillectomy combined with steroid pulse therapy in patients with immunoglobulin a nephropathy. Nephrol Dial Transplant. 2014;29(8):1546–53.

Abstract

Background: The study aim was, for the first time, to conduct a multicenter randomized controlled trial to evaluate the effect of tonsillectomy in patients with IgA nephropathy (IgAN).

Methods: Patients with biopsy-proven IgAN, proteinuria and low serum creatinine were randomly allocated to receive tonsillectomy combined with steroid pulses (group A; $n=33$) or steroid pulses alone (group B; $n=39$). The primary endpoints were urinary protein excretion and the disappearance of proteinuria and/or hematuria.

Results: During 12 months from baseline, the percentage decrease in urinary protein excretion was significantly larger in group A than that in group B ($P<0.05$). However, the frequency of the disappearance of proteinuria, hematuria, or both (clinical remission) at 12 months was not statistically different between the groups. Logistic regression analyses revealed the assigned treatment was a significant, independent factor contributing to the disappearance of proteinuria (odds ratio 2.98, 95 % CI 1.01–8.83, $P=0.049$), but did not identify an independent factor in achieving the disappearance of hematuria or clinical remission.

Conclusions: The results indicate tonsillectomy combined with steroid pulse therapy has no beneficial effect over steroid pulses alone to attenuate hematuria and to increase the incidence of clinical remission. Although the antiproteinuric effect was significantly greater in combined therapy, the difference was marginal, and its impact on the renal functional outcome remains to be clarified.

Critical Appraisal

Parameters	Yes	No	Comment
Validity			
Is the **randomization** procedure well described?	+1		
Double **blinded**?	0		But bias cannot be excluded
Is the **sample size** calculation described/ adequate?	+3		
Does it have a hard primary **endpoint**?		−1	Proteinuria/hematuria remission
Is the endpoint surrogate?	−2		
Is the follow-up appropriate?		−1	Only 12 months
Was there a **bias**?		+1	Except study limited to Asians
Is the dropout >25 %?		+1	
Is the analysis **ITT**?	+3		
Utility/usefulness			
Can the findings be generalized?	+1		But limited to Asians
Was the NNT <100?		N/A	
Score	**40 %**		

Comments and Discussion

This is the first RCT in the study of glomerular disease that has been performed to evaluate the effect of tonsillectomy on IgAN. Our Japanese colleagues need to be commended for designing and executing this trial.

The sample size increases the risk for a β error, and the rather short follow-up and the surrogate outcome measures used further reduce the level of confidence that the findings can be unambiguously interpreted. In addition, only 50 % of the subjects enrolled were treated with RAS inhibition. This is a peculiarity unique to Japanese medical care, since government rules prohibit use of RAS inhibitors in non-hypertensive patients, even if proteinuria >1.0 g is persistently present. The decrease in average proteinuria in the tonsillectomy plus pulse-steroid group is encouraging but only marginally statistically significant ($p = 0.047$) and very possibly not biologically significant at all. As expected, due to the patient characteristics at baseline and the short follow-up (1 year), no differences in renal function could be ascertained between the two groups post-randomization, but

the study was severely underpowered to detect such a difference even it existed (β error). Clinical remissions of proteinuria and/or hematuria were not different between the groups as had been previously claimed in observational studies [47–51].

Conclusion

Altogether, this trial provides insufficient evidence to alter the current KDIGO suggestion that tonsillectomy *not* be performed for treatment of IgA N [1]. It is possible that post hoc analysis of histology obtained in the course of this trial might identify a potentially responsive subset of individuals, but this would be hypothesis generating and require a further RCT for confirmation (Tomino Y; personal communication).

Membranoproliferative Glomerulonephritis

Trial # 23

Tarshish P, Bernstgein J, Tobin J, Edelmann CM Jr. Treatment of mesangiocapillary glomerulonephritis with alternate-day prednisone: a report of the international study of kidney disease in children. Pediatr Nephrol. 1992;6:123–30.

Abstract

It has been claimed that long-term prednisone treatment ameliorates the course of children with mesangiocapillary glomerulonephritis (MCGN). The International Study of Kidney Disease in Children conducted a randomized, double-blinded, placebo-controlled clinical trial in 80 children with idiopathic MCGN, including 42 patients with type I disease, 14 with type II disease, 17 with type III disease, and 7 with nontypable disease. Criteria for admission included heavy proteinuria and a glomerular filtration rate of greater than or equal to 70 ml/min/1.73 m². Prednisone or lactose, 40 mg/m², was given every other day as a single morning dose. The mean duration of treatment was 41 months, renal failure being the most common reason for termination of therapy. Treatment failure was defined as an increase from baseline of 30 % or more in serum creatinine or more than 35 μmol/l. Overall, treatment failure occurred in 55 % of patients treated with lactose, compared with 40 % in the prednisone group. Life-table analysis showed a renal survival rate (i.e., stable renal function) at 130 months of 61 % among patients receiving prednisone and 12 % among patients receiving lactose ($P = 0.07$). Of patients with type I or III MCGN, 33 % treated with prednisone were treatment failures, compared with 58 % in the lactose group.

Long-term treatment with prednisone appears to improve the outcome of children with MCGN.

Critical Appraisal

Parameters	Yes	No	Comment
Validity			
Is the **randomization** procedure well described?	+1		
Double **blinded**?	+2		
Is the **sample size** calculation described/ adequate?		−3	Sample size calculation not given
			Likely to be underpowered to answer the trial question
Does it have a hard primary **endpoint**?		−1	Changes in serum creatinine
			GFR not measured
Is the endpoint surrogate?	−2		
Is the follow-up appropriate?	+1		
Was there a **bias**?		−2	Very heterogeneous population. Not analysis of secondary MCGN (HCV, HBV)
Is the dropout >25 %?		−1	
Is the analysis **ITT**?	+3		
Utility/usefulness			
Can the findings be generalized?		−1	Probably not generalizable due to the heterogeneity of patient enrolled mostly pediatric
Was the NNT <100?	+1		
Score	**0 %**		

Comments and Discussion

Randomized trials of treatment of membranoproliferative glomerulonephritis (MPGN; often also called mesangiocapillary glomerulonephritis) that appeared in the literature before 2000 are difficult to interpret because of the changes that have occurred in identifying the underlying cause of the lesion, often classified as "primary" or idiopathic MPGN before 2000 (see 1 for a recent Review). Disorders of complement regulation and a growing array of infectious diseases (e.g., chronic hepatitis C infection) and neoplastic disease (e.g., plasma cell dyscrasias) have now been identified as causing what was previously called primary.

These developments led the KDIGO work groups to simply recommend that all patients with a lesion of MPGN be evaluated for underlying disease, and no evidence-based recommendations were made (except for crescentic lesions superimposed on MPGN [1]).

Thus, this RCT suffers from all of the criticisms of an obsolete classification system for MPGN but in addition has other flaws, such as small sample sizes not compensated for

by its strength of double-blind placebo design. No benefits of the active treatment could be found for the entire group for decreasing treatment failures when status was known ($p=0.087$, one tailed), and this declined (to $p=0.154$ one-tailed) when analyzed by a modified ITT.

A sub-analysis (not clearly prespecified) suggested a benefit on treatment failures in "type I or type III MPGN" when analyzed by a modified ITT ($p=0.054$), but no benefits at all on treatment failure in type II MPGN (now known as dense deposit disease, a part of the spectrum of C3 glomerulopathy ($p=0.657$, one tailed)). Renal survival at 130 months was also not statistically significant between active drug treatment and placebo ($p=0.07$), but the sample size makes it unreasonable to draw any firm conclusions.

Conclusion

In sum, the very weak evidence provided by this trial (that randomized the subjects in 1980 but was not published until 1991) is insufficient to make any suggestions or recommendations concerning the use of long-term alternate-day prednisone for renoprotection in children (or adults) with the lesion of MPGN.

Trial #24

Donadio JV Jr, Anderson CF, Mitchell JC 3rd, Holley KE, Ilstrup DM, Fuster V, Chesebro JH. Membranoproliferative glomerulonephritis. A prospective clinical trial of platelet-inhibitor therapy. N Engl J Med. 1984;310:1421–6.

Abstract

Forty patients with type I membranoproliferative glomerulonephritis were treated for 1 year with dipyridamole, 225 mg/day, and aspirin, 975 mg/day, in a prospective, randomized, double-blind, placebo-controlled study. At the baseline, the half-life of ^{51}Cr-labeled platelets was reduced in 12 of 17 patients. The platelet half-life became longer, and renal function stabilized in the treated group, as compared with the placebo group, suggesting a relation between platelet consumption and the glomerulopathy. The glomerular filtration rate, determined by iothalamate clearance, was better maintained in the treated group (average decrease, 1.3 ml/min/1.73 m^2 of body surface area per 12 months) than in the placebo group (average decrease, 19.6). Fewer patients in the treated group than in the placebo group had progression to end-stage renal disease (3 of 21 after 62 months as compared with 9 of 19 after 33 months). The data suggest that dipyridamole and aspirin slowed the deterioration of renal function and the development of end-stage renal disease.

Critical Appraisal

Parameters	Yes	No	Comment
Validity			
Is the **randomization** procedure well described?	+1		
Double **blinded**?	+2		
Is the **sample size** calculation described/adequate?		−3	Grossly underpowered study: 21 patients on treatment 19 placebo
Does it have a hard primary **endpoint**?	+1		GFR measured (iothalamate clearance)
Is the endpoint surrogate?		0	
Is the follow-up appropriate?		−1	12 months far too short
Was there a **bias**?		−2	But mainly MPGN type I according to conventional classification at the time of the RCT Population heterogeneity is bound to generate bias in such a small sample size
Is the dropout >25 %?		−1	
Is the analysis **ITT**?		−3	Not mentioned
Utility/usefulness			
Can the findings be generalized?		−1	Huge population heterogeneity in terms of age: 6–72 years GFR:15–130 ml/min and proteinuria: 0.8–19.4 g/day
Was the NNT <100?		−1	
Score	**0 %**		

Comments and Discussion

This historical study has been included in this review as many nephrologists, mostly in emerging countries, are still questioning the use of antiplatelet agents in MPGN.

The study claimed that antiplatelet therapy with aspirin (325 mg/day) and dipyridamole (75 mg) administered thrice daily slowed the progression (measured GFR) of MPGN.

This study is at best inconclusive in view of its serious flaws and limitations including the small sample size and inadequate power as well as the short follow-up time. This is compounded by the very large heterogeneity of such a small population with patients with age ranging from 6 to 72 years, GFR ranging from of 15 to 130 ml/min, and proteinuria from 0.8–19.4 g/day. These serious design flaws preclude any conclusion regarding efficacy of the regimen in MPGN.

The misleading nature of the study conclusion and the inconclusive nature of subsequent trials were challenged subsequently by the authors' own analysis of the data with emphasis on longer follow-up period of observation. Overall, they noted that survival was improved in patients treated with aspirin and dipyridamole when survival was plotted against time after clinical onset. However, when the data were replotted and the platelet inhibitor-treated group was compared with a contemporary randomized control group, no difference in either patient survival or survival free of renal disease was demonstrated [52, 53].

Also of concern is the high dose of anti platelet agents (including aspirin 325 mg/day) given to patients in CKD stages 3b and 4.

Conclusion

There is no place for aspirin and dipyridamole in the current management of MPGN.

When one views the substantial progress that has been made after almost 50 years of prospective randomized clinical trials (RCT) in primary glomerular disease, one cannot help to be impressed. Compared to the early, pioneering trials, contemporary RCTs are much better designed, executed, and analyzed. Nonetheless, many such trials still suffer from small size and short-term follow-up precluding any analysis of the impact if treatment on "hard" endpoints of doubling of serum creatinine needs for renal replacement therapy or death. As better surrogate biomarkers for these "hard" patient-centered outcomes are developed and refined, this situation may improve. The relative rarity and underlying pathogenetic heterogeneity of the primary glomerular diseases remain as major stumbling blocks. As the primary glomerular diseases are further subdivided into unique "biotypes," RCT for interventions will require large, multi-institutional, and international collaborative efforts and economical design with high generalizability. This evolution in the RCT enterprise will be profoundly challenging, in my opinion, and will take a concerted effort over several decades to achieve.

References

1. Improving Global Outcomes (KDIGO) Glomerulonephritis Work Group. KDIGO clinical practice guidelines for glomerulonephritis. Kidney Int Suppl. 2012;2:1–274.
2. Glassock RJ, Cattran DC. Evaluation of observational and controlled trials of therapy. In: Ponticelli C, Glassock R, editors. Treatment of primary glomerular disease. 2nd ed. Oxford: Oxford Medical Publishers; 2009. p. 127–77.
3. Rich AR. A hitherto undescribed vulnerability of the juxtamedullary glomeruli in lipoid nephrosis. Bull Johns Hopkins Hosp. 1957;100:173–86.
4. Brodehl J. Conventional therapy for minimal change disease. Clin Nephrol. 1991;35 Suppl 1:s8–15.
5. Arbeitgemeinschaft fur Padiatrische Nephrologie. Cyclophosphamide treatment of steroid dependent nephrotic syndrome: comparison of 8 week with 12 week course. Arch Dis Child. 1987;62:1102–6.

6. Coppo R, Ponticelli C. Minimal change nephropathy. In: Ponticelli C, Glassock R, editors. Treatment of primary glomerular disease. 2nd ed. Oxford: Oxford Medical Publishers; 2009. p. 180–231.

7. Waldman M, Crew RJ, Valeri A, Busch J, Stokes B, Markowitz G, D'Agati V, Appel G. Adult minimal-change disease: clinical characteristics, treatment, and outcomes. Clin J Am Soc Nephrol. 2007;2:445–53.

8. Korbet SM, Schwartz MM, Lewis EJ. Minimal-change glomerulopathy of adulthood. Am J Nephrol. 1988;8:291–7.

9. Jennette JC, Falk RJ. Adult minimal change glomerulopathy with acute renal failure. Am J Kidney Dis. 1990;16:432–7.

10. Niaudet P, The French Society of Paediatric Nephrology. Comparison of cyclosporin and chlorambucil in the treatment of steroid-dependent idiopathic nephrotic syndrome: a multicentre randomized controlled trial. Pediatr Nephrol. 1992;6:1–3.

11. Ishikura K, Yoshikawa N, Nakazato H, Sasaki S, Iijima K, Nakanishi K, Matsuyama T, Ito S, Yata N, Ando T, Honda M, Japanese Study Group of Renal Disease in Children. Two-year follow-up of a prospective clinical trial of cyclosporine for frequently relapsing nephrotic syndrome in children. Clin J Am Soc Nephrol. 2012;7:1576–83.

12. Pesavento TE, Bay WH, Agarwal G, Hernandez Jr RA, Hebert LA. Mycophenolate therapy in frequently relapsing minimal change disease that has failed cyclophosphamide therapy. Am J Kidney Dis. 2004;43:e3–6.

13. Kronbichler A, Kerschbaum J, Fernandez-Fresnedo G, Hoxha E, Kurschat CE, Busch M, Bruchfeld A, Mayer G, Rudnicki M. Rituximab treatment for relapsing minimal change disease and focal segmental glomerulosclerosis: a systematic review. Am J Nephrol. 2014;39(4):322–30.

14. Fornoni A, Sageshima J, Wei C, Merscher-Gomez S, Aguillon-Prada R, Jauregui AN, Li J, Mattiazzi A, Ciancio G, Chen L, Zilleruelo G, Abitbol C, Chandar J, Seeherunvong W, Ricordi C, Ikehata M, Rastaldi MP, Reiser J, Burke 3rd GW. Rituximab targets podocytes in recurrent focal segmental glomerulosclerosis. Sci Transl Med. 2011;3(85):85ra46.

15. van de Veerdonk FL, Lauwerys B, Marijnissen RJ, Timmermans K, Di Padova F, Koenders MI, Gutierrez-Roelens I, Durez P, Netea MG, van der Meer JW, van den Berg WB, Joosten LA. The anti-CD20 antibody rituximab reduces the Th17 cell response. Arthritis Rheum. 2011;63:1507–16.

16. Lieberman KV, Tejani A. A randomized double-blind placebo-controlled trial of cyclosporine in steroid-resistant idiopathic focal segmental glomerulosclerosis in children. J Am Soc Nephrol. 1996;7(1):56–63.

17. Sethi S, Glassock RJ, Fervenza FC. Focal segmental glomerulosclerosis: towards a better understanding for the practicing nephrologist. Nephrol Dial Transplant. 2015;30(3):375–84.

18. Hogan J, Bomback AS, Mehta K, Canetta PA, Rao MK, Appel GB, Radhakrishnan J, Lafayette RA. Treatment of idiopathic FSGS with adrenocorticotropic hormone gel. Clin J Am Soc Nephrol. 2013;8:2072–81.

19. Yu CC, Fornoni A, Weins A, Hakroush S, Maiguel D, Sageshima J, Chen L, Ciancio G, Faridi MH, Behr D, Campbell KN, Chang JM, Chen HC, Oh J, Faul C, Arnaout MA, Fiorina P, Gupta V, Greka A, Burke 3rd GW, Mundel P. Abatacept in B7-1-positive proteinuric kidney disease. N Engl J Med. 2013;369:2416–23.

20. Cattran DC, Delmore T, Roscoe J, Cole E, Cardella C, Charron R, Ritchie S. A randomized controlled trial of prednisone in patients with idiopathic membranous nephropathy. N Engl J Med. 1989;320:210–5.

21. Cameron JS, Healy MJ, Adu D. The Medical Research Council trial of short-term high-dose alternate day prednisolone in idiopathic membranous nephropathy with nephrotic syndrome in adults. The MRC Glomerulonephritis Working Party. Q J Med. 1990;74:133–56.

22. Kaasik P, Umnova M, Pehme A, Alev K, Aru M, Selart A, Seene T. Ageing and dexamethasone associated sarcopenia: peculiarities of regeneration. J Steroid Biochem Mol Biol. 2007;105:85–90.

23. Ponticelli C, Altieri P, Scolari F, Passerini P, Roccatello D, Cesana B, Melis P, Valzorio B, Sasdelli M, Pasquali S, Pozzi C, Piccoli G, Lupo A, Segagni S, Antonucci F, Dugo M, Minari M, Scalia A, Pedrini L, Pisano G, Grassi C, Farina M, Bellazzi R. A randomized study comparing methylprednisolone plus chlorambucil versus methylprednisolone plus cyclophosphamide in idiopathic membranous nephropathy. J Am Soc Nephrol. 1998;9:444–50.

24. Ponticelli C, Zucchelli P, Passerini P, Cesana B, Locatelli F, Pasquali S, Sasdelli M, Redaelli B, Grassi C, Pozzi C, et al. A 10-year follow-up of a randomized study with methylprednisolone and chlorambucil in membranous nephropathy. Kidney Int. 1995;48:1600–4.

25. Jha V, Ganguli A, Saha TK, Kohli HS, Sud K, Gupta KL, Joshi K, Sakhuja V. A randomized, controlled trial of steroids and cyclophosphamide in adults with nephrotic syndrome caused by idiopathic membranous nephropathy. J Am Soc Nephrol. 2007;18:1899–904.

26. Ponticelli C, Zucchelli P, Passerini P, Cesana B. The Italian Idiopathic Membranous Nephropathy Treatment Study Group. Methylprednisolone plus chlorambucil as compared with methylprednisolone alone for the treatment of idiopathic membranous nephropathy. N Engl J Med. 1992;327:599–603.

27. Polanco N, Gutiérrez E, Covarsí A, Ariza F, Carreño A, Vigil A, Baltar J, Fernández-Fresnedo G, Martín C, Pons S, Lorenzo D, Bernis C, Arrizabalaga P, Fernández-Juárez G, Barrio V, Sierra M, Castellanos I, Espinosa M, Rivera F, Oliet A, Fernández-Vega F, Praga M, Grupo de Estudio de las Enfermedades Glomerulares de la Sociedad Española de Nefrología. Spontaneous remission of nephrotic syndrome in idiopathic membranous nephropathy. J Am Soc Nephrol. 2010;21:697–704.

28. Praga M, Barrio V, Juárez GF, Luño J, Grupo Español de Estudio de la Nefropatía Membranosa. Tacrolimus monotherapy in membranous nephropathy: a randomized controlled trial. Kidney Int. 2007;71:924–30.

29. Branten AJ, du Buf-Vereijken PW, Vervloet M, Wetzels JF. Mycophenolate mofetil in idiopathic membranous nephropathy: a clinical trial with comparison to a historic control group treated with cyclophosphamide. Am J Kidney Dis. 2007;50:248–56.

30. Dussol B, Morange S, Burtey S, Indreies M, Cassuto E, Mourad G, Villar E, Pouteil-Noble C, Karaaslan H, Sichez H, Lasseur C, Delmas Y, Nogier MB, Fathallah M, Loundou A, Mayor V, Berland Y. Mycophenolate mofetil monotherapy in membranous nephropathy: a 1-year randomized controlled trial. Am J Kidney Dis. 2008;52:699–705.

31. Ruggenenti P, Cravedi P, Chianca A, Perna A, Ruggiero B, Gaspari F, Rambaldi A, Marasà M, Remuzzi G. Rituximab in idiopathic membranous nephropathy. J Am Soc Nephrol. 2012;23:1416–25.

32. Hladunewich MA, Cattran D, Beck LH, Odutayo A, Sethi S, Ayalon R, Leung N, Reich H, Fervenza FC. A pilot study to determine the dose and effectiveness of adrenocorticotrophic hormone (H.P. Acthar® Gel) in nephrotic syndrome due to idiopathic membranous nephropathy. Nephrol Dial Transplant. 2014;29:1570–7.

33. Lindskog A, Ebefors K, Johansson ME, Stefánsson B, Granqvist A, Arnadottir M, Berg AL, Nyström J, Haraldsson B. Melanocortin 1 receptor agonists reduce proteinuria. J Am Soc Nephrol. 2010;21:1290–8.

34. Donadio Jr JV, Grande JP, Bergstralh EJ, Dart RA, Larson TS, Spencer DC. The long-term outcome of patients with IgA nephropathy treated with fish oil in a controlled trial. Mayo Nephrology Collaborative Group. J Am Soc Nephrol. 1999;10:1772–7.

35. Hogg RJ, Lee J, Nardelli N, Julian BA, Cattran D, Waldo B, Wyatt R, Jennette JC, Sibley R, Hyland K, Fitzgibbons L, Hirschman G, Donadio Jr JV, Holub BJ, Southwest Pediatric Nephrology Study Group. Clinical trial to evaluate omega-3 fatty acids and alternate

day prednisone in patients with IgA nephropathy: report from the Southwest Pediatric Nephrology Study Group. Clin J Am Soc Nephrol. 2006;1:467–74.

36. Liu LL, Wang LN. ω-3 fatty acids therapy for IgA nephropathy: a meta-analysis of randomized controlled trials. Clin Nephrol. 2012;77:119–25.

37. Moriyama T, Iwasaki C, Tanaka K, Ochi A, Shimizu A, Shiohira S, Itabashi M, Takei T, Uchida K, Tsuchiya K, Nitta K. Effects of combination therapy with renin-angiotensin system inhibitors and eicosapentaenoic acid on IgA nephropathy. Intern Med. 2013;52:193–9.

38. Pozzi C, Andrulli S, Del Vecchio L, Melis P, Fogazzi GB, Altieri P, Ponticelli C, Locatelli F. Corticosteroid effectiveness in IgA nephropathy: long-term results of a randomized, controlled trial. J Am Soc Nephrol. 2004;15:157–63.

39. Coppo R. Is a legacy effect possible in IgA nephropathy? Nephrol Dial Transplant. 2013;28:1657–62.

40. TESTING STUDY- NCT01560052. Clinicaltrials.gov.

41. Praga M, Gutiérrez E, González E, Morales E, Hernández E. Treatment of IgA nephropathy with ACE inhibitors: a randomized and controlled trial. J Am Soc Nephrol. 2003;14:1578–83.

42. Lv J, Zhang H, Chen Y, Li G, Jiang L, Singh AK, Wang H. Combination therapy of prednisone and ACE inhibitor versus ACE-inhibitor therapy alone in patients with IgA nephropathy: a randomized controlled trial. Am J Kidney Dis. 2009;53:26–32.

43. Tang S, Leung JC, Chan LY, Lui YH, Tang CS, Kan CH, Ho YW, Lai KN. Mycophenolate mofetil alleviates persistent proteinuria in IgA nephropathy. Kidney Int. 2005;68:802–12.

44. Frisch G, Lin J, Rosenstock J, Markowitz G, D'Agati V, Radhakrishnan J, Preddie D, Crew J, Valeri A, Appel G. Mycophenolate mofetil (MMF) vs placebo in patients with moderately advanced IgA nephropathy: a double-blind randomized controlled trial. Nephrol Dial Transplant. 2005;20:2139–45.

45. Pozzi C, Andrulli S, Pani A, Scaini P, Del Vecchio L, Fogazzi G, Vogt B, De Cristofaro V, Allegri L, Cirami L, Procaccini AD, Locatelli F. Addition of azathioprine to corticosteroids does not benefit patients with IgA nephropathy. J Am Soc Nephrol. 2010;21:1783–90.

46. STOP-IgA N. NCT-00554502.Clinicaltrials.gov.

47. Yamamoto Y, Hiki Y, Nakai S, Yamamoto K, Takahashi K, Koide S, Murakami K, Tomita M, Hasegawa M, Kawashima S, Sugiyama S, Yuzawa Y. Comparison of effective impact among tonsillectomy alone, tonsillectomy combined with oral steroid and with steroid pulse therapy on long-term outcome of immunoglobulin A nephropathy. Clin Exp Nephrol. 2013;17:218–24.

48. Maeda I, Hayashi T, Sato KK, Shibata MO, Hamada M, Kishida M, Kitabayashi C, Morikawa T, Okada N, Okumura M, Konishi M, Konishi Y, Endo G, Imanishi M. Tonsillectomy has beneficial effects on remission and progression of IgA nephropathy independent of steroid therapy. Nephrol Dial Transplant. 2012;27:2806–13.

49. Wang Y, Chen J, Wang Y, Chen Y, Wang L, Lv Y. A meta-analysis of the clinical remission rate and long-term efficacy of tonsillectomy in patients with IgA nephropathy. Nephrol Dial Transplant. 2011;26:1923–31.

50. Piccoli A, Codognotto M, Tabbi MG, Favaro E, Rossi B. Influence of tonsillectomy on the progression of mesangioproliferative glomerulonephritis. Nephrol Dial Transplant. 2010;25:2583–9.

51. Ponticelli C. Tonsillectomy and IgA nephritis. Nephrol Dial Transplant. 2012;27:2610–3.

52. Sethi S, Fervenza FC. Membranoproliferative glomerulonephritis– a new look at an old entity. N Engl J Med. 2012;366:1119–31.

53. Donadio Jr JV, Offord KP. Reassessment of treatment results in membranoproliferative glomerulonephritis, with emphasis on life-table analysis. Am J Kidney Dis. 1989;14:445–51.

Hemodialysis Clinical Trials: A Critical Appraisal

Charles Chazot

General Introduction

Hemodialysis therapy has been one of the major breakthroughs in medicine in the twentieth century, allowing end-stage renal failure (ESRD) patients to remain alive for years or decades and to restore and continue their social and professional life and for some of them to wait for kidney transplantation. There has been since a tremendous effort in both clinical and engineering research to improve the burden of dialysis therapy and make it safer, easier, and more acceptable. In 50 years since Clyde Shields was started on chronic hemodialysis by Scribner et al. [1], a number of significant progresses have emerged such as the control of ultrafiltration, allowing to optimize convection, the way to assess the dialysis dose, the knowledge on uremic toxins, the release of more biocompatible and selectively permeable membranes, and the importance of nutrition for these patients. However despite all these significant improvements, we all face a persisting huge challenge because of the high mortality rate among dialysis patients, and questioning the current practices in the field of hemodialysis must be a continuous process: When to start dialysis therapy? How long and how frequent hemodialysis should be? Is high-volume convection the key? We owe the answers of these questions to our patients and their families and also to the healthcare authorities to provide the most cost-effective therapy.

Timing of Start of RRT

IDEAL Study

A randomized, controlled trial of early versus late initiation of dialysis

C. Chazot, MD
NephroCare Tassin-Charcot, 7 Avenue Marechal Foch,
Sainte Foy Les Lyon, Lyon, France
chchazot@gmail.com

Authors: Bruce A. Cooper, M.B., B.S., Ph.D., Pauline Branley, B. Med., Ph.D., Liliana Bulfone, B.Pharm., M.B.A., John F. Collins, M.B., Ch.B., Jonathan C. Craig, M.B., Ch.B., Ph.D., Margaret B. Fraenkel, B.M., B.S., Ph.D., Anthony Harris, M.A., M.Sc., David W. Johnson, M.B., B.S., Ph.D., Joan Kesselhut, Jing Jing Li, B.Pharm., B.Com., Grant Luxton, M.B., B.S., Andrew Pilmore, B.Sc., David J. Tiller, M.B., B.S., David C. Harris, M.B., B.S., M.D., and Carol A. Pollock, M.B., B.S., Ph.D. for the IDEAL Study

Abstract

In clinical practice, there is considerable variation in the timing of the initiation of maintenance dialysis for patients with stage V chronic kidney disease, with a worldwide trend toward early initiation. In this study, conducted at 32 centers in Australia and New Zealand, we examined whether the timing of the initiation of maintenance dialysis influenced survival among patients with chronic kidney disease.

Methods: We randomly assigned patients 18 years of age or older with progressive chronic kidney disease and an estimated glomerular filtration rate (GFR) between 10.0 and 15.0 ml/min/1.73 m^2 of body-surface area (calculated with the use of the Cockcroft–Gault equation) to planned initiation of dialysis when the estimated GFR was 10.0–14.0 ml/min (early start) or when the estimated GFR was 5.0–7.0 ml/min (late start). The primary outcome was death from any cause.

Results: Between July 2000 and November 2008, a total of 828 adults (mean age, 60.4 years; 542 men and 286 women; 355 with diabetes) underwent randomization, with a median time to the initiation of dialysis of 1.80 months (95 % confidence interval [CI], 1.60–2.23) in the early-start group and 7.40 months (95 % CI, 6.23–8.27) in the late-start group. A total of 75.9 % of the patients in the late-start group initiated dialysis when the estimated GFR was above the target of 7.0 ml/min, owing to the development of symptoms. During a median follow-up period of 3.59 years, 152 of 404 patients in the early-start group (37.6 %) and 155 of 424 in the late-start group (36.6 %) died (hazard ratio with early initiation, 1.04; 95 % CI, 0.83–1.30; $P = 0.75$). There was no significant difference between the groups in the frequency of adverse events (cardiovascular events, infections, or complications of dialysis).

Conclusions: In this study, planned early initiation of dialysis in patients with stage V chronic kidney disease was not associated with an improvement in survival or clinical outcomes. (Funded by the National Health and Medical Research Council of Australia and others; Australian New Zealand Clinical Trials Registry number, 12609000266268.)

Reference: *N Engl J Med*. 2010;363:609–19

Critical Appraisal

Parameters	Yes	No	Comment
Validity			
Is the **Randomization** Procedure well described?	+1		Yes. Permuted-block design stratified according to center
Double **blinded**?		−2	No
Is the **sample size** calculation described/adequate?	+3		Yes. Power of 80 % for a 10 % death reduction led to the need of 800 patients
Does it have a hard primary **end point**?	+1		Yes
Is the end point surrogate?		0	No
Is the follow-up appropriate?	+1		Yes. 3 years
Was there a **Bias**?	−2		Not blinded
Is the dropout >25 %?		+1	No
Is the analysis **ITT**?	+3		Yes
Utility/usefulness			
Can the findings be generalized?	+1		Yes. See the summary below
Are the findings easily translatable?	+1		Yes
Was the NNT <100?		−1	No
Score	**41 %**		

Summary and Conclusions

The IDEAL study has brought an important answer to the recurrent question of the best timing to start dialysis therapy. Several guidelines recommended the start at thresholds from 10 to 15 ml/min of estimated GFR [2–5]. The consequence was that in 2005 45 % of patients in the USA started hemodialysis therapy above 10 ml/min of eGFR [6]. The IDEAL study brings an answer for both peritoneal dialysis and hemodialysis showing no difference in outcome between early and late start. However, the patients were younger and with less comorbidities than in the USA and Europe, and these findings

may not apply in other parts of the world [7]. However subgroup analysis did not find any difference according to age and comorbidities. Also, it can be argued that the difference between groups was small (2.2 ml/min/1.73 m² difference for eGFR and 6-month delay between groups), but i shows that clinical management beyond eGFR value allow to safely postpone renal replacement therapy [8].

Adequacy of Hemodialysis

NCD Study

Effect of the hemodialysis prescription of patient morbidity report from the National Cooperative Dialysis Study
Authors: Lowrie EG, Laird NM, Parker TF, Sargent JA.
Reference: *N Engl J Med*. 1981 Nov 12;305(20):1176–81

Abstract

This report summarizes morbidity in 151 patients in a cooperative trial designed to evaluate the clinical effects of different dialysis prescriptions. Four treatment groups were divided along two dimensions: dialysis treatment time (long or short), and blood urea nitrogen (BUN) concentration averaged with respect to time (TACurea) (high or low). Dietary protein was not restricted. There was no difference in mortality between the groups. Withdrawal of patient from the high-BUN groups for medical reasons was significantly greater than withdrawal from the low-BUN groups. Hospitalization was also greater in the high-BUN groups but dialysis treatment time had no significant effects. The data indicate that the occurrence of morbid events is affected by the dialysis prescription. Increased morbidity appears to accompany prescriptions associated with a relatively high BUN. Conversely, morbidity may be decreased by prescriptions associated with more efficient removal of urea if the dietary intake of protein and other nutrients is adequate.

Critical Appraisal

Parameters	Yes	No	Comment
Validity			
Is the **Randomization** Procedure well described?	+1		Yes, done by a LEAD Center
Double **blinded**?		−2	No
Is the **sample size** calculation described/adequate?		−3	Not easily available. The authors refer to two references that the authors of this review could not retrieve

Parameters	Yes	No	Comment
Does it have a hard primary **end point**?		−1	Yes. Morbidity
Is the end point surrogate?	−2		Yes. Mortality was not different between groups
Is the follow-up appropriate?	+1		Yes. 22 months
Was there a **Bias**?	−2		Yes. See the Summary section below
Is the dropout >25 %?	−1		Yes
Is the analysis **ITT**?	+3		Yes
Utility/usefulness			
Can the findings be generalized?	+1		Yes
Are the findings easily translatable?	+1		Yes
Was the NNT <100?		−1	No
Score	**0 %**		

Summary and Conclusions

This is the first randomized control trial in hemodialysis therapy relating patients' outcomes and surrogates of dialysis dose (BUN level and treatment time). Its mechanistic interpretation [9] has opened the track for dialysis quantification with the K_t/V concept, allowing physician to quantify small-molecule clearance. The dialysis adequacy was born and has influenced dialysis prescriptions for the following decades. However, the interpretation of the NCDS has since been largely criticized. Treatment time was not retained as significantly influencing outcomes. In the subgroups with high BUN, the P value comparing outcomes according to treatment times (3 h versus 4.5 h) was 0.056. Ignoring this important factor was questionable [10, 11], leading to the idea that increasing K with a fixed T could reach dialysis adequacy. This approach has focused the prescription on small-molecule clearance, whereas important factors more "T dependent" have since emerged such as phosphate balance [12], fluid management [13], or middle-molecule removal [14]. Moreover, BUN as a marker of uremic toxicity reflects the protein intake. The range of protein intake in the study was wide, from 0.8 to 1.4 g/kg/day and then a source of confounding factor.

The implementation of new trials on alternative dialysis strategy on time and frequency (see elsewhere) is the evidence that the NCDS conclusions did not solve all aspects of dialysis adequacy. However, it has given the practitioner the key of the minimum requirements of dialysis treatment.

HEMO Study

Effect of dialysis dose and membrane flux in maintenance hemodialysis

Authors: Garabed Eknoyan, M.D., Gerald J. Beck, Ph.D., Alfred K. Cheung, M.D., John T. Daugirdas, M.D., Tom Greene, Ph.D., John W. Kusek, Ph.D., Michael Allon, M.D., James Bailey, M.D., James A. Delmez, M.D., Thomas A. Depner, M.D., Johanna T. Dwyer, D.Sc., R.D., Andrew S. Levey, M.D., Nathan W. Levin, M.D., Edgar Milford, M.D., Daniel B. Ornt, M.D., Michael V. Rocco, M.D., Gerald Schulman, M.D., Steve J. Schwab, M.D., Brendan P. Teehan, M.D., and Robert Toto, M.D. for the Hemodialysis (HEMO) Study Group

Reference: *N Engl J Med*. 2002; 347:2010–9

Abstract

Background: The effects of the dose of dialysis and the level of flux of the dialyzer membrane on mortality and morbidity among patients undergoing maintenance hemodialysis are uncertain.

Methods: We undertook a randomized clinical trial in 1,846 patients undergoing thrice-weekly dialysis, using a two-by-two factorial design to assign patients randomly to a standard or high dose of dialysis and to a low-flux or high-flux dialyzer.

Results: In the standard-dose group, the mean (±SD) urea-reduction ratio was 66.3 ± 2.5 %, the single-pool K_t/V was 1.32 ± 0.09, and the equilibrated K_t/V was 1.16 ± 0.08; in the high-dose group, the values were 75.2 ± 2.5 %, 1.71 ± 0.11, and 1.53 ± 0.09, respectively. Flux, estimated on the basis of beta$_2$-microglobulin clearance, was 3 ± 7 ml/min in the low-flux group and 34 ± 11 ml/min in the high-flux group. The primary outcome, death from any cause, was not significantly influenced by the dose or flux assignment: the relative risk of death in the high-dose group as compared with the standard-dose group was 0.96 (95 % confidence interval, 0.84–1.10; $P=0.53$), and the relative risk of death in the high-flux group as compared with the low-flux group was 0.92 (95 % confidence interval, 0.81–1.05; $P=0.23$). The main secondary outcomes (first hospitalization for cardiac causes or death from any cause, first hospitalization for infection or death from any cause, first 15 % decrease in the serum albumin level or death from any cause, and all hospitalizations not related to vascular access) also did not differ significantly between either the dose groups or the flux groups. Possible benefits of the dose or flux interventions were suggested in two of seven prespecified subgroups of patients.

Conclusion: Patients undergoing hemodialysis thrice weekly appear to have no major benefit from a higher dialysis dose than that recommended by current US guidelines or from the use of a high-flux membrane.

Critical Appraisal

Parameters	Yes	No	Comment
Validity			
Is the **Randomization** Procedure well described?	+1		Yes. Central assignment

Parameters	Yes	No	Comment
Double **blinded**?		−2	No
Is the **sample size** calculation described/ adequate?	+3		Yes. Calculated for a 25 % reduction of mortality [15]
Does it have a hard primary **end point**?	+1		Yes. Mortality
Is the end point surrogate?		0	No
Is the follow-up appropriate?	+1		Yes. 2.84 years and 5,237 patient-years
Was there a **Bias**?		+2	No
Is the dropout >25 %?	0	+1	No
Is the analysis **ITT**?	+3		Yes
Utility/usefulness			
Can the findings be generalized?	+1		Yes
Are the findings easily translatable?	+1		Yes
Was the NNT <100?		−1	No
Score	**68 %**		

Summary and Conclusions

The HEMO study was well designed, with an acceptable dropout rate and a substantial follow-up. This trial has shaken the thoughts of many nephrologists, providing no support for better survival with higher small-molecule clearance and for high-flux membrane (and then increased middle-molecule clearance). Interactions with baseline characteristics found a benefit of high-flux membrane in patients treated for more than 3.7 years and that women benefited of higher K_t/V [16]. Regarding this last finding, the in-depth analysis of the dialysis dose according to gender has pointed out that when K_t was related to body surface area rather than to "V," women were receiving a lower dialysis dose than men [17]. This might explain the better outcome of women in the high-dose group. It also questions the K_t/V paradigm and the way to normalize K_t. This study also highlights the fact that survival is multifactorial in hemodialysis patients and cannot be limited to small- and middle-molecule clearances. Especially bone mineral metabolism and fluid balance are important factors for outcome and were not covered by the HEMO trial. This has been well underlined by Twardowski and Misra [18], pointing a type III statistical error (wrong hypothesis and correct answer): the beneficial effect of the increase in K_t/V may be blunted when obtained only from its "K" component.

Type of Dialysis Membrane

MPO Study

Effect of membrane permeability on survival of hemodialysis patients

Authors: Locatelli F, Martin-Malo A, Hannedouche T, Loureiro A, Papadimitriou M, Wizemann V, Jacobson SH, Czekalski S, Ronco C, Vanholder R; Membrane Permeability Outcome (MPO) Study Group.
Reference: *J Am Soc Nephrol*. 2009 Mar;20(3):645–54

Abstract

The effect of high-flux hemodialysis membranes on patient survival has not been unequivocally determined. In this prospective, randomized clinical trial, we enrolled 738 incident hemodialysis patients, stratified them by serum albumin ≤4 and >4 g/dl, and assigned them to either low-flux or high-flux membranes. We followed patients for 3–7.5 years. Kaplan-Meier survival analysis showed no significant difference between high-flux and low-flux membranes, and a Cox proportional hazards model concurred. Patients with serum albumin ≤4 g/dl had significantly higher survival rates in the high-flux group compared with the low-flux group ($P=0.032$). In addition, a secondary analysis revealed that high-flux membranes may significantly improve survival of patients with diabetes. Among those with serum albumin ≤4 g/dl, slightly different effects among patients with and without diabetes suggested a potential interaction between diabetes status and low serum albumin in the reduction of risk conferred by high-flux membranes. In summary, we did not detect a significant survival benefit with either high-flux or low-flux membranes in the population overall, but the use of high-flux membranes conferred a significant survival benefit among patients with serum albumin ≤4 g/dl. The apparent survival benefit among patients who have diabetes and are treated with high-flux membranes requires confirmation given the post hoc nature of our analysis.

Critical Appraisal

Parameters	Yes	No	Comment
Validity			
Is the **Randomization** Procedure well described?	+1		Yes. Central block randomization
Double **blinded**?		−2	No
Is the **sample size** calculation described/ adequate?	+3		Yes. A 10 % decrease of mortality was expected and an expected mortality of 30–50 % during the 3-year follow-up

Parameters	Yes	No	Comment
Does it have a hard primary **end point**?	+1		Yes. Mortality
Is the end point surrogate?		0	No
Is the follow-up appropriate?	+1		Yes. 3.0 ± 1.9 years
Was there a **Bias**?	0	+2	No
Is the drop out >25 %?	−1		Yes. 41.7 %
Is the analysis **ITT**?	+3		Yes
Utility/usefulness			
Can the findings be generalized?	+1		Yes
Are the findings easily translatable?	+1		Yes
Was the NNT <100?		−1	No
Score	**52.9 %**		

Summary and Conclusions

The MPO study is the second negative study on membrane flux after the HEMO study. It included incident patients, ruling out selection of survivors and the effects of previous treatment. The subgroup analysis has shown a survival advantage in patients with serum albumin(S-Alb) below 40 g/l and in diabetic patients. The main issue is that the design has changed during the study because of the slow pace of inclusions. Initially recruitment involved patients with S-Alb <40 g/l. Thereafter inclusion was widened to patients with normal S-Alb. The sample size calculation was adapted to this change. But it may explain the negative results and it has blurred the message. However, it confirms the beneficial effect of high-flux membranes reported in diabetic patients reported from the 4-D trial [19].

Dialysis Frequency

FHN Study

In-center hemodialysis six times per week versus three times per week

Authors: The FHN Trial Group

Reference: *N Engl J Med*. 2010; 363:2287–300. December 9, 2010. doi:10.1056/NEJMoa1001593

Abstract

Background: In this randomized clinical trial, we aimed to determine whether increasing the frequency of in-center hemodialysis would result in beneficial changes in left ventricular mass, self-reported physical health, and other intermediate outcomes among patients undergoing maintenance hemodialysis.

Methods: Patients were randomly assigned to undergo hemodialysis six times per week (frequent hemodialysis, 125 patients) or three times per week (conventional hemodialysis, 120 patients) for 12 months. The two coprimary composite outcomes were death or change (from baseline to 12 months) in left ventricular mass, as assessed by cardiac magnetic resonance imaging, and death or change in the physical-health composite score of the RAND 36-item health survey. Secondary outcomes included cognitive performance; self-reported depression; laboratory markers of nutrition, mineral metabolism, and anemia; blood pressure; and rates of hospitalization and of interventions related to vascular access.

Results: Patients in the frequent-hemodialysis group averaged 5.2 sessions per week; the weekly standard K_t/V_{urea} (the product of the urea clearance and the duration of the dialysis session normalized to the volume of distribution of urea) was significantly higher in the frequent-hemodialysis group than in the conventional-hemodialysis group (3.54 ± 0.56 vs. 2.49 ± 0.27). Frequent hemodialysis was associated with significant benefits with respect to both coprimary composite outcomes (hazard ratio for death or increase in left ventricular mass, 0.61; 95 % confidence interval [CI], 0.46–0.82; hazard ratio for death or a decrease in the physical-health composite score, 0.70; 95 % CI, 0.53–0.92). Patients randomly assigned to frequent hemodialysis were more likely to undergo interventions related to vascular access than were patients assigned to conventional hemodialysis (hazard ratio, 1.71; 95 % CI, 1.08–2.73). Frequent hemodialysis was associated with improved control of hypertension and hyperphosphatemia. There were no significant effects of frequent hemodialysis on cognitive performance, self-reported depression, serum albumin concentration, or use of erythropoiesis-stimulating agents.

Conclusions: Frequent hemodialysis, as compared with conventional hemodialysis, was associated with favorable results with respect to the composite outcomes of death or change in left ventricular mass and death or change in a physical-health composite score but prompted more frequent interventions related to vascular access. (Funded by the National Institute of Diabetes and Digestive and Kidney Diseases and others; ClinicalTrials.gov number, NCT00264758.)

Critical Appraisal

Parameters	Yes	No	Comment
Validity			
Is the **Randomization** Procedure well described?	+1		Yes. Stratified randomization by clinical centers and diabetic status with randomly permuted blocks
Double **blinded**?		−2	No

Parameters	Yes	No	Comment
Is the **sample size** calculation described/adequate?	+3		Yes. Based on the hypothesis of a 20 % reduction in mortality with frequent dialysis with a 90 % power leading to 250 patients
Does it have a hard primary **end point**?		−1	No. 2 combined coprimary end points: mortality and left ventricular mass and mortality and physical-health composite score
Is the end point surrogate?	−2		Yes
Is the follow-up appropriate?		−1	No. Only 1 year
Was there a **Bias**?	−2		Yes. See the summary
Is the dropout >25 %?		+1	No
Is the analysis **ITT**?	+3		Yes
Utility/usefulness			
Can the findings be generalized?	+1		Yes
Are the findings easily translatable?		−1	No because implementing daily dialysis faces many barriers
Was the NNT <100?		−1	No
Score	0 %		

Summary and Conclusions

The FHN daily trial has highlighted the benefits of daily dialysis after 1 year on composite coprimary outcomes, death and left ventricular mass, and death and physical-health composite score. The authors explained the choice of these end points in a preliminary article about the FHN methodology [20]. Analyzing mortality per se would have been a hard challenge, requiring 1,500 patients and several years of follow-up [20]. Several concerns have been raised after the study release. The death rate was unusually low in the two groups and the use of coprimary outcomes is questionable [21]. Moreover, the frequent group received a 23 % extra time of dialysis treatment, introducing a serious bias regarding the frequency benefit [22]. The high frequency of blood access complications and the economic issues make the finding not easily translatable. The FHN trial is a good illustration of the huge difficulties in implementing an RCT to compare standard and alternative dialysis techniques.

FHN Nocturnal Study

The effects of frequent nocturnal home hemodialysis: the Frequent Hemodialysis Network Nocturnal Trial

Authors: Michael V Rocco, Robert S Lockridge Jr, Gerald J Beck, Paul W Eggers, Jennifer J Gassman, Tom Greene, Brett Larive, Christopher T Chan, Glenn M Chertow, Michael Copland, Christopher D Hoy, Robert M Lindsay, Nathan W Levin, Daniel B Ornt, Andreas Pierratos, Mary F Pipkin, Sanjay Rajagopalan, John B Stokes, Mark L Unruh, Robert A Star, Alan S Kliger and the Frequent Hemodialysis Network (FHN) Trial Group
Reference: *Kidney Int.* 2011;80:1080–91

Abstract

Prior small studies have shown multiple benefits of frequent nocturnal hemodialysis compared to conventional three times per week treatments. To study this further, we randomized 87 patients to three times per week conventional hemodialysis or to nocturnal hemodialysis six times per week, all with single-use high-flux dialyzers. The 4. patients in the frequent nocturnal arm had a 1.82-fold higher mean weekly std K_t/V_{urea}, a 1.74-fold higher average number of treatments per week, and a 2.45-fold higher average weekly treatment time than the 42 patients in the conventional arm. We did not find a significant effect o nocturnal hemodialysis for either of the two coprimary outcomes (death or left ventricular mass (measured by MRI) with a hazard ratio of 0.68, or of death or RAND Physical Health Composite with a hazard ratio of 0.91). Possible explanations for the left ventricular mass result include limited sample size and patient characteristics. Secondary outcomes included cognitive performance, self-reported depression, laboratory markers of nutrition, mineral metabolism and anemia, blood pressure and rates of hospitalization, and vascular access interventions. Patients in the nocturnal arm had improved control of hyperphosphatemia and hypertension, but no significant benefit among the other main secondary outcomes. There was a trend for increased vascular access events in the nocturnal arm. Thus, we were unable to demonstrate a definitive benefit o more frequent nocturnal hemodialysis for either coprimary outcome.

Critical Appraisal

Parameters	Yes	No	Comment
Validity			
Is the **Randomization** Procedure well described?	+1		Yes. Stratified randomization by clinical centers and diabetic status with randomly permuted blocks

Parameters	Yes	No	Comment
Double **blinded**?		−2	No
Is the **sample size** calculation described/ adequate?		−3	Yes. Major difficulties in recruitment led to several adjustments in the sample size. It was the size of the cohort that dictated the outcome changes calculations then the reverse
Does it have a hard primary **end point**?		−1	No. 2 combined coprimary end points: mortality and left ventricular mass and mortality and physical-health composite score
Is the end point surrogate?	−2		Yes
Is the follow-up appropriate?		−1	No. Only 1 year
Was there a **Bias**?	−2		Yes. See the summary
Is the dropout >25 %?		+1	No
Is the analysis **ITT**?	+3		Yes
Utility/usefulness			
Can the findings be generalized?		−1	No. The study is negative
Are the findings easily translatable?		−1	No
Was the NNT <100?		−1	No
Score	0 %		

Summary and Conclusions

The FHN nocturnal trial failed to show an advantage of daily long nocturnal dialysis on the coprimary end points (the same as the FHN daily trial). The disappointment has to be tempered by the many flaws and limitations of the study. First, the limited size, because of difficulties in recruitment, has favored a high risk of type 1 error. Second, many patients were incident ones with persistent diuresis that might have blunted the improvement in left ventricular mass [23]. Third, other biases were present such as a very low mortality rate in the conventional arm (seven times less than the usual one) and the fact that there was overlap of dialysis frequency between the two groups [24]. These flaws and limitations allow us to nuance the *Kidney International* cover of the issue in which the study was published stating bluntly "No benefit from frequent nocturnal HD" [25] – a misleading and unfair statement.

Type of Dialysis Trials

The effect of on-line high-flux hemofiltration versus low-flux hemodialysis on mortality in chronic kidney failure: a small randomized controlled trial

Authors: Santoro A, Mancini E, Bolzani R, Boggi R, Cagnoli L, Francioso A, Fusaroli M, Piazza V, Rapanà R, Strippoli GF.

Reference: *Am J Kidney Dis.* 2008;52(3):507–18. doi:10.1053/j.ajkd.2008.05.011. Epub 2008 Jul 9.

Abstract

Background: Given the paucity of prospective randomized controlled trials assessing comparative performances of different dialysis techniques, we compared on-line high-flux hemofiltration (HF) with ultrapure low-flux hemodialysis (HD), assessing survival and morbidity in patients with end-stage renal disease (ESRD).

Study Design: An investigator-driven, prospective, multicenter, 3-year follow-up, centrally randomized study with no blinding and based on the intention-to-treat principle.

Setting & Participants: Prevalent patients with ESRD (age, 16–80 years; vintage >6 months) receiving renal replacement therapy at 20 Italian dialysis centers.

Interventions: Patients were centrally randomly assigned to HD ($n=32$) or HF ($n=32$).

Outcomes & Measurements: All-cause mortality, hospitalization rate for any cause, prevalence of dialysis hypotension, standard biochemical indexes, and nutritional status. Analyses were performed using the multivariate analysis of variance and Cox proportional hazard method.

Results: There was significant improvement in survival with HF compared with HD (78 % HF versus 57 %, HD) at 3 years of follow-up after allowing for the effects of age ($P=0.05$). End-of-treatment K_t/V was significantly higher with HD (1.42 ± 0.06 versus 1.07 ± 0.06 with HF), whereas beta(2)-microglobulin levels remained constant in HD patients (33.90 ± 2.94 mg/dl at baseline and 36.90 ± 5.06 mg/dl at 3 years), but decreased significantly in HF patients (30.02 ± 3.54 mg/dl at baseline versus 23.9 ± 1.77 mg/dl; $P<0.05$). The number of hospitalization events for each patient was not significantly different (2.36 ± 0.41 versus 1.94 ± 0.33 events), whereas length of stay proved to be significantly shorter in HF patients compared with HD patients ($P<0.001$). End-of-treatment body mass index decreased in HD patients, but increased in HF patients. Throughout the study period, the difference in trends of intradialytic acute hypotension was statistically significant, with a clear decrease in HF ($P=0.03$).

Limitations: This is a small preliminary intervention study with a high dropout rate and problematic generalizability.

Conclusion: On-line HF may improve survival independent of K_t/V in patients with ESRD, with a significant decrease in plasma beta(2)-microglobulin levels and increased body mass index. A larger study is required to confirm these results.

Critical Appraisal

Parameters	Yes	No	Comment
Validity			
Is the **Randomization** Procedure well described?	+1		Yes. Random central 1:1 assignment
Double **blinded**?		−2	No
Is the **sample size** calculation described/ adequate?	+1		Power is only 60 %. Risk of type 2 error
Does it have a hard primary **end point**?	+1		Yes. Mortality
Is the end point surrogate?		0	No
Is the follow-up appropriate?	+1		Yes. 3 years
Was there a **Bias**?		+2	No
Is the dropout >25 %?	−1		Yes. 23 dropouts (37.1 %)
Is the analysis **ITT**?	+3		Yes
Utility/usefulness			
Can the findings be generalized?		−1	No. Only patients with high comorbidities (Charlson ≥3) were enrolled
Are the findings easily translatable?		−1	No. This technique is not easily implemented
Was the NNT <100?	+1		Yes. Switching five patients to hemofiltration would spare one death
Score	29 %		

Summary and Conclusions

This trial is very interesting by its results. It is the first positive RCT reporting a survival advantage with an online convective therapy. Whereas the sample size calculation increased the risk of a type 2 error, the trial ended positive. It can be considered as strength. However, this trial has two limitations. First, it included only "at-risk" patients, i.e., with a high Charlson comorbidity index and compromised hemodynamic stability. Patients with a body weight over 75 k were excluded. So the generalization does not apply. Moreover, the control group was treated with low-flux

membrane. Even if the HEMO and the MPO studies are negative [26, 27], the question that nephrologists may have "does online hemofiltration provide better outcomes than high flux hemodialysis?" remains unknown.

Hemofiltration and hemodiafiltration reduce intradialytic hypotension in ESRD

Authors: Francesco Locatelli, Paolo Altieri, Simeone Andrulli, Piergiorgio Bolasco, Giovanna Sau, Luciano A. Pedrini, Carlo Basile, Salvatore David, Mariano Feriani, Giovanni Montagna, Biagio Raffaele Di Iorio, Bruno Memoli, Raffaella Cravero, Giovanni Battaglia, and Carmine Zoccali

Reference: *J Am Soc Nephrol.* 2010 October 21(10):1798–807.

Abstract

Symptomatic intradialytic hypotension is a common complication of hemodialysis (HD). The application of convective therapies to the outpatient setting may improve outcomes, including intradialytic hypotension. In this multicenter, open-label, randomized controlled study, we randomly assigned 146 long-term dialysis patients to HD ($n=70$), online predilution hemofiltration (HF; $n=36$), or online predilution hemodiafiltration (HDF; $n=40$). The primary end point was the frequency of intradialytic symptomatic hypotension (ISH). Compared with the run-in period, the frequency of sessions with ISH during the evaluation period increased for HD (7.1–7.9 %) and decreased for both HF (9.8–8.0 %) and HDF (10.6–5.2 %) ($P<0.001$). Mean predialysis systolic BP increased by 4.2 mmHg among those who were assigned to HDF compared with decreases of 0.6 and 1.8 mmHg among those who were assigned to HD and HF, respectively ($P=0.038$). Multivariate logistic regression demonstrated significant risk reductions in ISH for both HF (odds ratio 0.69; 95 % confidence interval 0.51–0.92) and HDF (odds ratio 0.46; 95 % confidence interval 0.33–0.63). There was a trend toward higher dropout for those who were assigned to HF ($P=0.107$). In conclusion, compared with conventional HD, convective therapies (HDF and HF) reduce ISH in long-term dialysis patients.

Critical Appraisal

Parameters	Yes	No	Comment
Validity			
Is the **Randomization** Procedure well described?	+1		Yes. Central computer-generated randomization

Parameters	Yes	No	Comment
Double **blinded**?		−2	No
Is the **sample size** calculation described/adequate?	+3		Yes. However, the calculation ends at 246 patients for a 3 % reduction of intradialytic hypotension, whereas the trial includes 146 patients
Does it have a hard primary **end point**?	+1		Yes. The end point is the prevalence of intradialytic symptomatic hypotension. See the Summary section
Is the end point surrogate?	−2		Yes
Is the follow-up appropriate?	+1		Yes. 1.5 years (IQR: 0.8–2.2) including 28,950 dialysis sessions
Was there a **Bias**?		+2	No
Is the dropout >25 %?		+1	No. The dropout is 22.5 %
Is the analysis **ITT**?	+3		Yes
Utility/usefulness			
Can the findings be generalized?	+1		Yes
Are the findings easily translatable?		−1	No, because convective therapies are not available or authorized in important areas
Was the NNT <100?	+1		Switching 37 patients from HD to HDF will avoid one session with symptomatic hypotension
Score	**47 %**		

Summary and Conclusions

The benefit of convective therapies has been questioned since their implementation in the late 1970s [28]. Other RCTs on hemodiafiltration are discussed later in this chapter. This study confirms improvement of hemodynamic stability in hemodialysis patients. Even if disputed by cohort study [29], another RCT recently confirmed this finding [30]. Because circulatory stress and hemodynamic stability is related to cardiovascular stress with potential organ damage [31], this end point is of primary importance. It must be mentioned that with convective therapies in this trial, there was a slight and significant increase in systolic blood pressure. The relationship between this hemodynamic effect and the reduction of symptomatic blood pressure drop is possible. It also questions the sodium balance with convective therapies.

Effect of online hemodiafiltration on all-cause mortality and cardiovascular outcomes

Authors: Muriel P.C. Grooteman, Marinus A. van den Dorpel, Michiel L. Bots, E. Lars Penne, Neelke C. van der Weerd, Albert H.A. Mazairac, Claire H. den Hoedt, Ingeborg van der Tweel, Renée Lévesque, Menso J. Nubé, Piet M. ter Wee, Peter J. Blankestijn and for the CONTRAST Investigators
Reference: *JASN*. June 1, 2012;23(6):1087–96

Abstract

In patients with ESRD, the effects of online hemodiafiltration on all-cause mortality and cardiovascular events are unclear. In this prospective study, we randomly assigned 714 chronic hemodialysis patients to online postdilution hemodiafiltration ($n = 358$) or to continue low-flux hemodialysis ($n = 356$). The primary outcome measure was all-cause mortality. The main secondary endpoint was a composite of major cardiovascular events, including death from cardiovascular causes, nonfatal myocardial infarction, nonfatal stroke, therapeutic coronary intervention, therapeutic carotid intervention, vascular intervention, or amputation. After a mean 3.0 years of follow-up (range, 0.4–6.6 years), we did not detect a significant difference between treatment groups with regard to all-cause mortality (121 versus 127 deaths per 1,000 person-years in the online hemodiafiltration and low-flux hemodialysis groups, respectively; hazard ratio, 0.95; 95 % confidence interval, 0.75–1.20). The incidences of cardiovascular events were 127 and 116 per 1,000 person-years, respectively (hazard ratio, 1.07; 95 % confidence interval, 0.83–1.39). Receiving high-volume hemodiafiltration during the trial associated with lower all-cause mortality, a finding that persisted after adjusting for potential confounders and dialysis facility. In conclusion, this trial did not detect a beneficial effect of hemodiafiltration on all-cause mortality and cardiovascular events compared with low-flux hemodialysis. On-treatment analysis suggests the possibility of a survival benefit among patients who receive high-volume hemodiafiltration, although this subgroup finding requires confirmation.

Critical Appraisal

Parameters	Yes	No	Comment
Validity			
Is the **Randomization** Procedure well described?	+1		Yes. Computer-based randomization into a 1:1 ratio stratified per participating center (permuted blocks)

Parameters	Yes	No	Comment
Double **blinded**?		−2	No
Is the **sample size** calculation described/adequate?	+3		Yes. Designed to have 80 % statistical power to detect a relative risk reduction of 20 % for online hemodiafiltration with a two-sided level of 5 %. Expected number of 772
Does it have a hard primary **end point**?	+1		Yes
Is the end point surrogate?		0	No
Is the follow-up appropriate?	+1		Yes. Mean follow-up of 3.04 years
Was there a **Bias**?		+2	No
Is the dropout >25 %?	−1		Yes. 33 %
Is the analysis **ITT**?	+3		Yes
Utility/usefulness			
Can the findings be generalized?		−1	No
Are the findings easily translatable?		−1	No
Was the NNT <100?		−1	No
Score	**29 %**		

Summary and Conclusions

This is the first RCT analyzing the effect of online hemodiafiltration (OL-HDF) on dialysis patients' outcomes (mortality and fatal and nonfatal cardiovascular events). At first sight and because of the absence of superiority of the convective technique when compared to low-flux dialysis, this study was disappointing for the convective technique upholders and did not justify the burden and extra costs of OL-HDF. However, the study has clearly highlighted the importance of the convection dose with a survival advantage when the convection volume was above 22 l. The study was designed before the DOPPS report describing the importance of the convective volume [32]. The convection volume was arbitrarily fixed at 24 l, given as an indication of the maximum volume expected. It was clearly not a target and one third of the cohort remained below 18 l. This volume matched closely the results of the Turkish study reported a few months later [33] (see elsewhere). As stated by Martin Kuhlmann in the *JASN* accompanying editorial

"On-line HDF is not a self-fulfilling prophecy; it must be used wisely" [34].

Turkish Online Hemofiltration Study

Mortality and cardiovascular events in online haemodiafiltration (OL-HDF) compared with high-flux dialysis: results from the Turkish OL-HDF Study

Authors: Ok E, Asci G, Toz H, Ok ES, Kircelli F, Yilmaz M, Hur E, Demirci MS, Demirci C, Duman S, Basci A, Adam SM, Isik IO, Zengin M, Suleymanlar G, Yilmaz ME, Ozkahya M; Turkish Online Haemodiafiltration Study.

Reference: *Nephrol Dial Transplant.* 2013 Jan;28(1):192–202.

Abstract

Background: Online haemodiafiltration (OL-HDF) is considered to confer clinical benefits over haemodialysis (HD) in terms of solute removal in patients undergoing maintenance HD. The aim of this study was to compare postdilution OL-HDF and high-flux HD in terms of morbidity and mortality.

Methods: In this prospective, randomized, controlled trial, we enrolled 782 patients undergoing thrice-weekly HD and randomly assigned them in a 1:1 ratio to either postdilution OL-HDF or high-flux HD. The mean age of patients was 56.5 ± 13.9 years, time on HD 57.9 ± 44.6 months with a diabetes incidence of 34.7 %. The follow-up period was 2 years, with the mean follow-up of 22.7 ± 10.9 months. The primary outcome was a composite of death from any cause and nonfatal cardiovascular events. The major secondary outcomes were cardiovascular and overall mortality, intradialytic complications, hospitalization rate, changes in several laboratory parameters and medications used.

Results: The filtration volume in OL-HDF was 17.2 ± 1.3 l. Primary outcome was not different between the groups (event-free survival of 77.6 % in OL-HDF versus 74.8 % in the high-flux group, $P = 0.28$), as well as cardiovascular and overall survival, hospitalization rate and number of hypotensive episodes. In a post hoc analysis, the subgroup of OL-HDF patients treated with a median substitution volume >17.4 l per session (high-efficiency OL-HDF, $n = 195$) had better cardiovascular ($P = 0.002$) and overall survival ($P = 0.03$) compared with the high-flux HD group. In adjusted Cox-regression analysis, treatment with high-efficiency OL-HDF was associated with a 46 % risk reduction for overall mortality and a 71 % risk reduction for cardiovascular mortality [RR = 0.29 (95 % CI 0.12–0.65), $P = 0.003$] compared with high-flux HD.

Conclusions: The composite of all-cause mortality and nonfatal cardiovascular event rate was not different in the OL-HDF and in the high-flux HD groups. In a post hoc analysis, OL-HDF treatment with substitution volumes over 17.4 l was associated with better cardiovascular and overall survival.

Critical Appraisal

Parameters	Yes	No	Comment
Validity			
Is the **Randomization** Procedure well described?	+1		Yes. Central randomization in a 1:1 ratio
Double **blinded**?		−2	No
Is the **sample size** calculation described/ adequate?	+3		Yes. 780 patients needed for a 35 % reduction of the primary end point with OL-HDF with a 80 % power
Does it have a hard primary **end point**?	+1		Yes. Death and nonfatal cardiovascular event
Is the end point surrogate?		0	No
Is the follow-up appropriate?	+1		Yes. 2 years
Was there a **Bias**?		+2	No
Is the dropout >25 %?	−1		Yes. 200 patients dropped out, that is, 25.6 %
Is the analysis **ITT**?	+3		Yes
Utility/usefulness			
Can the findings be generalized?		−1	No
Are the findings easily translatable?		−1	No
Was the NNT <100?		−1	No
Score	**17 %**		

Summary and Conclusions

This is the second negative RCT regarding OL-HDF. The authors point the risk of a type 2 error because the frequency of mortality and major cardiovascular events, composite primary end point, used for sample size calculation was 30 % lower than expected. As in the CONTRAST study [35], the convective volume analyzed in subgroups was found critical. In patients with more than 17.4 l per session, a 30 % decrease was found for the risk of reaching the end point. The study was designed from DOPPS [36] with a minimal target volume of 15 l. A posteriori appraisal with the knowledge of CONTRAST data may suggest this target was too low as CONTRAST showed survival advantage when con-

vective volume is above 22 l [35]. However, and like in CONTRAST, a selection bias cannot be ruled out from reaching high convective volumes. Patients with convective volume above 17.4 l had less diabetes, higher blood flow rates, higher serum albumin and lower hemoglobin levels, lower interdialytic weight gain, and lower phosphate levels.

ESHOL Study

High-efficiency postdilution online hemodiafiltration reduces all-cause mortality in hemodialysis patients

Authors: Maduell F, Moreso F, Pons M, Ramos R, Mora-Macià J, Carreras J, Soler J, Torres F, Campistol JM, Martinez-Castelao A; ESHOL Study Group.
Reference: *J Am Soc Nephrol.* 2013;24(3):487–97

Abstract

Retrospective studies suggest that online hemodiafiltration (OL-HDF) may reduce the risk of mortality compared with standard hemodialysis in patients with ESRD. We conducted a multicenter, open-label, randomized controlled trial in which we assigned 906 chronic hemodialysis patients either to continue hemodialysis ($n=450$) or to switch to high-efficiency postdilution OL-HDF ($n=456$). The primary outcome was all-cause mortality, and secondary outcomes included cardiovascular mortality, all-cause hospitalization, treatment tolerability, and laboratory data. Compared with patients who continued on hemodialysis, those assigned to OL-HDF had a 30 % lower risk of all-cause mortality (hazard ratio [HR], 0.70; 95 % confidence interval [95 % CI], 0.53–0.92; $P=0.01$), a 33 % lower risk of cardiovascular mortality (HR, 0.67; 95 % CI, 0.44–1.02; $P=0.06$), and a 55 % lower risk of infection-related mortality (HR, 0.45; 95 % CI, 0.21–0.96; $P=0.03$). The estimated number needed to treat suggested that switching eight patients from hemodialysis to OL-HDF may prevent one annual death. The incidence rates of dialysis sessions complicated by hypotension and of all-cause hospitalization were lower in patients assigned to OL-HDF. In conclusion, high-efficiency postdilution OL-HDF reduces all-cause mortality compared with conventional hemodialysis.

Critical Appraisal

Parameters	Yes	No	Comment
Validity			
Is the **Randomization** Procedure well described?	+1		Yes. Randomization by a central computerized random generator stratified by center
Double **blinded**?		−2	No

Parameters	Yes	No	Comment
Is the **sample size** calculation described/adequate?	+3		Yes. 800 patients needed for 80 % power to detect an HR at 0.63 with OL-HDF
Does it have a hard primary **end point**?	+1		Yes. All-cause mortality
Is the end point surrogate?		0	No
Is the follow-up appropriate?	+1		Yes. 3 years
Was there a **Bias**?	−2		Yes
Is the dropout >25 %?	−1		Yes. 39 %
Is the analysis **ITT**?	+3		Yes
Utility/usefulness			
Can the findings be generalized?	+1		Yes
Are the findings easily translatable?		−1	No
Was the NNT <100?	+1		Yes. 1 annual spared death with eight patients switched from high-flux dialysis to OL-HDF
Score	**41 %**		

Summary and Conclusions

The ESHOL study is the first RCT who found that OL-HDF provides a survival advantage compared to high-flux hemodialysis with a 30 % reduction of overall mortality, mainly from reduction of fatal stroke and infection. Among secondary end points, the cardiovascular mortality was not significantly reduced, whereas hospitalization rate and intradialytic hypotensive episodes were significantly lower in the OL-HDF group. The major difference of the ESHOL trial with the negative CONTRAST and Turkish studies [37, 38] (see elsewhere) was the amount of convection that was delivered to the patients (>18 l) with exclusion of patients not reaching this target. The best survival was observed with convection volume above 23.1 l. According to PJ Blankestijn in his accompanying editorial, this study is the important breakthrough that should drive authorization of convective therapies in the USA [39]. However, the big issue of the trial is that despite the randomization stratified by center, the patients assigned to OL-HDF were slightly younger, with less diabetes and with significantly less catheters as blood access [40]. Adjustments for these parameters did not change the advantage of OL-HDF. The other question raised by K. Farrington and A. Davenport [41] is related to β2-microglobulin that was not different between groups, like in the Turkish trial [38] and even increased in both groups along time. The role of residual renal function could not be analyzed because the information was not collected. Also, as

OL-HDF theoretical superiority is related to middle-molecul removal, this finding questions the mechanisms of the sur vival advantage found with high-volume convection. The the community needs other trials on hemodiafiltration to address these questions.

Nutrition in HD

Intradialytic parenteral nutrition does not improve sur vival in malnourished hemodialysis patients: a 2-year multicenter, prospective, randomized study

Authors: Noël J.M. Cano, Denis Fouque, Hubert Roth Michel Aparicio, Raymond Azar, Bernard Canaud, Philippe Chauveau, Christian Combe, Maurice Laville, Xavier M. Leverve and the French Study Group for Nutrition in Dialysis

Reference: *JASN*. 2007;18(9):2583–91

Abstract

Although intradialytic parenteral nutrition (IDPN) is a method used widely to combat protein-calorie malnutrition in hemodialysis patients, its effect on survival has not been thoroughly studied. We conducted a prospective, random ized trial in which 186 malnourished hemodialysis patients received oral nutritional supplements with or without 1 year of IDPN. IDPN did not improve 2-year mortality (primary end point), hospitalization rate, Karnofsky score, body mass index, or laboratory markers of nutritional status. Instead both groups demonstrated improvement in body mass index and the nutritional parameters serum albumin and prealbu min ($P < 0.05$). Multivariate analysis showed that an increase in prealbumin of >30 mg/l within 3 months, a marker of nutritional improvement, independently predicted a 54 % decrease in 2-year mortality, as well as reduced hospitaliza tions and improved general well-being as measured by the Karnofsky score. Therefore, although we found no definite advantage of adding IDPN to oral nutritional supplementa tion, this is the first prospective study demonstrating that an improvement in prealbumin during nutritional therapy is associated with a decrease in morbidity and mortality in malnourished hemodialysis patients.

Critical Appraisal

Parameters	Yes	No	Comment
Validity			
Is the **Randomization** Procedure well described?	+1		Yes. Central randomization stratified by center
Double **blinded**?		−2	No

Parameters	Yes	No	Comment
Is the **sample size** calculation described/adequate?	+3		Yes. 204 patients needed to identify a 10 % reduction in mortality with α and â error types of 5 and 20 %
Does it have a hard primary **end point**?	+1		Yes. Overall mortality
Is the end point surrogate?	−2		
Is the follow-up appropriate?	+1		Yes. 2 years
Was there a **Bias**?	−2		Yes (see the summary below)
Is the dropout >25 %?		+1	No. 22.6 %
Is the analysis **ITT**?	+3		Yes
Utility/usefulness			
Can the findings be generalized?	+1		Yes
Are the findings easily translatable?	+1		Yes
Was the NNT <100?		−1	No
Score	**29 %**		

Summary and Conclusions

The goal of this study was to evaluate the beneficial effect of intradialytic parenteral nutrition (IDPN) on patients' survival to confirm cohort data [42]. However, the design of the study has biased the evaluation. For ethical reasons, all the patients selected on malnutrition criteria received daily oral supplements during the study, allocated or not to IDPN. That means that the effect of IDPN per se was not possible to analyze without a true control group [43]. The first finding was that IDPN did not change the mortality in malnourished patients receiving oral supplements. As reported by the authors and according to the nutritional effects of oral supplements, the study was then clearly underpowered. However, nutritional parameters improved in nondiabetic patients under the effects of nutritional supplements whatever the route. And importantly, the increase in serum prealbumin during nutritional therapy was an independent predictor of mortality and hospitalization risk during a 2-year follow-up. The final conclusion of this study is that the nutritional support, oral or IV, improves nutritional markers and that this improvement is related with patients' outcomes.

General Discussion

More than twenty years have been necessary between the first patient treated with maintenance hemodialysis therapy and the publication of the first RCT in the field. No RCT was necessary to prove the efficacy of chronic dialysis in prolonging life of ESRD patients (the well-defined "traumatic interocular test" described by Twardowski and Misra [44], meaning that the "difference (was) so profound and obvious that, metaphorically, it hits one between the eyes" and does not require a P value to be confirmed significant). After that "honeymoon" time in the 1960s, and with changes in practices, such as reducing treatment time to treat more patients, a number of clinical issues emerged questioning the way of treating patients, and trials were required.

For instance, along decades, doubts have been raised regarding the adequate timing for dialysis start. The IDEAL trial [45] has answered that question and supports the concept that with adequate predialysis care, starting dialysis therapy may be postponed until the patient presents uremic burden that may happen late even when estimated GFR is below 10 ml/min. This study (re)places the clinician as the key person to counsel the patient.

The NCD study [46] has provided us the first step of dialysis adequacy with K_t/V_{urea}. The HEMO study [47] failed to show a survival advantage by increasing K_t/V_{urea} beyond the standard dose (single-pool K_t/V at 1.32). The nephrologist has to know that this K_t/V value is a "minimum" that is easily jeopardized by reduced treatment time and the use of catheters [48]. Every nephrologist now knows that the real adequacy goes far beyond small-molecule clearance.

The membrane issue is puzzling. Beta2-microglobulin, the surrogate marker of middle molecule, has been shown independently associated with mortality in HD patients in two studies [49, 50]. Then the failure at first sight of the HEMO and MPO trials [47, 51] to show a survival advantage with highly permeable membrane is surprising. Complementary analysis found superiority of these membranes in subgroups, but this is not an undisputable answer to the question supposed to be answered. Despite that, the use of highly permeable membrane is now worldwide, and it is highly probable that the community will be reluctant to go back to low-permeability membranes. The progressive disappearance of β2-related amyloidosis supports this choice [52].

The issue of membrane permeability has been switched to flux and convection with the development of convective therapies. The study by Santoro et al. [53] is spectacular in the sense that despite the relatively small number of patients has led to a very significant result, but in selected patients. However, it supports the importance of convection in at-risk patients. Locatelli et al. [54] have demonstrated a better hemodynamic tolerance with convective therapies. However, in that trial patient survival according to the techniques was not addressed. It was the case in three subsequent studies. The two first negative trials (CONTRAST and Turkish [55, 56]) have been important in highlighting the critical issue of infusion volume. They were very useful for the design of the ESHOL study [57] that found a significant survival advantage with online hemodiafiltration. This study, however, suffers from limitations with higher risk in the hemodialysis group. It is then not the end of the story to convince nephrologists and healthcare authorities to implement this technique for all patients.

Very early since the beginning of chronic dialysis, nutrition has been a key issue and emerged as an important prognostic factor. It was necessary to understand how to advise patients coming from low-protein diet before dialysis start. A significant protein intake appeared to be necessary to maintain nitrogen balance [58]. Despite counseling, the HEMO study showed that prevalent HD patients display progressive nutritional impairment [59] during the 3-year follow-up. Then the question of nutritional support has become important for HD patients with malnutrition criteria. The FINE study [60] wanted to demonstrate the beneficial effect of intradialytic parenteral nutrition (IDPN) on malnourished patients outcomes. The answer was different as the control group had to receive oral supplements for ethical reasons. There was no superiority of IDPN compared to oral supplements. But the study clearly demonstrates the usefulness of nutritional support.

Last but not least, more than 50 years after the first patient was treated with chronic HD, we still do not know the optimal dialysis frequency and time. The FHN trials [61, 62] tried to answer the question but the expected number of patients to be recruited appeared very high and out of reach. Coprimary end points were proposed to limit the number of required patients. The FHN short daily [61] showed significantly better coprimary end points at 1 year, but with a real threat on blood access complications. Since then a cohort study has shown increased mortality with daily short HD and caution in the implementation of such dialysis alternative is necessary.

Hence, a number of RCTs have addressed important issues in HD therapy. Some of the answers are still pending. None of them have directly addressed quality of life. This is an important point, especially at a time when the dialysis question is raised for the elderly. It will be one of the important challenges in the future at least in countries proposing dialysis therapy since the 1960s.

References

1. Scribner BH, Buri R, Caner JE, Hegstrom R, Burnell JM. The treatment of chronic uremia by means of intermittent hemodialysis: a preliminary report. Trans Am Soc Artif Intern Organs. 1960;6:114–22.
2. Peritoneal Dialysis Adequacy Work Group. Clinical practice guidelines for peritoneal dialysis adequacy. Am J Kidney Dis. 2006;48 Suppl 1:S98–129.
3. Hemodialysis Adequacy 2006 Work Group. Clinical practice guidelines for hemodialysis adequacy, update 2006. Am J Kidney Dis. 2006;48 Suppl 1:S2–90.
4. Churchill DN, Blake PG, Jindal KK, Toffelmire EB, Goldstei MB. Clinical practice guidelines for initiation of dialysis. Canadia Society of Nephrology. J Am Soc Nephrol. 1999;10 Suppl 1: S289–291.
5. Kelly J, Stanley M, Harris D. The CARI guidelines. Acceptanc into dialysis guidelines. Nephrology (Carlton). 2005;10 Suppl 4 S46–60.
6. Rosansky SJ, Clark WF, Eggers P, Glassock RJ. Initiation of dialysis at higher GFRs: is the apparent rising tide of early dialysis harmful or helpful? Kidney Int. 2009;76(3):257–61.
7. Brunkhorst R. Early versus late initiation of dialysis. N Engl J Mec 2010;363(24):2368; author reply 2369–70.
8. Lameire N, Van Biesen W. The initiation of renal-replacement ther apy – just-in-time delivery. N Engl J Med. 2010;363(7):678–80.
9. Gotch FA, Sargent JA. A mechanistic analysis of the Nationa Cooperative Dialysis Study (NCDS). Kidney Int. 1985;28(3):526–34
10. Saran R, Canaud BJ, Depner TA, et al. Dose of dialysis: key lesson from major observational studies and clinical trials. Am J Kidne Dis. 2004;44(5 Suppl 2):47–53.
11. Twardowski ZJ, Misra M, Singh AK. Con: Randomized controlle trials (RCT) have failed in the study of dialysis methods. Nephro Dial Transplant. 2013;28(4):826–32; discussion 832.
12. Block GA, Hulbert-Shearon TE, Levin NW, Port FK. Associatio of serum phosphorus and calcium x phosphate product with mortal ity risk in chronic hemodialysis patients: a national study. Am Kidney Dis. 1998;31(4):607–17.
13. Flythe J, Kimmel SE, Brunelli SM. Rapid fluid removal durin dialysis is associated with cardiovascular morbidity and mortality Kidney Int. 2011;79:250–7.
14. Cheung AK, Rocco MV, Yan G, et al. Serum beta-2 microglobuli levels predict mortality in dialysis patients: results of the HEMC study. J Am Soc Nephrol. 2006;17(2):546–55.
15. Greene T, Beck GJ, Gassman JJ, et al. Design and statistical issue of the hemodialysis (HEMO) study. Control Clin Trials. 200C 21(5):502–25.
16. Depner T, Daugirdas J, Greene T, et al. Dialysis dose and the effec of gender and body size on outcome in the HEMO Study. Kidne Int. 2004;65(4):1386–94.
17. Daugirdas JT, Greene T, Chertow GM, Depner TA. Can rescalin, dose of dialysis to body surface area in the HEMO study explain th different responses to dose in women versus men? Clin J Am So Nephrol. 2010;5(9):1628–36.
18. Twardowski ZJ, Misra M, Singh AK. Con: Randomized controlle trials (RCT) have failed in the study of dialysis methods. Nephro Dial Transplant. 2013;28(4):826–32; discussion 832.
19. Krane V, Krieter DH, Olschewski M, et al. Dialyzer membran characteristics and outcome of patients with type 2 diabetes o maintenance hemodialysis. Am J Kidney Dis. 2007;49(2):267–75
20. Suri RS, Garg AX, Chertow GM, et al. Frequent Hemodialysi Network (FHN) randomized trials: study design. Kidney Int 2007;71(4):349–59.
21. Badve SV, Hawley CM, Johnson DW. Frequent versus standar hemodialysis. N Engl J Med. 2011;364(10):975; author reply 976
22. Chazot C, Ok E, Lacson E, Kerr PG, Jean G, Misra M. Thrice-weekl nocturnal hemodialysis: the overlooked alternative to improve patien outcomes. Nephrol Dial Transplant. 2013;28(10):2447–55.
23. Stokes JB. Nocturnal hemodialysis: analysis following the Frequen Hemodialysis Network trial. Semin Dial. 2012;24(6):614–20.
24. Misra M, Twardowski ZJ. Benefits of frequent nocturnal hom hemodialysis. Kidney Int. 2012;82:114–5.
25. Twardowski ZJ, Misra M, Singh AK. Con: Randomized controlle trials (RCT) have failed in the study of dialysis methods. Nephro Dial Transplant. 2013;28(4):826–32; discussion 832.
26. Eknoyan G, Beck GJ, Cheung AK, et al. Effect of dialysis dose an membrane flux in maintenance hemodialysis. N Engl J Med 2002;347(25):2010–9.

27. Locatelli F, Martin-Malo A, Hannedouche T, et al. Effect of membrane permeability on survival of hemodialysis patients. J Am Soc Nephrol. 2009;20(3):645–54.

28. Henderson LW. Current status of hemofiltration. Artif Organs. 1978;2(2):120–4.

29. Caplin B, Alston H, Davenport A. Does online haemodiafiltration reduce intra-dialytic patient symptoms? Nephron. 2013;124(3–4):184–90.

30. Maduell F, Moreso F, Pons M, et al. High-efficiency postdilution online hemodiafiltration reduces all-cause mortality in hemodialysis patients. J Am Soc Nephrol. 2013;24(3):487–97.

31. McIntyre CW. Recurrent circulatory stress: the dark side of dialysis. Semin Dial. 2010;23(5):449–51.

32. Canaud B, Bragg-Gresham JL, Marshall MR, et al. Mortality risk for patients receiving hemodiafiltration versus hemodialysis: European results from the DOPPS. Kidney Int. 2006;69(11):2087–93.

33. Ok E, Asci G, Toz H, et al. Mortality and cardiovascular events in online haemodiafiltration (OL-HDF) compared with high-flux dialysis: results from the Turkish OL-HDF Study. Nephrol Dial Transplant. 2013;28(1):192–202.

34. Kuhlmann MK. On-line hemodiafiltration: not a self-fulfilling prophecy. J Am Soc Nephrol. 2012;23(6):974–5.

35. Grooteman MPC, van den Dorpel MA, Bots ML, et al. Effect of online hemodiafiltration on all-cause mortality and cardiovascular outcomes. J Am Soc Nephrol. 2012;23(6):1087–96.

36. Canaud B, Bragg-Gresham JL, Marshall MR, et al. Mortality risk for patients receiving hemodiafiltration versus hemodialysis: European results from the DOPPS. Kidney Int. 2006;69(11):2087–93.

37. Grooteman MPC, van den Dorpel MA, Bots ML, et al. Effect of online hemodiafiltration on all-cause mortality and cardiovascular outcomes. J Am Soc Nephrol. 2012;23(6):1087–96.

38. Ok E, Asci G, Toz H, et al. Mortality and cardiovascular events in online haemodiafiltration (OL-HDF) compared with high-flux dialysis: results from the Turkish OL-HDF Study. Nephrol Dial Transplant. 2013;28(1):192–202.

39. Blankestijn PJ. Has the time now come to more widely accept hemodiafiltration in the United States? J Am Soc Nephrol. 2013;24(3):332–4.

40. Mann JF. How does hemodiafiltration improve survival? Kidney Int. 2013;84(6):1287–8.

41. Farrington K, Davenport A. The ESHOL study: hemodiafiltration improves survival-but how? Kidney Int. 2013;83(6):979–81.

42. Chertow GM, Ling J, Lew NL, Lazarus JM, Lowrie EG. The association of intradialytic parenteral nutrition administration with survival in hemodialysis patients. Am J Kidney Dis. 1994;24(6):912–20.

43. Dukkipati R, Kalantar-Zadeh K, Kopple JD. Is there a role for intradialytic parenteral nutrition? A review of the evidence. Am J Kidney Dis. 2010;55(2):352–64.

44. Twardowski ZJ, Misra M, Singh AK. Con: Randomized controlled trials (RCT) have failed in the study of dialysis methods. Nephrol Dial Transplant. 2013;28(4):826–32; discussion 832.

45. Cooper BA, Branley P, Bulfone L, et al. A randomized, controlled trial of early versus late initiation of dialysis. N Engl J Med. 2010;363(7):609–19.

46. Lowrie EG, Laird NM, Parker TF, Sargent JA. Effect of the hemodialysis prescription of patient morbidity: report from the National Cooperative Dialysis Study. N Engl J Med. 1981;305(20):1176–81.

47. Eknoyan G, Beck GJ, Cheung AK, et al. Effect of dialysis dose and membrane flux in maintenance hemodialysis. N Engl J Med. 2002;347(25):2010–9.

48. Chand DH, Teo BW, Fatica RA, Brier M, Medical Review Board of The Renal Network Inc. Influence of vascular access type on outcome measures in patients on maintenance hemodialysis. Nephron. 2008;108(2):c91–98.

49. Cheung AK, Rocco MV, Yan G, et al. Serum beta-2 microglobulin levels predict mortality in dialysis patients: results of the HEMO study. J Am Soc Nephrol. 2006;17(2):546–55.

50. Okuno S, Ishimura E, Kohno K, et al. Serum β2-microglobulin level is a significant predictor of mortality in maintenance haemodialysis patients. Nephrol Dial Transplant. 2009;24(2):571–7.

51. Locatelli F, Martin-Malo A, Hannedouche T, et al. Effect of membrane permeability on survival of hemodialysis patients. J Am Soc Nephrol. 2009;20(3):645–54.

52. Floege J, Ketteler M. beta2-microglobulin-derived amyloidosis: an update. Kidney Int Suppl. 2001;78:S164–171.

53. Santoro A, Mancini E, Bolzani R, et al. The effect of on-line high-flux hemofiltration versus low-flux hemodialysis on mortality in chronic kidney failure: a small randomized controlled trial. Am J Kidney Dis. 2008;52(3):507–18.

54. Locatelli F, Altieri P, Andrulli S, et al. Hemofiltration and hemodiafiltration reduce intradialytic hypotension in ESRD. J Am Soc Nephrol. 2010;21(10):1798–807.

55. Grooteman MP, van den Dorpel MA, Bots ML, et al. Effect of online hemodiafiltration on all-cause mortality and cardiovascular outcomes. J Am Soc Nephrol. 2012;23(6):1087–96.

56. Ok E, Asci G, Toz H, et al. Mortality and cardiovascular events in online haemodiafiltration (OL-HDF) compared with high-flux dialysis: results from the Turkish OL-HDF Study. Nephrol Dial Transplant. 2013;28(1):192–202.

57. Maduell F, Moreso F, Pons M, et al. High-efficiency postdilution online hemodiafiltration reduces all-cause mortality in hemodialysis patients. J Am Soc Nephrol. 2013;24(3):487–97.

58. Borah MF, Schoenfeld PY, Gotch FA, Sargent JA, Wolfsen M, Humphreys MH. Nitrogen balance during intermittent dialysis therapy of uremia. Kidney Int. 1978;14(5):491–500.

59. Rocco MV, Dwyer JT, Larive B, et al. The effect of dialysis dose and membrane flux on nutritional parameters in hemodialysis patients: results of the HEMO Study. Kidney Int. 2004;65(6):2321–34.

60. Cano N, Fouque D, Roth H, et al. The french intradialytic nutrition evaluation study (FineS) (Abstract). Paper presented at: American Society of Nephrology, Philadelphia, 2005.

61. Chertow GM, Levin NW, Beck GJ, et al. In-center hemodialysis six times per week versus three times per week. N Engl J Med. 2010;363(24):2287–300.

62. Rocco MV, Lockridge Jr RS, Beck GJ, et al. The effects of frequent nocturnal home hemodialysis: the Frequent Hemodialysis Network Nocturnal Trial. Kidney Int. 2011;80(10):1080–91.

Simon J. Davies

Introduction

As is frequently pointed out, the record for clinical trials in patients treated with dialysis is poor, and this is especially the case for peritoneal dialysis. The reasons are complex and include a relatively small patient population, a lack of critical mass (with some exceptions) in trial methodology and infrastructure leading to an overreliance on industry support, the relatively complex outcomes and endpoints that affect patients treated with the modality, and a low repertoire of novel interventions. It would also be fair to say that the outcomes of patients treated with peritoneal dialysis over the last 30 years have improved considerably without these trials, largely because we have learned a lot about the therapy from a number of key observational studies and registry data analyses.

In selecting the "top" trials in peritoneal dialysis, the approach taken was initially to undertake a literature search using PubMed, Embase, and the Thompson Reuters Web of Science, incorporating the terms "peritoneal dialysis" and either "randomized trial" or "Cochrane." As a measure of impact, the studies were ranked in order of total citations and citation rate; although these were generally highly correlated, the citation rate (>10/year) was taken at the final cutoff so that important trials published more recently were given equal weight. Studies that included a randomized design to answer a scientific question but did not have implications for current clinical practice were excluded, as were studies published before 1990. In using this approach, the majority of trials identified were those looking at different dialysis fluid

interventions, usually industry funded but in some cases investigator led. There were disappointingly few studies addressing infection management (none on treatment of infection made the grade – see Cochrane review) or how PD is best practiced, the exception being the ADEMEX study investigating dialysis dose. The NECOSAD study, designed to compare outcomes on PD versus hemodialysis, was included here not just because it fulfilled the impact criteria, but because it was conceived mainly to demonstrate that outcomes on PD were equivalent and thus of more clinical significance to this modality.

The order chosen to present the studies is not chronological but grouped by type of intervention (e.g., studies on preserving residual kidney function and biocompatible solutions) and where possible reflects the patient pathway in the order of events they address.

Comparison of Dialysis Modality

Trial 1

Publication: Effect of starting with hemodialysis compared with peritoneal dialysis in patients new on dialysis treatment: a randomized controlled trial

Authors: Korevaar JC, Feith GW, Dekker FW, van Manen JG, Boeschoten EW, Bossuyt PM, Krediet RT; NECOSAD Study Group

Reference: *Kidney Int*. 2003 Dec;64(6):2222–8

Abstract

Background: Up until now, the survival and health-related quality of life of hemodialysis and peritoneal dialysis patients has only been compared in observational studies. These studies have reported small and opposing differences between both modalities. The aim of this study was to compare the outcome of hemodialysis as initial chronic dialysis treatment with that of peritoneal dialysis in a randomized controlled trial.

S.J. Davies, BSc, MD, FRCP
Department of Nephrology, University Hospital
of North Staffordshire, Newcastle Road, Stoke-On-Trent,
Staffordshire ST4 6QG, UK
e-mail: simondavies1@compuserve.com;
simonj.davies@uhns.nhs.uk

M. El Kossi, A. Khwaja, and M. El Nahas (eds.), *Informing Clinical Practice in Nephrology: The Role of RCTs*,
DOI 10.1007/978-3-319-10292-4_12, © Springer International Publishing Switzerland 2015

Methods: All new dialysis patients from 38 dialysis centers in the Netherlands without indications against either modality were invited to participate. Patients were assigned to start with hemodialysis or peritoneal dialysis. The primary outcome was mean quality-adjusted life year (QALY) score. Secondary outcome was survival.

Results: Due to the low inclusion rate, the trial was prematurely stopped after which 38 patients had been randomized: 18 patients to hemodialysis and 20 to peritoneal dialysis. The mean QALY score in the first 2 years was 59.1 (SD 12) for hemodialysis patients versus 54.0 (SD 19) for peritoneal dialysis patients, which constitutes a small difference in favor of hemodialysis of 5.1 (95 % CI −7.3 to 17.6). After 5 years of follow-up, nine hemodialysis and five peri-

toneal dialysis patients had died, a significant difference in survival; hazard ratio of hemodialysis versus peritoneal dialysis is 3.8 (95 % CI 1.1–12.6). After adjustment for age, comorbidity, and primary kidney disease, the hazard ratio was 3.6 (0.8–15.4).

Conclusion: Only a small difference in QALY score was observed between patients who started with hemodialysis compared to patients who started with peritoneal dialysis, lending support for the equivalence hypothesis. The significant difference in longer-term survival, which favored peritoneal dialysis in this small group of patients, could be used to posit that incident dialysis patients might benefit from starting on peritoneal dialysis.

Critical Appraisal

Parameters	Yes	No	Comment
Validity			
Is the **Randomization** Procedure well described?	+1		Central process, block randomization in which block size also varied randomly, with stratification for center and diabetic status. Offered to all eligible patients starting dialysis sequentially at 38 Dutch dialysis centers during inclusion period (1997–2000)
Double **blinded**?		0	Open study, neither investigator nor patient blinded as this would not have been possible
Is the **sample size** calculation described/ adequate?	+3		The study was designed to demonstrate equivalence between dialysis modalities. As a maximal difference of 10 points in QALY score is considered as indicating equivalence and given a mean QALY score of 62 points (SD 17.8), expected in both groups, 50 patients per group were needed to refute the null hypothesis
Does it have a hard primary **endpoint**?	+1		The primary outcome measure was the mean quality-adjusted life year (QALY) score in the first 2 years after the start of dialysis. Secondary endpoint was survival
Is the endpoint surrogate?		0	The QALY is a well-accepted endpoint but should probably be considered as a surrogate
Is the follow-up appropriate?	+1		Follow-up to primary endpoint was 2 years; survival follow-up to 5 years
Was there a **Bias**?	−1		Despite 773 patients fulfilling the inclusion criteria, the study did not recruit to target (just 38 randomized) which caused selection bias
Is the dropout >25 %?	−1		26 % drop-out for the primary endpoint; all patients included in the secondary survival endpoint
Is the analysis **ITT**?	+1		Primary analyses were ITT, with a secondary "as treated" analysis, which may be more important
Utility/usefulness			
Can the findings be generalized?		−1	The failure to recruit to target (reducing power to 36 %) and the very low proportion of patients willing to be randomized is the main limitation of this otherwise well-conducted study
Are the findings easily translatable?	+1		The findings are reassuring in that no big differences were seen supporting current practice. The main translational message is that patients value choice and have strong modality preferences
Was the NNT <100?		0	Not applicable as this was a negative study trying to show equivalence
Score	**30 %**		

Summary and Conclusions

Equivalence of patient survival between the dialysis modalities has been a major issue since peritoneal dialysis was introduced in the late 1970s. Several registry analyses, themselves often flawed [1], suggested that survival on peritoneal dialysis was inferior. This was a strong stimulus to undertake a definitive RCT and was the underpinning rationale for setting up the Netherlands Cooperative Study on the Adequacy Dialysis

(NECOSAD). This study had many strong points including the high level of participation of Dutch dialysis centers (making it effectively a national registry) and enrollment of sequential patients using a pragmatic study design, combined with a high quality of organization and research methodology team. The study also enabled a large number of powerful secondary analyses when treated as an observational cohort. The fact that they found it impossible to randomly allocate many patients is of course a problem for the trial – in fact those patients willing to be randomized must in some sense be quite atypical – but it also shows us what is most important for patients. Given that the choice they were presented with had such important ramifications for their everyday life, it is completely understandable that they did not wish to be randomized, but this needed to be demonstrated with rigor in a formal trial setting. The study also illustrated another challenge when undertaking trials of this type in the kidney failure population which is that there is differential movement of patients from one modality to another, including transplantation. Although the numbers were too small to be certain, there was a tendency for more patients to switch from PD to HD than vice versa, in keeping with the known higher technique failure rate associated with this modality. This is important for interpretation as the borderline significant survival advantage for PD was only present on ITT analysis and disappeared on the "as treated" analysis.

So what can be concluded from this trial? First and foremost, the implication is that patient choice over their modality matters greatly and how dialysis affects everyday life is rightly the focus of increased research activity, something that the NECOSAD group should take credit for. The choice of their primary endpoint is also worthy of comment. The attempt to combine survival with the quality of life by using the QALY is in many ways commendable as it recognizes that dialysis treatment is about more than just staying alive but intuitively problematic. Is living for 1 year with good quality of life (score 80) followed by a premature death giving an overall 2-year score of 40 really equivalent to living for 2 years with a below typical median score of 40 throughout? Taken in context with more recent and sophisticated analyses of registries, this study corroborates the overall picture that survival by modality is now equivalent [2–5]. There is at present another RCT in progress in China (NCT01413074) which may in time shed further light on the equivalence of these modalities.

Peritoneal Dialysis Adequacy

Trial 2

Publication: Effects of increased peritoneal clearances on mortality rates in peritoneal dialysis: ADEMEX, a prospective, randomized, controlled trial

   Authors: Ramón Paniagua, Dante Amato, Edward Vonesh, Ricardo Correa-Rotter, Alfonso Ramos, John Moran, Salim Mujais for the Mexican Nephrology Collaborative Study Group

   Reference: *J Am Soc Nephrol*. 2002 May;13(5):1307–20

Abstract

Small-solute clearance targets for peritoneal dialysis (PD) have been based on the tacit assumption that peritoneal and renal clearances are equivalent and therefore additive. Although several studies have established that patient survival is directly correlated with renal clearances, there have been no randomized, controlled, interventional trials examining the effects of increases in peritoneal small-solute clearances on patient survival. A prospective, randomized, controlled, clinical trial was performed to study the effects of increased peritoneal small-solute clearances on clinical outcomes among patients with end-stage renal disease who were being treated with PD. A total of 965 subjects were randomly assigned to the intervention or control group (in a 1:1 ratio). Subjects in the control group continued to receive their preexisting PD prescriptions, which consisted of four daily exchanges with 2 l of standard PD solution. The subjects in the intervention group were treated with a modified prescription, to achieve a peritoneal creatinine clearance (pCrCl) of 60 l/week/1.73 m^2. The primary endpoint was death. The minimal follow-up period was 2 years. The study groups were similar with respect to demographic characteristics, causes of renal disease, prevalence of coexisting conditions, residual renal function, peritoneal clearances before intervention, hematocrit values, and multiple indicators of nutritional status. In the control group, peritoneal creatinine clearance (pCrCl) and peritoneal urea clearance (K_t/V) values remained constant for the duration of the study. In the intervention group, pCrCl and peritoneal K_t/V values predictably increased and remained separated from the values for the control group for the entire duration of the study ($P < 0.01$). Patient survival was similar for the control and intervention groups in an intent-to-treat analysis, with a relative risk of death (intervention/control) of 1.00 [95 % confidence interval (CI), 0.80–1.24]. Overall, the control group exhibited a 1-year survival of 85.5 % (CI, 82.2–88.7 %) and a 2-year survival of 68.3 % (CI, 64.2–72.9 %). Similarly, the intervention group exhibited a 1-year survival of 83.9 % (CI, 80.6–87.2 %) and a 2-year survival of 69.3 % (CI, 65.1–73.6 %). An as-treated analysis revealed similar results (overall relative risk = 0.93; CI, 0.71–1.22; $P = 0.6121$). Mortality rates for the two groups remained similar even after adjustment for factors known to be associated with survival for patients undergoing PD (e.g., age, diabetes mellitus, serum albumin levels, normalized protein equivalent of total nitrogen appearance, and anuria). This study provides evidence that increases in peritoneal small-solute clearances within the range studied have a neutral effect on patient survival, even when the groups are stratified according to a variety of factors (age, diabetes mellitus, serum albumin levels, normalized protein equivalent of total nitrogen appearance, and anuria) known to affect survival. No clear survival advantage was obtained with increases in peritoneal small-solute clearances within the range achieved in this study.

Critical Appraisal

Parameters	Yes	No	Comment
Validity			
Is the **Randomization** Procedure well described?	+1		Yes, centralized with stratification
Double **blinded**?		−1	This would have been difficult to achieve; clinician blinding would have improved the study
Is the **sample size** calculation described/adequate?	+3		Study over-recruited so it had more power than originally planned, with 90 % to detect a 30 % reduction in mortality at 2 years. However, death rate was lower (18 rather than 23 deaths/100 years) leading to an extension in the trial length and a final observed 85 % power to detect a 30 % reduction of mortality in the higher dialysis dose group
Does it have a hard primary **endpoint**?	+1		Yes – death
Is the endpoint surrogate?		0	
Is the follow-up appropriate?	+1		2 years (extended for up to 3 years)
Was there a **Bias**?	−1		Withdrawal bias is likely (more dropout due to uremic symptoms in the control group)
Is the dropout >25 %?		+1	Dropout is low but reasons are different according to randomization (see bias)
Is the analysis **ITT**?	+3		All primary analyses were ITT including preplanned subgroup analyses. Censoring at transplantation. As treated analyses gave similar results
Utility/usefulness			
Can the findings be generalized?	+1		There are limitations – for example, the lack of automated peritoneal dialysis as undertaken in many countries (possible because average size of patients was) and exclusion of patients with heart failure
Are the findings easily translatable?	+1		The message is simple
Was the NNT <100?		0	Not applicable as this was a useful negative study
Score	**59 %**		

Summary and Conclusions

This was a well-conducted, industry-sponsored study addressing an important question. There was good separation of the delivered peritoneal dialysis dose (expressed as either K_t/V or creatinine clearance) throughout the study; the power was similar to that of the HEMO study [6] and the effect of the intervention so well centered around a hazard ratio of 1.00 (95 % CI: 0.8–1.24) that the level of certainty of the lack of effect of increasing peritoneal clearances within the prescribed range can be considered as very high.

Although there was some bias, mainly attributed to the unblinded nature of the intervention, which did lead to some differences in reasons for dropout, this was <5 % and cannot account for the lack of treatment effect. There are real issues associated with generalizability, in that the methods of dialysis available – most notably automated peritoneal dialysis (as opposed to an assist device which gives a single extra exchange per day), now the most common form of PD in many countries – were not tested. This is also the case for the only RCT comparing the effects of dialysis dose on survival in PD (the Hong Kong study [7]). However, there are no a priori reasons for thinking that this invalidates the central question of the study, i.e., that increasing the peritoneal dialysis dose is PD modality specific. It would be wrong to conclude from this study that 4×2 l exchanges should be a standard prescription in all settings given the relatively small body size of the Mexican PD population. The exclusion of patients with cardiac failure is potentially a problem, especially as the presence of ischemic heart disease is not given.

Overall the message from the study is clear – there is no reason to increase peritoneal dialysis dose in an attempt to achieve the higher clearance values associated with preserved residual kidney function and better survival as seen in the CANUSA study. The results also sit well with other observational studies which have only been able to show that the increased survival associated with higher total small solute clearances is related to residual kidney function [8–10].

Prevention of Infection

Trial 3

Publication: Randomized, double-blind trial of antibiotic exit site cream for prevention of exit site infection in peritoneal dialysis patients

Authors: Bernardini J, Bender F, Florio T, Sloand J, PalmMontalbano L, Fried L, Piraino B.

Reference: *J Am Soc Nephrol*. 2005;16(2):539–45

Abstract

Infection is the Achilles heel of peritoneal dialysis. Exit site mupirocin prevents *Staphylococcus aureus* peritoneal dialysis (PD) infections but does not reduce *Pseudomonas aeruginosa* or other Gram-negative infections, which are associated with considerable morbidity and sometimes death. Patients from three centers (53 % incident to PD and 47 % prevalent) were randomized in a double-blinded manner to daily mupirocin or gentamicin cream to the catheter exit site. Infections were tracked prospectively by organism and expressed as episodes per dialysis-year at risk. A total of 133 patients were randomized, 67 to gentamicin and 66 to mupirocin cream. Catheter infection rates were 0.23/year with gentamicin cream versus 0.54/year with mupirocin ($P = 0.005$). Time to first catheter infection was longer using gentamicin ($P = 0.03$). There were no *P. aeruginosa* catheter infections using gentamicin compared with 0.11/year using mupirocin ($P < 0.003$). *S. aureus* exit site infections were infrequent in both groups (0.06 and 0.08/year; $P = 0.44$). Peritonitis rates were 0.34/year versus 0.52/year ($P = 0.03$), with a striking decrease in Gram-negative peritonitis (0.02/year versus 0.15/year; $P = 0.003$) using gentamicin compared with mupirocin cream, respectively. Gentamicin use was a significant predictor of lower peritonitis rates (relative risk, 0.52; 95 % confidence interval, 0.29–0.93; $P < 0.03$), controlling for center and incident versus prevalent patients. Gentamicin cream applied daily to the peritoneal catheter exit site reduced *P. aeruginosa* and other Gram-negative catheter infections and reduced peritonitis by 35 %, particularly Gram-negative organisms. Gentamicin cream was as effective as mupirocin in preventing *S. aureus* infections. Daily gentamicin cream at the exit site should be the prophylaxis of choice for PD patients.

Critical Appraisal

Parameters	Yes	No	Comment
Validity			
Is the **Randomization** Procedure well described?	+1		Central randomization was undertaken, computer generated, 1:1
Double **blinded**?	+2		Patients and investigators were blinded
Is the **sample size** calculation described/adequate?	+3		A sample size calculation was made on the basis of known exit-site infection rates due to *P. aeruginosa*. To get sufficient endpoints to show a 50 % reduction, it was calculated that 140 patient-years follow-up would be required
Does it have a hard primary **endpoint**?	+1		The primary study outcome was *P. aeruginosa* and *S. aureus* catheter infection rates in the groups, with the hypothesis that gentamicin cream would be equally effective in preventing *S. aureus* exit-site infections but more effective in preventing *P. aeruginosa* exit-site infections. Exit-site infection is an important "hard" endpoint in its own right
Is the endpoint surrogate?		0	Catheter-related infection is also a surrogate endpoint for treatment failure as it is still the primary cause of PD technique failure worldwide
Is the follow-up appropriate?	+1		Follow-up was event driven and the study stopped after 114 patient-years follow-up as determined from 3-monthly interim analyses due to observation of a significant treatment effect
Was there a **Bias**?		+2	Randomization is well balanced. Low risk of selection/performance bias. Possible detection bias
Is the dropout >25 %?		+1	Overall dropout was <15 % and well balanced between intervention groups
Is the analysis **ITT**?	+3		Analyses were both ITT and as treated with no difference in the outcomes seen
Utility/usefulness			
Can the findings be generalized?	+1		In principle generalizable but some limitations mainly due to different local factors (e.g., bacterial resistance) and infection rates which can vary significantly. Prevention of exit-site infection is likely achieved through several practices
Are the findings easily translatable?		−1	This can be problematic. Any antibacterial prophylaxis strategy has to be compatible with local bacteriological practice and antibacterial resistance patterns. Many bacteriologists in different countries will not sanction use of these agents – especially gentamicin
Was the NNT <100?	+1		Yes
Score	**88 %**		

Summary and Conclusions

Catheter-related infection does continue to be a major cause of treatment dropout globally, and a significant proportion of these are precipitated by exit-site infection that are associated with preexisting or contemporary skin carriage of *S. aureus* [11]. The Pittsburgh group has contributed a number of research studies over the years, pioneering the use of local antibacterial creams – in particular the use of mupirocin to be applied at the exit site – to prevent *S. aureus* infection [12, 13]. One of the criticisms of this approach has been the increased incidence of *P. aeruginosa* infection replacing *S. aureus*, also predisposing to high-risk peritonitis and subsequently documented in the global pediatric peritonitis registry [14]. This well-designed and well-executed study was undertaken to address this problem and has led to changes in practice in some centers. However, the concerns related to bacterial resistance has been a major limiting factor in the adoption of this practice, especially for gentamicin which remains the mainstay antibiotic for Gram-negative infections in many countries and dialysis units. Other alternatives, such as the use of honey with antibacterial properties, have unfortunately not been shown to be superior [15].

Icodextrin: (1) Safety and Efficacy

Trial 4

Publication: A randomized multicenter clinical trial comparing iso-osmolar icodextrin with hyperosmolar glucose solutions in CAPD. MIDAS Study Group. Multicenter Investigation of Icodextrin in Ambulatory Peritoneal Dialysis

   Authors: Mistry CD, Gokal R, Peers E for the MIDAS Group

   Reference: *Kidney Int.* 1994;46(2):496–503

Abstract

The osmotic effectiveness of a large molecular weight glucose polymer fraction (icodextrin) as a novel "colloid" osmotic agent in peritoneal dialysis was established, but the long-term safety remained undetermined. A randomized, controlled multicenter investigation of icodextrin in ambulatory peritoneal dialysis (MIDAS) was undertaken to evaluate the long-term safety and efficacy by comparing daily overnight (8–12 h dwell) use of isosmolar icodextrin (282 mOsm/kg) with conventional 1.36 % (346 mOsm/kg) and 3.86 % (484 mOsm/kg) glucose exchanges over 6 months. Two hundred and nine patients were randomized from 11 centers, with 106 allocated to receive icodextrin (D) and 103 to remain on glucose (control group; C); 138 patients completed the 6-month study (71 C, 67 D). All patients were divided into weak (1.36 % or strong (3.86 %) subgroups based on their use of glucose solutions overnight during the pretreatment baseline period. The mean (±SEM) overnight ultrafiltration (UF) with D was 3.5 times greater than 1.36 % glucose at 8 h [527 ± 36 vs. 150 ± 47 ml; 95 % confidence interval (CI) for the difference +257 to +497 ml; $P < 0.0001$] and 5.5 times greater at 12 h (561 ± 44 vs. 101 ± 48 ml, 95 % CI for the difference +329 to +590; $P < 0.0001$) and no different from that of 3.86 % glucose at 8 h (510 ± 48 vs 448 ± 60 ml, 95 % CI for the difference -102 to +226 ml $P = 0.44$) and at 12 h (552 ± 44 vs. 414 ± 78 ml, 95 % CI for the difference −47 to +325 ml; $P = 0.06$). The biochemical profiles were no different in the two groups except for a small fall in serum sodium (140–136 mmol/l and chloride (103–99 mmol/l) concentrations in the icodextrin group. The mean serum maltose increased from a pre-dialysis value of 0.04 g/l to a steady-state level of 1.20 g/l within 2 weeks and remained stable throughout the study. This was not associated with any adverse clinical effects, and the overall CAPD-related symptom score was significantly better for D than C. This study demonstrates that the daily overnight use of an isosmolar icodextrin solution was safe and effective up to 6 months and could replace the overnight use of hyperosmolar glucose solutions. Longer-term data will be necessary to establish further safety and efficacy.

Critical Appraisal

Parameters	Yes	No	Comment
Validity			
Is the **Randomization** Procedure well described?	+0.5		Central randomization was undertaken, but it is not clear if this was stratified by usual overnight glucose concentration
Double **blinded**?		−1	No (blinded product not available)
Is the **sample size** calculation described/adequate?	+1		Prior single-center studies had shown efficacy from which a sample size calculation could have been undertaken. Despite lack of sample size calculation, the power of the study was ample for the primary endpoint; power calculations related to safety are notoriously unreliable and thus not appropriate for designing an RCT

Parameters	Yes	No	Comment
Does it have a hard primary **endpoint**?	+1		The study endpoint was the achieved overnight ultrafiltration compared with icodextrin versus the usual, referred to as the "main parameter." Safety was also an important objective of the study
Is the endpoint surrogate?	−1		Yes
Is the follow-up appropriate?	+1		6 months for a surrogate endpoint is reasonable
Was there a **Bias**?		0	Randomization is well balanced despite apparent lack of stratification. Lack of blinding could cause performance and detection bias
Is the dropout >25 %?	−1		Overall dropout was 34 % (28 % of those who started treatment) although the main reason was transplantation, and this was well balanced after starting study product
Is the analysis **ITT**?	+3		All primary analyses were ITT. As treated analyses gave identical results not presented
Utility/usefulness			
Can the findings be generalized?	+1		Main limitation is the lack of automated peritoneal dialysis (APD) patients so the benefits cannot be generalized to these regimes
Are the findings easily translatable?	+1		Yes. This study was critical for the establishment of icodextrin as an alternative dialysis solution
Was the NNT <100?	+1		Preventing fluid reabsorption is a key objective for using icodextrin. This study showed that for every 100 patients reabsorbing overnight with 1.36 % glucose, this would reduce to 15 with icodextrin
Score	**38 %**		

Summary and Conclusions

The establishment of icodextrin as an alternative solution to glucose for the long dialysis exchange (overnight in CAPD, day dwell for APD patients) has been one of the key developments of the therapy since its inception [16]. The MIDAS study showed that it would work – was safe in the short term – especially as blood icodextrin metabolite levels were shown to be stable over the study period (key secondary endpoint) while efficacy was maintained. Further analyses also reported peritonitis outcomes [17]. Although it does not score strongly on critical appraisal, its findings have been reproduced many times and the intervention is highly effective. The lack of a defined power calculation is diluted by the fact that the treatment effect is very powerful when compared to low strength (1.36/1.5 % glucose), and in fact in this regard, the study is overpowered due to the desire to demonstrate safety using a multicenter study design. The comparison between icodextrin and hypertonic glucose (3.86/4.25 %) is more one of noninferiority.

Ultrafiltration is a key objective of dialysis treatment albeit a surrogate endpoint. Preventing fluid reabsorption is also important, and there is a powerful body of evidence to suggest that the increased mortality seen in patients with rapid solute transport membranes treated with CAPD, especially in the 1990s, was due to poor ultrafiltration and fluid reabsorption in the long dwell [18]. There have been more trials done using icodextrin than any other nonstandard non-biocompatible dialysis fluid (see Cochrane review [19]), and although there are no large trials to link the use of icodextrin to a hard endpoint such as patient or technique survival, a propensity-matched study of observational cohort data indicates that its use is associated with reduced mortality [20].

Icodextrin: (2) Efficacy on Fluid Status

Trial 5

Publication: Icodextrin improves the fluid status of peritoneal dialysis patients: results of a double-blind randomized controlled trial

Authors: Davies SJ, Woodrow G, Donovan K, Plum J, Williams P, Johansson AC, Bosselmann HP, Heimbürger O, Simonsen O, Davenport A, Tranaeus A, Divino Filho JC.

Reference: *J Am Soc Nephrol*. 2003;14(9):2338–44

Abstract

Worsening fluid balance results in reduced technique and patient survival in peritoneal dialysis. Under these conditions, the glucose polymer icodextrin is known to enhance ultrafiltration in the long dwell. A multicenter, randomized, double-blind, controlled trial was undertaken to compare icodextrin *versus* 2.27 % glucose to establish whether icodextrin improves fluid status. Fifty patients with urine output <750 ml/day, high solute transport, and either treated hypertension or untreated BP >140/90 mmHg, or a requirement for the equivalent of all 2.27 % glucose exchanges, were randomized 1:1 and evaluated at 1, 3, and 6 months. Members of the icodextrin group lost weight, whereas the control group gained weight. Similar differences in total body water were observed, largely explained by reduced extracellular fluid volume in those receiving icodextrin, who also achieved better ultrafiltration and total sodium losses at 3 months ($P<0.05$) and had better maintenance of urine volume at 6 months ($P=0.039$). In patients fulfilling the study's inclu-sion criteria, the use of icodextrin, when compared with 2.27 % glucose, in the long exchange improves fluid removal and status in peritoneal dialysis. This effect is apparent within 1 month of commencement and was sustained for 6 months without harmful effects on residual renal function.

Critical Appraisal

Parameters	Yes	No	Comment
Validity			
Is the **Randomization** Procedure well described?	+0.5		Stratified for country, PD modality, and presence of cardiovascular disease, not specified how random sequence generated
Double **blinded**?	+2		Double-blind design using specially made opaque fluid bags
Is the **sample size** calculation described/adequate?	+3		Study was powered to detect a change in weight of 1.6 kg from baseline
Does it have a hard primary **endpoint**?	+1		Fall in weight of the patient
Is the endpoint surrogate?	−1		Change in weight was a surrogate for improved fluid status and body composition confirmed by bioimpedance as secondary endpoint
Is the follow-up appropriate?	+1		Follow-up was for 6 months so as to confirm that the weight change was sustained rather than just a short-term benefit
Was there a **Bias**?		+2	Randomization is well balanced. Low risk of selection/performance bias. Despite double-blind design, the patients likely noticed the treatment effect
Is the dropout >25 %?		+1	Overall dropout by 6 months was 20 % (10 % at 1 month). Dropout balanced
Is the analysis **ITT**?	+2		Both ITT and as treated analyses (carefully defined) were undertaken with similar results so only ITT shown
Utility/usefulness			
Can the findings be generalized?	+1		Inclusion criteria excluded diabetics and patient with less than average peritoneal solute transport rates; subsequent RCTs in these groups show that the results are generalizable
Are the findings easily translatable?	+1		If available the use of icodextrin in the long exchange is easily translated into clinical practice. Population studies using propensity matching suggest that the use of icodextrin is safe and associated with better survival, but there is no RCT of sufficient power to determine whether icodextrin affects patient or technique survival
Was the NNT <100?			Not applicable as endpoint is a continuous variable, but whole study size is $n=50$
Score	**79 %**		

Summary and Conclusions

Whereas MIDAS (see Trial 4) demonstrated that icodextrin can improve ultrafiltration and prevent fluid reabsorption across the peritoneal membrane, it was important to demonstrate that this translates into an improvement in fluid status and understand the implications for body composition. There were concerns that the presence of icodextrin metabolites in plasma (which cause a very slightly hyperosmolar hyponatremia) might increase thirst, so negating the benefits on fluid status, and it was hoped that the reduced glucose exposure might prevent body fat accumulation. It was also important to determine the effects of an improvement in fluid status on residual kidney function.

This multicenter European study addressed these questions looking at changes in weight and body composition employing bioimpedance and deuterium dilution to obtain relative and absolute estimates of fluid status, respectively. It was unique to trials investigating the effects of dialysis fluids in using a double-blind design.

Weight did fall in the icodextrin group, not quite as much as predicted, but body water reduced by 1.5 kg and yet there was significant weight gain in the control group that could be attributed to a gain of body fat, supporting the hypothesis that its use has a double benefit. A similarly designed trial also found that fluid status improved using icodextrin but differed in that residual renal function was adversely affected [21]

The recent Cochrane review found that overall icodextrin does not reduce residual renal function on meta-analysis [22].

The inclusion criteria focused on patients with above-average peritoneal solute transport rates due to the growing concern at that time (subsequently confirmed on meta-analysis [23]), that the increased mortality in this group reflected their worse ultrafiltration. Diabetics were excluded mainly because the equipoise of the European clinicians at that time was to use icodextrin preferentially in these patients to avoid excess glucose exposure, despite good evidence of benefit. Subsequent to the publication of this study, icodextrin has been shown effective in improving fluid status in diabetics as well as improving metabolic control [24, 25].

Preserving Residual Kidney Function: ACE Inhibitors

Trial 6

Publication: Effects of an angiotensin-converting enzyme inhibitor on residual renal function in patients receiving peritoneal dialysis. A randomized, controlled study

Authors: Li PK, Chow KM, Wong TY, Leung CB, Szeto CC

Reference: *Ann Intern Med.* 2003;139(2):105–12

Abstract

Background: Residual renal function is an important determinant of mortality and morbidity in patients receiving peritoneal dialysis. However, few studies have evaluated therapeutic approaches for preserving residual renal function after the initiation of dialysis.

Objective: To test the hypothesis that the angiotensin-converting enzyme (ACE) inhibitor ramipril slows the decline in residual renal function in patients with end-stage renal failure treated with peritoneal dialysis.

Design: Randomized, open-label, controlled trial.

Setting: Single-center study in the dialysis unit of a university teaching hospital.

Patients: 60 patients receiving peritoneal dialysis.

Measurements: Patients were randomly assigned to ramipril (5 mg daily) or no treatment. The target blood pressure was 135/85 mmHg or less. Rate of decline in residual glomerular filtration rate (GFR) and development of complete anuria were compared among groups.

Results: Over 12 months, average residual GFR declined by 2.07 ml/min/1.73 m^2 in the ramipril group versus 3.00 ml/min/1.73 m^2 in the control group ($P=0.03$). The difference between the average changes in residual GFR in the ramipril and control groups from baseline to 12 months was 0.93 ml/min/1.73 m^2 (95 % CI, 0.09–1.78 ml/min/1.73 m^2). At 12 months, 14 patients in the ramipril group and 22 in the control group developed anuria. With intention-to-treat multivariable analysis using the Cox model, it was estimated that at 3, 6, and 9 months, patients assigned to ramipril had a higher adjusted hazard of complete anuria than did patients assigned to no treatment. Of the 25 patients who still did not have complete anuria at 12 months, those assigned to ramipril had a better prognosis than did those assigned to no treatment (adjusted hazard ratio, 0.58 [CI, 0.36–0.94]). The rates of death from any cause, duration of hospitalization, and cardiovascular events did not differ significantly between groups.

Conclusions: Although the trial was small and had a limited ability to exclude effects of potential confounding factors, the angiotensin-converting enzyme inhibitor ramipril may reduce the rate of decline of residual renal function in patients with end-stage renal failure treated with peritoneal dialysis.

Critical Appraisal

Parameters	Yes	No	Comment
Validity			
Is the **Randomization** Procedure well described?	+1		Computer-generated randomization concealed from investigators at recruitment
Double **blinded**?		−2	Open study, neither investigator nor patient blinded. No placebo
Is the **sample size** calculation described/adequate?	+3		Yes, based on a control rate of decline in residual function of 0.3 ml/min/1.73 m^2, the study was powered to detect a 50 % reduction with the intervention
Does it have a hard primary **endpoint**?	+1		Both rate of decline ("change") in residual renal function and time to anuria are given as the endpoint, but see power calculation above. Anuria not specifically defined
Is the endpoint surrogate?		0	Residual kidney function is a hard clinical endpoint associated with many clinical advantages in its own right, but it is also a good surrogate for survival in dialysis patients
Is the follow-up appropriate?	+1		12-month follow-up was appropriate especially as the effect of being on ACE versus control appears to change over time

Parameters	Yes	No	Comment
Was there a **Bias**?	−1		Lack of blinding causing risk of performance bias. Randomization appears well balanced, but authors comment that some measures (e.g., diabetics status, baseline residual clearance) were "somewhat" different
Is the dropout >25 %?		+1	Overall dropout was 12 %. It is unclear why the numbers of patients at risk at the end of the study of developing anuria are different to those in the analysis of declining kidney function
Is the analysis **ITT**?	+1		The analyses are ITT but are complex; for the change in residual function, a repeated measures analysis of covariance was undertaken with adjustment for apparently unbalanced baseline measures. The time to anuria analysis is even more complex and necessitated constructing a propensity score for all patients as the primary randomization survival curves violated the Cox regression
Utility/usefulness			
Can the findings be generalized?		−1	A single-center study and requirement of complex analyses, essentially necessitated by the relatively small number of patients, there have to be concerns over generalizability
Are the findings easily translatable?	+1		The intervention is very easily translated into clinical practice. The lack of hyperkalemia in the study was an important safety outcome – potentially the most useful aspect given the desire to use ACE for many other indications in this patient population
Was the NNT <100?			Not applicable as endpoint is a continuous variable
Score	**30 %**		

Summary and Conclusions

This is an important and influential study that ideally should be repeated with larger numbers – although given the wide number of indications for ACE inhibition for cardiovascular risk in the dialysis population, this may prove difficult to do. Its importance is mainly related to the huge survival advantage associated with preserved residual kidney function seen in both PD and hemodialysis patients [26, 27], although it also has benefits of its own ranging from a reduced dialysis burden to improved well-being and quality of life [28]. The lack of using a blinded placebo is the major limitation of the trial design, especially as it was single center, as this opens it up to significant performance bias. It is also a concern that the authors had to resort to very complex analytic approaches, which it is difficult to imagine were all prespecified, given that they could not have anticipated the differential time effects of being in the ACE versus control group. Propensity scoring in such a small group of subjects is also to be treated with caution. The strong suggestion from the data analysis that the use of ACE in PD patients has a biphasic effect on residual function – an early increased risk of anuria which parallels the effects seen in other studies and may reflect an early hemodynamic effect, followed by a more sustained benefit in the longer term is of interest clinically and would certainly inform future trial design.

The lack of hyperkalemia in the intervention group is also an important safety message for the use of ACE in PD patients; given the many indications for use of ACE in this high-risk patient population, this trial's undoubted value is that overall it does not otherwise disadvantage patients and may potentially lead to survival benefits [29]. However, a recent meta-analysis could not confirm that this is the case; also concluded that the evidence of beneficial effects of ACE or ARBi in preserving residual kidney function is limited [30].

Biocompatible Dialysis Fluids (1): Membrane Effects

Trial 7

Publication: The Euro-Balance trial: the effect of a new biocompatible peritoneal dialysis fluid (balance) on the peritoneal membrane

Authors: Williams JD, Topley N, Craig KJ, Mackenzie RK, Pischetsrieder M, Lage C, Passlick-Deetjen J; Euro Balance Trial Group

Reference: *Kidney Int.* 2004 Jul;66(1):408–18

Abstract

Background: Although peritoneal dialysis (PD) is a widely accepted form of renal replacement therapy (RRT), concern remain regarding the bioincompatible nature of standard PD fluid. In order to evaluate whether a newly formulated fluid of neutral pH, and containing low levels of glucose degradation products (GDP), resulted in improved in vivo biocompatibility, it was compared in a clinical study to a standard PD fluid.

Methods: In a multicenter, open, randomized, prospective study with a crossover design and parallel arms, a conventional, acidic, lactate-buffered fluid (SPDF) was compared with a pH neutral, lactate-buffered, low GDP fluid (balance). Overnight effluent was collected and assayed for cancer antigen 125 (CA125), hyaluronic acid (HA), procollagen peptide (PICP), vascular endothelial growth factor (VEGF), and tumor necrosis factor alpha (TNFalpha). Serum samples were assayed for circulating advanced glycosylation end products (AGE), N(epsilon)-(carboxymethyl) lysine (CML), and imidazolone. Clinical end points were residual renal function (RRF), adequacy of dialysis, ultrafiltration, and peritoneal membrane function. Eighty-six patients were randomized to either group I starting with SPDF for 12 weeks (Phase I), then switching to "balance" for 12 weeks (phase II), or group II, which was treated vice versa. Seventy-one patients completed the study with data suitable for entry into the per-protocol analysis. Effluent and serum samples, together with peritoneal function tests and adequacy measurements, were undertaken at study centers on three occasions during the study: after the four-week run-in period, after phase I, and again after phase II.

Results: In patients treated with balance, there were significantly higher effluent levels of CA125 and PICP in both arms of the study. Conversely, levels of HA were lower in patients exposed to balance, while there was no change in the levels of either VEGF or TNF-alpha. Serum CML and imidazolone levels fell significantly in balance-treated patients. Renal urea and creatinine clearances were higher in both treatment arms after patients were exposed to balance. Urine volume was higher in patients exposed to balance. In contrast, peritoneal ultrafiltration was higher in patients on SPDF. When anuric patients were analyzed as a subgroup, there was no significant difference in peritoneal transport characteristics or in ultrafiltration on either fluid. There were no changes in peritonitis incidence on either solution.

Conclusion: This study indicates that the use of balance, a neutral pH, low GDP fluid, is accompanied by a significant improvement in effluent markers of peritoneal membrane integrity and significantly decreased circulating AGE levels. Clinical parameters suggest an improvement in residual renal function on balance, with an accompanying decrease in peritoneal ultrafiltration. It would appear that balance solution results in an improvement in local peritoneal homeostasis, as well as having a positive impact on systemic parameters, including circulating AGE and residual renal function.

Critical Appraisal

Parameters	Yes	No	Comment
Validity			
Is the **Randomization** Procedure well described?		−1	Method of randomization is not specified
Double **blinded**?		−1	Open study
Is the **sample size** calculation described/adequate?	+1		It is stated in the text that the study was "powered to examine in detail the biological parameters, principally CA125, in the effluent," but no power calculation is given
Does it have a hard primary **endpoint**?	+1		Primary endpoint is clearly defined as the concentration of CA125 in dialysate effluent
Is the endpoint surrogate?		−1	CA125 is used as a surrogate endpoint for membrane injury
Is the follow-up appropriate?	+1		This was a 3-month crossover study design which is appropriate for demonstrating short-term reversible effects of the biocompatible dialysis fluid on surrogate markers of membrane injury. Less appropriate for some of the secondary endpoints (e.g., residual kidney and membrane function)
Was there a **Bias**?	−1		Minor imbalance in the randomization in the cause of renal failure (more glomerulonephritis in the group receiving standard solution first). Possible detection bias as open study
Is the dropout >25 %?		+1	Overall dropout was 15 % and well balanced between intervention groups. Analysis of primary endpoint was made in 82.5 % of participants; complete clinical data available on 78 %
Is the analysis **ITT**?	+2		Analyses were "per protocol," i.e., in 82.5 % of participants, but not stated as being ITT but likely is
Utility/usefulness			
Can the findings be generalized?	+1		The primary endpoint has been used for several studies of biocompatible solutions, and they have all shown a similar effect – so this is likely generalizable
Are the findings easily translatable?		0	Switching patients to biocompatible solutions is straightforward. The problem with this study is knowing what the surrogate primary endpoint actually means
Was the NNT <100?			Not applicable as endpoint is a continuous variable
Score	**18 %**		

Summary and Conclusions

The primary objective of this study was to show that a low glucose degradation product containing dialysis solution with a normal pH is less harmful to the peritoneal membrane. The hypothesis is based on a large number of in vitro and ex vivo studies showing that conventional dialysis solutions cause various types of biological injury and the belief that certain soluble biomarkers can be measured in dialysate effluent that are surrogate indicators of membrane injury [31]. For example, CA125 is produced by mesothelial cells, so an increase in the effluent concentrations is considered as evidence that the mesothelial cell lining of the peritoneal cavity – a known casualty of prolonged exposure to incompatible dialysis fluid – is more healthy. Euro-Balance supports this view, and the finding of similar effects using other biocompatible solutions suggests that this is generalizable to all such solutions (see Trial 8 and Refs. [32, 33]). The clinical relevance of these biomarkers, however, remains very controversial [34]. This study did not find an effect on inflow pain, considered to be a clinical manifestation of biocompatibility and observed as a benefit in other studies (Trial 8 and Ref. [35]).

The findings of the secondary endpoints of this study, notably the effects on membrane function and residual renal function, have perhaps caused more interest and driven further investigations more than the primary analysis findings. This is likely because these are more clinically relevant endpoints although it should be pointed out that a crossover study design is not the ideal approach when investigating endpoints which are known to change over time in a way that is unlikely to be reversible. The observation that the low-GDP solution caused an increase in peritoneal solute transport rate, a change that has generally been associated with increasing membrane injury, is also difficult to reconcile, although this study does show that this effect is reversible. The apparent preservation of residual kidney function associated with the use of the low-GDP solutions was also of considerable interest even though the mechanism is unclear. These findings were the stimulus for subsequent studies examining the clinical benefits of biocompatible solutions (Trials 9 and 10), in particular the balANZ study (see Trial 11).

Biocompatible Dialysis Fluids (2): Membrane Effects

Trial 8

Publication: Long-term clinical effects of a peritoneal dialysis fluid with less glucose degradation products

Authors: Rippe B, Simonsen O, Heimbürger O, Christensson A, Haraldsson B, Stelin G, Weiss L, Nielsen FD, Bro S, Friedberg M, Wieslander A

Reference: *Kidney Int.* 2001 Jan;59(1):348–57

Abstract

Background: Glucose degradation products (GDPs) are cytotoxic in vitro and potentially toxic in vivo during peritoneal dialysis (PD). We are presenting the results of a 2-year randomized clinical trial of a new PD fluid, produced in a two-compartment bag and designed to minimize heat induced glucose degradation while producing a near-neutral pH. The effects of the new fluid over 2 years of treatment on membrane transport characteristics, ultrafiltration (UF) capacity, and effluent markers of peritoneal membrane integrity were investigated and compared with those obtained during treatment with a standard solution.

Design: A two-group parallel design with 80 continuous ambulatory peritoneal dialysis patients was used. The patients were randomly assigned to either the new fluid ($N=40$) or to a conventional one ($N=40$) and were stratified with respect to age, diabetes, and time on PD. Peritoneal transport characteristics were assessed by the Personal Dialysis Capacity (PDCtrade mark) test at 1, 6, 12, 18, and 24 months after inclusion and by weighing the overnight bag daily. Infusion pain and handling were evaluated using a questionnaire. Peritoneal mesothelial and interstitial integrity were evaluated by analyzing overnight effluent dialysate concentrations of CA 125, hyaluronan (HA), procollagen-1 C-terminal peptide (PICP), and procollagen-3-N-terminal peptide (PIIINP) at 1, 6, 12, 18, and 24 months.

Results: The handling of the new two-compartment bag was considered easy, and there were no indications of increased discomfort with the new system. Furthermore, no changes in peritoneal fluid or solute transport characteristics were observed during the study period for either fluid, and neither were there any differences with regard to peritonitis incidence. However, significantly higher dialysate CA 125 (73 ± 41 vs. 25 ± 18 U/ml), PICP (387 ± 163 vs. 244 ± 81 ng/ml), and PIIINP (50 ± 24 vs. 29 ± 13 ng/ml) and significantly lower concentrations of HA (395 ± 185 vs. 530 ± 298 ng/ml) were observed in the overnight effluent during treatment with the new fluid.

Conclusion: We conclude that the new fluid with a higher pH and less GDPs is safe and easy to use and has no negative effects on either the frequency of peritonitis or peritoneal transport characteristics as compared with conventional ones. Our results indicate that the new solution causes less mesothelial and interstitial damage than conventional ones; that is, it may be considered more biocompatible than a number of conventional PD solutions currently in use.

Critical Appraisal

Parameters	Yes	No	Comment
Validity			
Is the **Randomization** Procedure well described?	+1		The process of randomization was not clearly stated but was stratified by age, diabetic status, and time on PD, so it must have been centralized
Double **blinded**?		−1	Open study, neither investigator nor patient blinded as this would not have been possible
Is the **sample size** calculation described/adequate?	+1		None is shown in methods but is referred to in the results section
Does it have a hard primary **endpoint**?		−1	No primary endpoint is defined. The study states that the intention was to see the effects of the biocompatible solution on membrane function and residual kidney function and infusion pain
Is the endpoint surrogate?		0	The membrane biomarkers are clearly surrogate endpoints. Measures of membrane function and residual kidney function are
Is the follow-up appropriate?	+1		Initially designed at 1 year, this was extended to 2 years without increasing recruitment. This appears to have been decided after the trial commenced
Was there a **Bias**?	−2		Multiple biases; initial randomization balanced.
Is the dropout >25 %?	−1		At 1 year, dropout was 35 % and asymmetric between groups (NS). For some biomarkers, data was available in <50 % in the controls and 70 % of the active group. At 24 months, dropout was >80 %
Is the analysis **ITT**?		0	Not stated but likely to be "as treated" – at least for biomarkers
Utility/usefulness			
Can the findings be generalized?	+1		The biomarker findings are similar to other studies of biocompatible solutions
Are the findings easily translatable?	0		Given the lack of understanding of the clinical relevance of the surrogate endpoints, it is difficult to translate into clinical practice
Was the NNT <100?			Not applicable as this was not powered to a clinical endpoint
Score	**0 %**		

Summary and Conclusions

This study has to be considered more as an exploratory exercise than as testing a clearly defined primary endpoint. Despite the fact that it is subject to very significant bias, this study has been influential. The general hypothesis is that low-GDP solutions are good for the membrane, reduce infusion pain, and possibly preserve residual renal function. The impact on infusion pain was close to being statistically significant but was potentially biased due to the lack of blinding of the study product; it does, however, corroborate the findings of a crossover study done with the Baxter biocompatible solution [35], and both of these studies are in keeping with everyday experience, although this is not a common occurrence. There were no detectable differences between the solutions on membrane function parameters and residual kidney function in contrast to the Euro-Balance (Trial 7) and balANZ trials (Trial 11); this could either reflect a lack of statistical power, high dropout, or that these solutions have different physiological effects.

Significant differences were seen in the various measured dialysate biomarkers, for example, increases in cancer antigen (CA125), procollagen-1-C-terminal peptide (PICP), procollagen-3-N-terminal peptide (PIINP), and a reduction in hyaluronan. In the results section, there is mention of a power calculation which appears to refer to PIINP indicating that to demonstrate a 20 % difference in the dialysate concentration between the groups, it would have required 14 patients randomized to each group. It would therefore appear that the study was sufficiently powered to detect this sort of difference although the lack of a prerandomization baseline value is problematic. Despite being likely to be real and thus generalizable – the findings are similar to other studies of biocompatible solutions on membrane biomarkers – the difficulty is the interpretation as to what these surrogates actually mean clinically. They seem to imply better health of cells – e.g., the mesothelium, leukocytes [36], and fibroblasts [37] – but increased amounts of procollagen and reduced hyaluronan could be interpreted either way [38]. The value of this trial is usefully put in context in the Cochrane review of biocompatible solutions [39].

Biocompatible Dialysis Fluids (3): Residual Kidney Function

Trial 9

Publication: Randomized controlled study of biocompatible peritoneal dialysis solutions: effect on residual renal function

    Authors: Fan SL, Pile T, Punzalan S, Raftery MJ, Yaqoob MM

    Reference: *Kidney Int.* 2008;73(2):200–6

Abstract

Residual kidney function is important for patient and technique survival in peritoneal dialysis (PD). Biocompatible dialysis solutions are thought to improve function and viability of peritoneal mesothelial cells and to preserve residual renal function (RRF). We conducted a randomized controlled study comparing use of biocompatible (B) with standard (S) solutions in 93 incident PD patients during 1-year period. The demographics, comorbidities, and RRF of both groups were similar. At 3 and 12 months, 24-h urine samples were collected to measure volume and the mean of urea and creatinine clearance normalized to body surface area. Surrogate markers of fluid status, diuretic usage, C-reactive protein concentration, peritonitis episodes, survival data, and peritoneal equilibrium tests were also collected. Changes in the normalized mean urea and creatinine clearance were the same for both groups, with no significant differences in secondary end points. Despite nonrandomized studies suggesting benefits of these newer biocompatible solutions, we could not detect any clinically significant advantages. Additional studies are needed to determine if advantages are seen with longer-term use.

Critical Appraisal

Parameters	Yes	No	Comment
Validity			
Is the **Randomization** Procedure well described?		−1	The randomization procedure is not described
Double **blinded**?		−1	Open study, neither investigator nor patient blinded as this would not have been possible
Is the **sample size** calculation described/adequate?	+3		Based on extrapolation of 3-month data from the Euro-Balance study, the anticipated loss of kidney function was 60 % over follow-up. Sample size was that required to show that a halving in this rate of loss with biocompatible solutions. It should be noted that this was effectively a double comparison – i.e., of two different solutions and their biocompatible counterparts
Does it have a hard primary **endpoint**?	+1		The rate of decline ("change") in residual renal function as defined by (a) urine volume and (b) normalized creatinine clearance
Is the endpoint surrogate?	+1		Residual kidney function is a hard clinical endpoint associated with many clinical advantages in its own right, but it is also a good surrogate for survival in dialysis patients
Is the follow-up appropriate?	+1		9-month follow-up is reasonable, although short compared to balANZ in fact the differences observed in this study were evident before 12 months
Was there a **Bias**?	−1		Lack of blinding causing risk of performance bias
Is the dropout >25 %?		+1	Overall dropout was 21 %. Reasons for dropout were similar between groups
Is the analysis **ITT**?	+3		Both per-protocol and ITT analyses were undertaken. In addition, a predefined noninferiority analysis was used
Utility/usefulness			
Can the findings be generalized?	0		This was a negative study both for primary and secondary endpoints. The main difficulty in generalizing the findings is the mixed use of two different standard commercial solutions and their biocompatible counterparts. The pragmatic design is a strength
Are the findings easily translatable?	+1		The negative findings of the study help clinicians prioritize the value of using the newer biocompatible solutions if these have a cost implication
Was the NNT <100?			Not applicable as this was a negative study
Score	**47 %**		

Summary and Conclusions

This was an investigator-led study undertaken in incident PD patients at a single center and stimulated by the secondary findings of the Euro-Balance trial suggesting that biocompatible dialysate might preserve residual kidney function. It addresses an important question given the value of residual kidney function to dialysis patients and was generally well conducted. The difficulty in blinding patients and clinicians is essentially a practical problem, as biocompatible solutions necessitate a different bag design and require different actions by the patients in how they are used. The decision to include PD solutions made by more than one company was essentially a pragmatic one, as it reflected the local use of these two products by the center at the time, but does raise some difficulties when making comparison with other studies in terms of generalizability. In fact, the pragmatic design is also one of the strengths of this study as a high proportion of eligible patients were included. There are, therefore, pros and cons when it comes to generalizing these results which is reflected in the way this study has been scored. In reality, the proportion of patients using Baxter (92 %) was much higher than Fresenius fluids (8 %) in this study with relatively high proportion using APD (60 %), all of whom were on the Baxter product. If the impact of biocompatible solutions is different by manufacturer, this might explain the negative finding of this study compared with trials involving other manufacturers (Fresenius, Euro-Balance and balANZ; Gambro, DIUREST; see Trials 7, 10, and 11). However, PD modality may also be an important confounder as there are some studies suggesting that automated peritoneal dialysis leads to a more rapid loss in residual kidney function [40–42]. The study was included in the Cochrane review [43] which found overall that biocompatible solutions tend to preserve residual renal function in studies that are extended beyond 12 months (e.g., balANZ) and in the 2-year follow-up data of the bal-NET study [44]. This is somewhat paradoxical as the separation in the rate of loss of kidney function in these longer trials occurs within 12 months.

The significance of the study, given the overall negative findings and the secondary analysis suggesting that biocompatible solutions are not inferior, is that it helps clinicians plan the best use of resources. If the biocompatible solution comes at a cost premium, clinicians may prefer to use this finance to support other initiatives to improve patient outcomes.

Biocompatible Dialysis Fluid (4): Residual Kidney Function

Trial 10

Publication: Low-GDP fluid (Gambrosol trio) attenuates decline of residual renal function in PD patients: a prospective randomized study

Authors: Haag-Weber M, Krämer R, Haake R, Islam MS, Prischl F, Haug U, Nabut JL, Deppisch R; behalf of the DIUREST Study Group

Reference: *Nephrol Dial Transplant*. 2010;25(7):2288–96

Abstract

Background: Residual renal function (RRF) impacts outcome of peritoneal dialysis (PD) patients. Some PD fluids contain glucose degradation products (GDPs) which have been shown to affect cell systems and tissues. They may also act as precursors of advanced glycosylation end products (AGEs) both locally and systemically, potentially inflicting damage to the kidney as the major organ for AGE elimination. We conducted a clinical study in PD patients to see if the content of GDP in the PD fluid has any influence on the decline of the residual renal function.

Methods: In a multicenter approach, 80 patients (GFF ≥ 3 ml/min/1.732 or creatinine clearance ≥ 3 ml/min/1.73 m^2) were randomized to treatment with a PD fluid containing low levels of GDP or standard PD fluid for 18 months. RRF was assessed every 4–6 weeks. Fluid balance, mesothelial cell mass marker CA125, peritoneal membrane characteristics, C-reactive protein (CRP), total protein, albumin, electrolytes, and phosphate were measured repeatedly.

Results: Data from 69 patients revealed a significant difference in monthly RRF change: -1.5 % (95 % CI $=-3.07$ to $+0.03$ %) with low GDP (43 patients) vs -4.3 % (95 % CI $=-6.8$ to -2.06 %) with standard fluids (26 patients) ($P = 0.0437$), independent of angiotensin-converting enzyme (ACE) inhibitor or angiotensin receptor blocker medication. Twenty-four-hour urine volume declined more slowly with low-GDP fluid compared to standard fluids (12 vs 38 ml/month, $P = 0.0241$), and monthly change of phosphate level was smaller ($+0.013$ vs $+0.061$ mg/dl, $P = 0.0381$).

Conclusions: Our prospective study demonstrates for the first time a significant benefit concerning preservation of RRF and urine volume of using a PD fluid with low GDP levels. These findings suggest that GDPs might affect patient outcome related to RRF.

Critical Appraisal

Parameters	Yes	No	Comment
Validity			
Is the **Randomization** Procedure well described?	+1		Centrally managed list of random number blocks stratified for diabetic status; despite this there was poor randomization balance
Double **blinded**?		−1	Open study, neither investigator nor patient blinded as this would not have been possible
Is the **sample size** calculation described/adequate?	+2		Sample size was calculated to have sufficient power to show a difference between groups in the rate of loss of residual function of 1 ml/min/1.73 m²/year. It is implied that the power calculation was undertaken after an initial analysis of the first 11 patients
Does it have a hard primary **endpoint**?	+1		The rate of decline of residual renal function as defined by normalized creatinine clearance
Is the endpoint surrogate?	+1		Residual kidney function is a hard clinical endpoint associated with many clinical advantages in its own right, but it is also a good surrogate for survival in dialysis patients
Is the follow-up appropriate?	+1		18-month follow-up was reasonable but will have contributed to the high dropout
Was there a **Bias**?	−2		Lack of blinding causing risk of performance bias and dropout causing attrition bias. Poor randomization balance
Is the dropout >25 %?	−1		Dropout was complex and high. Of the 80 patients randomized, 69 (86 %) had baseline data; subsequent dropout was 42 % in the active group, 46 % in controls giving overall dropout of 51.3 %
Is the analysis **ITT**?		0	An "as treated" analysis was undertaken supplemented by a multivariate regression model
Utility/usefulness			
Can the findings be generalized?		−1	The high risk of bias associated with disproportionate dropout is a major concern
Are the findings easily translatable?	+1		If true, transfer to biocompatible solution is easily translated into practice
Was the NNT <100?			Not applicable to a continuous variable
Score	**12 %**		

Summary and Conclusions

Also inspired by the findings of the Euro-Balance study, this industry-sponsored trial was designed to determine whether a biocompatible solution (Gambrosol trio) might preserve residual kidney function. The main finding of the study was that Gambrosol trio was associated with a slower decline of 24-h urine volume, decreasing by 12 ml/month as compared to 38 ml/month with the standard fluid, $P=0.024$. There were no significant differences in blood pressure between the groups although it tended to be lower in the standard dialysate group. The authors were not able to calculate the relative achieved ultrafiltration in the two groups, a pity given the findings of Euro-Balance and balANZ, due to uncertainty over the overfill volume of the two solutions. Overfill is an important confounder in determining achieved ultrafiltration, and it is of obvious importance in a trial designed to assess preservation of residual kidney function [45–47].

The main criticisms of this trial are methodological. It seems that the power calculation was actually done after the study was commenced in an interim analysis of the first 3 patients which will likely have exacerbated any early bias. There is also the high dropout rate in the context of a randomization process that is well described but failed to achieve well-balanced groups in terms of size, with 44 patients in the active and 36 in the control arm, but baseline data for the primary endpoint only available on 43 and 26 patients, respectively. There was therefore a very disproportionate dropout of control subjects, and given the fact that the primary endpoint is associated with survival on PD, this may have resulted in informative bias [48, 49]. There was also unequal use of ACE or ARBi in the two groups as this was not stratified for although the authors claim to have accounted for this in their analysis. Finally, despite the dropout imbalance, an as treated rather than intention to treat analysis was undertaken.

Biocompatible Dialysis Fluid: (5) Residual Kidney Function and Membrane Effects

Trial 11

Publication: Effects of biocompatible versus standard fluid on peritoneal dialysis outcomes

Authors: Johnson DW, Brown FG, Clarke M, Boudville N, Elias TJ, Foo MW, Jones B, Kulkarni H, Langham R, Ranganathan D, Schollum J, Suranyi M, Tan SH, Voss D; balANZ Trial Investigators

Reference: *J Am Soc Nephrol*. 2012 Jun;23(6):1097–107

Abstract

The clinical benefits of using "biocompatible" neutral pH solutions containing low levels of glucose degradation products for peritoneal dialysis compared with standard solutions are uncertain. In this multicenter, open-label, parallel-group, randomized controlled trial, we randomly assigned 185 incident adult peritoneal dialysis patients with residual renal function to use either biocompatible or conventional solution for 2 years. The primary outcome measure was slope of renal function decline. Secondary outcome measures comprised time to anuria, fluid volume status, peritonitis-free survival, technique survival, patient survival, and adverse events. We did not detect a statistically significant difference in the rate of decline of renal function between the two groups as measured by the slopes of GFR: 20.22 and 20.28 ml/min/1.73 m²/month ($P=0.17$) in the first year in the biocompatible and conventional groups, respectively, and 20.09 and 20.10 ml/min/1.73 m²/month ($P=0.9$) in the second year. The biocompatible group exhibited significantly longer times to anuria ($P=0.009$) and to the first peritonitis episode ($P=0.01$). This group also had fewer patients develop peritonitis (30 % versus 49 %) and had lower rates of peritonitis (0.30 versus 0.49 episodes per year, $P=0.01$). In conclusion, this trial does not support a role for biocompatible fluid in slowing the rate of GFR decline, but it does suggest that biocompatible fluid may delay the onset of anuria and reduce the incidence of peritonitis compared with conventional fluid in peritoneal dialysis.

Critical Appraisal

Parameters	Yes	No	Comment
Validity			
Is the **Randomization** Procedure well described?	+1		Well described with central computer-generated randomization concealed from investigators and stratified by center and diabetic status
Double **blinded**?		−1	Open study, neither investigator nor patient blinded as this would not have been possible
Is the **sample size** calculation described/adequate?	+3		Yes, based on an expected difference in the rate of loss of residual renal function between groups of 0.067 ml/min/1.73 m²/month
Does it have a hard primary **endpoint**?	+1		Yes – rate of decline of residual renal function. Time to anuria designated a secondary endpoint alongside time to first peritonitis, fluid status of patients, and technique failure
Is the endpoint surrogate?	+1		Residual kidney function is an important clinical endpoint in dialysis patients
Is the follow-up appropriate?	+1		2 years is appropriate and longer than most studies
Was there a **Bias**?	−1		Open study, so there is some performance bias
Is the dropout >25 %?	−2		Overall dropout was high at 51 %; reasons are well balanced by group and are fully documented. This is concerning in the context of under-recruitment to the study – initially planned as 336 but stopped at 186 after prolongation of the recruitment window
Is the analysis **ITT**?	+1		Yes
Utility/usefulness			
Can the findings be generalized?	+1		Despite high dropout and under-recruitment the findings fit well with other studies of this fluid, the secondary endpoints are likely generalizable at least to CAPD patients (APD was poorly represented)
Are the findings easily translatable?	+1		Yes – substituting the test dialysis fluid for conventional dialysate is easily done
Was the NNT <100?	+1		Not applicable to the primary endpoint due to its being a continuous variable. True of time to anuria
Score	**42 %**		

Summary and Conclusions

The balANZ study was also stimulated by the findings of the Euro-Balance trial, especially the secondary observation in that study that the biocompatible solution under investigation (Balance, Fresenius) might lead to preservation in residual kidney function. Although balANZ was industry supported with representation on the study steering group, one of its strengths is that it was instigated and led by independent academic investigators. Generally, it is a high-quality study from a methodological perspective that was let down by the difficulty in recruiting to time and target. In retrospect, it can be seen that the investigators were unfortunate to pick the rate of decline of residual kidney function rather than time to anuria and their primary endpoint, as the latter led to significant difference, whereas the former only approached significance. However, taking the overview (especially as it could be argued that time to anuria is a more important clinical event [50]), this should be seen as a positive trial. This is strengthened by the other positive finding in the important secondary endpoint, time to first peritonitis episode, which on further analysis is shown to be clinically less severe [51].

The question we are left with is our understanding of the mechanism by which the intervention protects residual kidney function. Of those proposed, two merit further discussion here. In the Euro-Balance study, there was evidence that the use of a solution with ultralow levels of glucose degradation products (GDPs) translated into lower systemic levels, either by reducing their absorption from the peritoneal cavity or possibly enhancing their clearance (renal or peritoneal). Given that some GDPs are potentially nephrotoxic, then reduced systemic levels could preserve residual function better [52]. The main difficulties with this argument are the relatively small reduction in GDPs (which are already abundant in renal failure) and the chicken-and-egg problem of knowing which comes first: was residual kidney function preserved by another mechanism so lowering GDP, or vice versa? The other likely mechanism is volume homeostasis. It is clear from both the Euro-Balance and balANZ study that the two dialysis solutions being tested have different effects on membrane function, both in the short term where Balance is associated with a significant increase in the rate of small solute transport, so reducing ultrafiltration capacity of the membrane and in the long term by protecting against the increase in solute transport over time [53]. It is remarkable that in both studies, the total fluid removal (ultrafiltration plus urine volume) is identical between groups at all time points, suggesting that lower achieved ultrafiltration in the context of preserved kidney function is of benefit. In effect the balANZ group did a trial of ultrafiltration target which may be of more overall clinical significance than the original objective [54].

General Discussion

This collection of high impact clinical trials in PD enables some general points to be made regarding the challenges as well as benefits of doing this important type of research in this patient group. There can be no doubt that they have been major drivers in clinical practice in some cases, for example the setting of dialysis adequacy targets, preventing catheter associated infection, demonstrating the efficacy of icodextrin, and showing us the importance of how modality choice affects lives in ways that go beyond survival. It also shows that the quality of methodological approach is highly variable and that this does not necessarily equate to impact. On the positive side, the vast majority were multicenter, usually using central, concealed, and stratified randomization techniques.

Some of the methodological problems are common and to an extent dictated by the therapy. For example, almost all the studies discussed had difficulty in concealing the study label post randomization. This is largely because the dialysis fluids or interventions required patients and clinicians to do something different; manufacture of control solutions with otherwise similar connectology and bag construction techniques is extremely expensive for the purposes of a research study and requires the study to be industry led. Relatively high dropout is also a major problem in several of these studies once they go beyond 6 months duration. While dropout can be for good (e.g., transplantation) as well as bad reasons, it is well recognized that technique failure remains a serious problem for the modality. Also in terms of generalizability, too many studies did not adequately represent automated peritoneal dialysis either because this therapy was not available in the recruiting country (e.g., ADEMEX) or because the solution was not available in the correct bag size (e.g., DIUREST, Euro-Balance, balANZ).

In terms of choice of endpoint, it is notable that only one study was adequately powered in relation to patient survival (ADEMEX). The fact that the study was resoundingly negative still makes it a very valuable contribution to how the therapy is practiced although there is a risk that it feeds an attitude of therapeutic nihilism. It is clear that we need more trials that are sufficiently powered to address the "big" endpoints (patient and technique survival). Hemodialysis faces a similar problem, despite the fact that there are ten times as many patients using this modality; one of the solutions has been to develop different methodological approaches such as those developed by the Dialysis Outcomes and Practice Patterns Study, and this has now been extended to include peritoneal dialysis (PDOPPS). Although not a replacement for the randomized clinical trial, this will ensure that a much higher proportion of PD patients are participating in clinical studies that include these endpoints (PDOPPS will focus on practices that extend technique survival without detriment to patient survival) and hopefully identify the key interventions that should then be formally tested.

The other endpoints that were investigated and that are of clear importance to dialysis patients were peritonitis and preservation of residual kidney function. The poor number and quality of studies addressing the treatment of peritonitis such that none are represented in these high impact studies (see *Cochrane*

Review Database CD005284) is surprising, disappointing, and in need of rectifying. The lessons learned from choosing preservation of residual renal function as a primary endpoint are interesting and would benefit from an internationally agreed consensus statement. For example, each of the studies expresses the rate of loss of kidney function in a different way, ranging from nl of clearance over the study period of 9 months to ml/min/1.73 m^2/month which might be considered the clearest approach. Taking the studies together, it would seem that the initial rate of loss in control patients is typically 0.25–0.28 ml/min/1.73 m^2/month. It is also clear that investigators struggled to decide whether the rate of decline is more important than time to anuria, and there are very real technical issues to consider here. Once a patient becomes anuric, a rate of decline cannot be further calculated, which means that this patient is no longer informing the primary endpoint as they have effectively dropped out; however, this dropout is likely to be affected by informative censoring, potentially contributing bias to the study. The problem is further complicated by the fact that for many patients, the rate of loss of residual function is not linear over time. This can be dealt with by fitting individual logarithmic functions, but this is labor intensive and still subject to the number of observations available. It is suggested that in future studies treat these as equally important endpoints and present both.

Finally it is worth pointing out that there is an overrepresentation of these high impact studies testing biocompatible solutions compared to other potentially more clinically important or relevant endpoints. This is not a criticism of these studies which have recently been summarized in more detail than is possible here by an excellent meta-analysis by the Cochrane collaboration (Cochrane database CD007554), but of the PD practicing community that is responsible for driving the research agenda and in particular the barriers to taking part in clinical research faced by clinical teams which are often considerable. There are notable exceptions to this, such as the ANZ clinical trials registry, but it would be highly desirable to see more academic investigator-led trials that answer key questions relating to how PD is practiced in the future.

References

1. Bloembergen WE, Port FK, Mauger EA, Wolfe RA. A comparison of mortality between patients treated with hemodialysis and peritoneal dialysis. J Am Soc Nephrol. 1995;6(2):177–83.
2. Weinhandl ED, Foley RN, Gilbertson DT, Arneson TJ, Snyder JJ, Collins AJ. Propensity-matched mortality comparison of incident hemodialysis and peritoneal dialysis patients. J Am Soc Nephrol. 2010;21(3):499–506.
3. Mehrotra R, Chiu YW, Kalantar-Zadeh K, Vonesh E. The outcomes of continuous ambulatory and automated peritoneal dialysis are similar. Kidney Int. 2009;76(1):97–107.
4. Perl J, Wald R, McFarlane P, Bargman JM, Vonesh E, Na Y, Jassal SV, Moist L. Hemodialysis vascular access modifies the association between dialysis modality and survival. J Am Soc Nephrol. 2011;22(6):1113–21.
5. Yeates K, Zhu N, Vonesh E, Trpeski L, Blake P, Fenton S. Hemodialysis and peritoneal dialysis are associated with similar outcomes for end-stage renal disease treatment in Canada. Nephrol Dial Transplant. 2012;27(9):3568–75.
6. Eknoyan G, Beck GJ, Cheung AK, Daugirdas JT, Greene T, Kusek JW, et al. Hemodialysis (HEMO) Study Group. Effect of dialysis dose and membrane flux in maintenance hemodialysis. N Engl J Med. 2002;347(25):2010–9.
7. Lo WK, Ho YW, Li CS, Wong KS, Chan TM, Yu AW, Ng FS, Cheng IK. Effect of Kt/V on survival and clinical outcome in CAPD patients in a randomized prospective study. Kidney Int. 2003;64(2):649–56.
8. Bargman JM, Thorpe KE, Churchill DN, CANUSA Peritoneal Dialysis Study Group. Relative contribution of residual renal function and peritoneal clearance to adequacy of dialysis: a reanalysis of the CANUSA study. J Am Soc Nephrol. 2001;12(10):2158–62.
9. Brown EA, Davies SJ, Rutherford P, Meeus F, Borras M, Riegel W et al. EAPOS Group. Survival of functionally anuric patients on automated peritoneal dialysis: the European APD Outcome Study. J Am Soc Nephrol. 2003;14(11):2948–57.
10. Jansen MA, Termorshuizen F, Korevaar JC, Dekker FW, Boeschoten E, Krediet RT, NECOSAD Study Group. Predictors of survival in anuric peritoneal dialysis patients. Kidney Int. 2005;68(3):1199–205.
11. Davies SJ, Ogg CS, Cameron JS, Poston S, Noble WC. *Staphylococcus aureus* nasal carriage, exit-site infection and catheter loss in patients treated with continuous ambulatory peritoneal dialysis (CAPD). Perit Dial Int. 1989;9:61–4.
12. Piraino B, Bernardini J, Sorkin M. A five year study of the microbiologic results of exit site infections and peritonitis in continuous ambulatory peritoneal dialysis. Am J Kidney Dis. 1987;10:281–6.
13. Bernardini J, Piraino B, Holley J, Johnston JR, Lutes R. A randomized trial of *Staphylococcus aureus* prophylaxis in peritoneal dialysis patients: mupirocin calcium ointment 2% applied to the exit site versus cyclic oral rifampin. Am J Kidney Dis. 1996;27:695–700.
14. Schaefer F, Feneberg R, Aksu N, Donmez O, Sadikoglu B, Alexander SR, et al. Worldwide variation of dialysis-associated peritonitis in children. Kidney Int. 2007;72(11):1374–9.
15. Johnson DW, Badve SV, Pascoe EM, Beller E, Cass A, Clark C, et al. HONEYPOT Study Collaborative Group. Antibacterial honey for the prevention of peritoneal-dialysis-related infections (HONEYPOT): a randomised trial. Lancet Infect Dis. 2014;14(1):23–30.
16. Mistry CD. The beginning of icodextrin. Perit Dial Int. 2011;31 Suppl 2:S49–52.
17. Gokal R, Mistry CD, Peers EM. Peritonitis occurrence in a multicenter study of icodextrin and glucose in CAPD MIDAS Study Group. Multicenter Investigation of Icodextrin in Ambulatory Dialysis. Perit Dial Int. 1995;15(6):226–30.
18. Davies SJ. Mitigating peritoneal membrane characteristics in modern peritoneal dialysis therapy. Kidney Int Suppl. 2006;103:S76–83.
19. Cho Y, Johnson DW, Craig JC, Strippoli GF, Badve SV, Wiggins KJ. Biocompatible dialysis fluids for peritoneal dialysis. Cochrane Database Syst Rev. 2014;(3):CD007554.
20. Han SH, Ahn SV, Yun JY, Tranaeus A, Han DS. Effects of icodextrin on patient survival and technique success in patients undergoing peritoneal dialysis. Nephrol Dial Transplant. 2012;27(5):2044–50.
21. Konings CJ, Kooman JP, Schonck M, Gladziwa U, Wirtz J, van den Wall Bake AW, et al. Effect of icodextrin on volume status, blood pressure and echocardiographic parameters: a randomized study. Kidney Int. 2003;63(4):1556–63.
22. Cho Y, Johnson DW, Craig JC, Strippoli GF, Badve SV, Wiggins KJ. Biocompatible dialysis fluids for peritoneal dialysis. Cochrane Database Syst Rev. 2014;(3):CD007554.
23. Brimble KS, Walker M, Margetts PJ, Kundhal KK, Rabbat CG. Meta-analysis: peritoneal membrane transport, mortality, and technique failure in peritoneal dialysis. J Am Soc Nephrol. 2006;17(9):2591–8.
24. Paniagua R, Ventura MD, Avila-Díaz M, Cisneros A, Vicenté-Martínez M, Furlong MD, et al. Icodextrin improves metabolic and

fluid management in high and high-average transport diabetic patients. Perit Dial Int. 2009;29(4):422–32.

25. Li PK, Culleton BF, Ariza A, Do JY, Johnson DW, Sanabria M, Shockley TR, et al. IMPENDIA and EDEN Study Groups. Randomized, controlled trial of glucose-sparing peritoneal dialysis in diabetic patients. J Am Soc Nephrol. 2013;24(11):1889–900.

26. Bargman JM, Thorpe KE, Churchill DN, CANUSA Peritoneal Dialysis Study Group. Relative contribution of residual renal function and peritoneal clearance to adequacy of dialysis: a reanalysis of the CANUSA study. J Am Soc Nephrol. 2001;12(10):2158–62.

27. Termorshuizen F, Dekker FW, van Manen JG, Korevaar JC, Boeschoten EW, Krediet RT, NECOSAD Study Group. Relative contribution of residual renal function and different measures of adequacy to survival in hemodialysis patients: an analysis of the Netherlands Cooperative Study on the Adequacy of Dialysis (NECOSAD)-2. J Am Soc Nephrol. 2004;15(4):1061–70.

28. Termorshuizen F, Korevaar JC, Dekker FW, van Manen JG, Boeschoten EW, Krediet RT, NECOSAD Study Group. The relative importance of residual renal function compared with peritoneal clearance for patient survival and quality of life: an analysis of the Netherlands Cooperative Study on the Adequacy of Dialysis (NECOSAD)-2. Am J Kidney Dis. 2003;41(6):1293–302.

29. Fang W, Oreopoulos DG, Bargman JM. Use of ACE inhibitors or angiotensin receptor blockers and survival in patients on peritoneal dialysis. Nephrol Dial Transplant. 2008;23(11):3704–10.

30. Akbari A, Knoll G, Ferguson D, McCormick B, Davis A, Biyani M. Angiotensin-converting enzyme inhibitors and angiotensin receptor blockers in peritoneal dialysis: systematic review and meta-analysis of randomized controlled trials. Perit Dial Int. 2009;29(5):554–61.

31. Mackenzie R, Holmes CJ, Jones S, Williams JD, Topley N. Clinical indices of in vivo biocompatibility: the role of ex vivo cell function studies and effluent markers in peritoneal dialysis patients. Kidney Int Suppl. 2003;88:S84–93.

32. Jones S, Holmes CJ, Krediet RT, Mackenzie R, Faict D, Tranaeus A, Williams JD, Coles GA, Topley N, Bicarbonate/Lactate Study Group. Bicarbonate/lactate-based peritoneal dialysis solution increases cancer antigen 125 and decreases hyaluronic acid levels. Kidney Int. 2001;59(4):1529–38.

33. le Poole CY, Welten AG, ter Wee PM, Paauw NJ, Djorai AN, Valentijn RM, et al. A peritoneal dialysis regimen low in glucose and glucose degradation products results in increased cancer antigen 125 and peritoneal activation. Perit Dial Int. 2012;32(3):305–15.

34. Cheema H, Bargman JM. Cancer antigen 125 as a biomarker in peritoneal dialysis: mesothelial cell health or death? Perit Dial Int. 2013;33(4):349–52.

35. Mactier RA, Sprosen TS, Gokal R, Williams PF, Lindbergh M, Naik RB, et al. Bicarbonate and bicarbonate/lactate peritoneal dialysis solutions for the treatment of infusion pain. Kidney Int. 1998;53(4):1061–7.

36. Wieslander AP, Nordin MK, Martinson E, Kjellstrand PT, Boberg UC. Heat sterilized PD-fluids impair growth and inflammatory responses of cultured cell lines and human leukocytes. Clin Nephrol. 1993;39(6):343–8.

37. Wieslander AP, Nordin MK, Kjellstrand PT, Boberg UC. Toxicity of peritoneal dialysis fluids on cultured fibroblasts, L-929. Kidney Int. 1991;40(1):77–9.

38. Yung S, Chan TM. Pathophysiology of the peritoneal membrane during peritoneal dialysis: the role of hyaluronan. J Biomed Biotechnol. 2011;2011:180594.

39. Cho Y, Johnson DW, Craig JC, Strippoli GF, Badve SV, Wiggins KJ. Biocompatible dialysis fluids for peritoneal dialysis. Cochrane Database Syst Rev. 2014;(3):CD007554.

40. Michels WM, Verduijn M, Grootendorst DC, le Cessie S, Boeschoten EW, Dekker FW, Krediet RT, NECOSAD study group. Decline in residual renal function in automated compared with continuous ambulatory peritoneal dialysis. Clin J Am Soc Nephrol. 2011;6(3):537–42.

41. Kim CH, Oh HJ, Lee MJ, Kwon YE, Kim YL, Nam KH, Park KS, An SY, Ko KI, Koo HM, Doh FM, Han SH, Yoo TH, Kim BS, Kang SW, Choi KH. Effect of peritoneal dialysis modality on the 1-year rate of decline of residual renal function. Yonsei Med J. 2014;55(1): 141–8.

42. Bieber SD, Burkart J, Golper TA, Teitelbaum I, Mehrotra R. Comparative outcomes between continuous ambulatory and automated peritoneal dialysis: a narrative review. Am J Kidney Dis. 2014;63:1027–37. doi:10.1053/j.ajkd.2013.11.025. pii: S0272-6386(13)01620-X. PubMed PMID: 24423779.

43. Cho Y, Johnson DW, Craig JC, Strippoli GF, Badve SV, Wiggins KJ. Biocompatible dialysis fluids for peritoneal dialysis. Cochrane Database Syst Rev. 2014;(3):CD007554.

44. Kim SG, Kim S, Hwang YH, Kim K, Oh JE, Chung W, et al. Could solutions low in glucose degradation products preserve residual renal function in incident peritoneal dialysis patients? A 1-year multicenter prospective randomized controlled trial (Balnet study). Perit Dial Int. 2008;28 Suppl 3:S117–22.

45. McCafferty K, Fan SL. Are we underestimating the problem of ultrafiltration in peritoneal dialysis patients? Perit Dial Int. 2006;26(3):349–52.

46. Davies SJ. Overfill or ultrafiltration? We need to be clear. Perit Dial Int. 2006;26(4):449–51.

47. La Milia V, Pozzoni P, Crepaldi M, Locatelli F. Overfill of peritoneal dialysis bags as a cause of underestimation of ultrafiltration failure. Perit Dial Int. 2006;26(4):503–5.

48. Misra M, Vonesh E, Van Stone JC, Moore HL, Prowant B, Nolph KD. Effect of cause and time of dropout on the residual GFR: a comparative analysis of the decline of GFR on dialysis. Kidney Int. 2001;59(2):754–63.

49. Misra M, Vonesh E, Churchill DN, Moore HL, Van Stone JC, Nolph KD. Preservation of glomerular filtration rate on dialysis when adjusted for patient dropout. Kidney Int. 2000;57(2): 691–6.

50. van der Wal WM, Noordzij M, Dekker FW, Boeschoten EW, Krediet RT, Korevaar JC, Geskus RB, Netherlands Cooperative Study on the Adequacy of Dialysis Study Group (NECOSAD). Full loss of residual renal function causes higher mortality in dialysis patients; findings from a marginal structural model. Nephrol Dial Transplant. 2011;26(9):2978–83.

51. Johnson DW, Brown FG, Clarke M, Boudville N, Elias TJ, Foo MW, et al. balANZ Trial Investigators. The effects of biocompatible compared with standard peritoneal dialysis solutions on peritonitis microbiology, treatment, and outcomes: the balANZ trial. Perit Dial Int. 2012;32(5):497–506.

52. Justo P, Sanz AB, Egido J, Ortiz A. 3,4-Dideoxyglucosone-3-ene induces apoptosis in renal tubular epithelial cells. Diabetes. 2005;54:2424–9.

53. Johnson DW, Brown FG, Clarke M, Boudville N, Elias TJ, Foo MW, et al. balANZ Trial Investigators. The effect of low glucose degradation product, neutral pH versus standard peritoneal dialysis solutions on peritoneal membrane function: the balANZ trial. Nephrol Dial Transplant. 2012;27(12):4445–53.

54. Davies SJ. What has balANZ taught us about balancing ultrafiltration with membrane preservation? Nephrol Dial Transplant. 2013;28(8):1971–4.

Renal Transplantation Clinical Trials: A Critical Appraisal

13

Lionel Rostaing and Richard J. Baker

Introduction

In kidney transplantation, the major step forward has been, in the 1970s and 1980s, the use of calcineurin inhibitors (CNIs), which dramatically reduces the number of acute rejections within the first year posttransplantation. However, beyond this first year, the half-life of the kidney does not increase significantly compared to that in the pre-CNI era.

The first CNI to be used in 1984 was cyclosporine in association with azathioprine. Because daily doses of cyclosporine were very high in those days, cyclosporine led to irreversible nephrotoxicity in some recipients. Hence, there is the belief that CNIs are nephrotoxic. Indeed, Nankivell et al.'s study showed, over a 10-year period, that there were changes in renal histopathology in kidney-pancreas-transplant recipients treated with cyclosporine-based immunosuppression, with evidence of chronic nephrotoxicity such as fibrosis and arteriolar hyalinosis [1] . In the early 1990s, tacrolimus was released on the market. While another CNI, it proved to be more powerful than cyclosporine. At the same time, azathioprine was replaced by more powerful anti-metabolite mycophenolate mofetil (MMF). The association of tacrolimus plus MMF achieved very good long-term results by substantially decreasing tacrolimus trough levels (<7 ng/mL) and avoiding, to some extent, nephrotoxicity when compared to the association between cyclosporine plus MMF (as demonstrated in the SYMPHONY study). The DIRECT study compared de novo kidney-transplant recipients receiving cyclosporine-based immunosuppression versus tacrolimus-based immunosuppression, in addition to MMF, steroids, and an induction therapy. The DIRECT study showed that, by 1 year posttransplantation, the two CNIs had the same immunosuppressive potency, but that cyclosporine was associated with significantly less new-onset diabetes after transplantation and less BKV replication.

The immunosuppressive power of tacrolimus plus MMF also allows us to avoid the long-term use of steroids, which are associated with detrimental side effects. In the 5-year double-blind, placebo-controlled study of Woodle et al., steroid avoidance after postoperative day 7 was safe, even though there was significantly more acute cellular rejection; however, this had no adverse consequences on long-term allograft survival or function.

Because CNIs are potentially nephrotoxic, this led to the development of non-nephrotoxic drugs, including a range of monoclonal antibodies to enhance induction therapy and minimize the use/dose of CNIs. This included in the 1990s the introduction of monoclonal anti-interleukin-2 receptor (IL-2R) (basiliximab and daclizumab) as well as more recently anti-CD52 (Campath). These have nowadays replaced to a large extent the use of antithymocyte globulin (ATG)/antilymphocyte globulin (ALG).

Also, belatacept, which is a fusion protein that blocks the second signal within lymphocytes, has been introduced in the last decade. Belatacept is infused every 4 weeks and is very well tolerated, and no anti-belatacept-blocking antibodies develop. Two phase III trials have compared belatacept-based immunosuppression with cyclosporine-based immunosuppression in de novo recipients of either a standard kidney (BENEFIT) or a kidney from an extended-criteria deceased donor (BENEFIT-EXT). It was shown that at 3 and 5 years posttransplantation, when compared to cyclosporine, belatacept resulted in significantly and sustained allograft function (a difference of more than 10 mL/min), with improved cardiovascular parameters, very few de novo donor-specific alloantibodies(DSA), and the same rates of de novo cancers and infections as compared to

L. Rostaing, MD, PhD (✉)
Department of Nephrology, University Hospital of Toulouse, 1 avenue Jean Poulhès TSA 50032, Toulouse 31059, France
e-mail: rostaing.l@chu-toulouse.fr

R.J. Baker, MB, BChir, PhD, FRCP
Renal Unit, St. James's University Hospital, Lincoln Wing, Beckett Street, Leeds, West Yorkshire LS9 7TP, UK
e-mail: Richard.baker@leedsth.nhs.uk

cyclosporine-treated patients. The only point of concern was that there was a higher risk of developing a posttransplant lymphoproliferative disorder (PTLD) in EBV-seronegative recipients; thus, these recipients should not receive belatacept.

The prevalence of de novo DSAs after kidney transplantation is high and is mainly the result of suboptimal immunosuppression and poor patient compliance. When DSAs are present, we can optimize immunosuppression but, so far, there is no efficient therapy that can alter their negative impacts on short-term allograft function. However, the recent study by [2] has shown that the most deleterious DSAs are those that bind complement, whereas those that do not may just be bystanders. This finding is of utmost importance because, if this effect is universal, therapies that interfere with the complement pathway, such as eculizumab (a monoclonal antibody that blocks C5a), could be of huge value.

In the setting where DSAs are already present at the time of transplantation, desensitization protocols based on plasmapheresis and rituximab and/or IVIg have been shown to be efficient, i.e., they allow successful kidney transplantation. An induction therapy with rituximab in these patients may be associated with (i) less occurrence of antibody-mediated rejection and (ii) significantly less occurrence of de novo DSAs [3]. However, in this setting, despite adapted pre- and posttransplant immunosuppressive therapies, some patients will develop very severe acute antibody-mediated rejection (aAMR) that, if treated successfully, might nonetheless evolve to chronic antibody-mediated rejection (cAMR). In this field, the prophylactic use of eculizumab immediately after kidney transplantation may effectively prevent AAMR and maybe, ultimately, CAMR [4].

Chronic immunosuppression, particularly when it is very powerful, may result in opportunistic infections and in de novo virus-driven cancers. With regard to infections, the IMPACT study has shown that valganciclovir prophylaxis in D+/R− patients significantly decreased the rates of CMV infection and CMV disease and that 200 days of prophylaxis was significantly more efficient in terms of preventing CMV infection than 100 days of prophylaxis. Thus, the longer period of prophylaxis may decrease the long-term detrimental indirect effects of CMV.

BKV virus infection can occur within the first months posttransplantation and ultimately result in BKV-associated nephropathy, which may eventually destroy the allograft. Hirsch et al. have shown that BKV replication is a relatively frequent event and that monitoring for it in the urine and blood using PCR is important [5]. Above a certain cutoff level, immunosuppression has to be modified, i.e., to be decreased if one wants to halt the replication of BKV. Alternatively, the use of m-TOR inhibitors as immunosuppressants may reduce the risk of BKV replication [6].

Virus-induced de novo cancers, such as skin cancers Kaposi sarcoma, PTLDs, and cervical carcinoma, increase in prevalence posttransplantation by 10- to 100-fold. Dantal et al. reported, in a prospective randomized trial, implemented at 1 year posttransplantation that decreasing daily doses of cyclosporine by 50 % significantly decreased de novo skin cancers [7]. More recently, Euvrard et al. have shown that kidney-transplant patients receiving CNI-based immunosuppression and presenting with relapsing cutaneous squamous cell carcinomas (SCC) had less relapsing SCC and less (pre)neoplastic cutaneous lesions when CNI therapy was stopped under the umbrella of mTOR inhibitors, i.e., sirolimus (The TUMORAPA study discussed below).

The key clinical studies mentioned above that shaped current management of renal transplantation are discussed and critically appraised in this chapter.

Original Cyclosporine, tacrolimus, and Mycophenolate Trials

Cyclosporine in Renal Transplantation

The discovery of the calcineurin inhibitor, cyclosporine, by Borel and his colleagues at Sandoz (now Novartis) [8], as a more selective immunosuppressive agent opened a new era in organ transplantation including renal transplantation. Cyclosporine binds to the cytosolic protein cyclophilin in T cells and consequently inhibits calcineurin that activates the transcription of interleukin-2 (IL-2), a potent T-cell activator.

N Engl J Med. 1986 May 8;314(19):1219–25.

A randomized clinical trial of cyclosporine in cadaveric renal transplantation. Analysis at three years. The Canadian Multicenter Transplant Study Group.

[No authors listed]

Abstract

In a multicenter trial, we investigated the effect of immunosuppressive therapy on graft and patient survival, renal function, and complications in 291 recipients of cadaveric renal transplants. One hundred and forty-two patients were randomly assigned to treatment with cyclosporine and prednisone, and 149 to control immunosuppressive therapy (azathioprine and prednisone, with or without antilymphocyte globulin). At 3 years, graft survival was 69 % in the cyclosporine-treated patients and 58 % in the control. (P=0.05). The number of episodes of graft rejection was similar in the two groups, but the severity of rejection was significantly worse among the controls. Patients surviva after 3 years was 90 % in the cyclosporine group and 82 % in the control group ($P=0.04$). Acute tubular necrosis was an important risk factor for graft loss in both groups. Risk factors for death included diabetes and older age of the recipient. Renal function as indicated by the serum creatinine concentration or creatinine clearance was poorer in the cyclosporine-treated patients than in the controls but has remained stable in both groups since the sixth month after transplantation. We conclude that, among recipients of cadaveric renal transplants, those treated with cyclosporine, despite having poorer (but stable) renal function, have better graft and patient survival at 3 years than those treated with alternative forms of immunosuppressive therapy.

Critical Appraisal

Parameters	Yes	No	Comment
Validity			
Is the **randomization** procedure well described?	+1		142 on cyclosporine + steroids versus 149 best therapy at the time mostly azathioprine + steroids
Double **blinded**?		−2	Unblinded trial, thus raising potential of observer bias
Is the **sample size** calculation described/adequate?	+3		Power of 90 % to detect a 20 % difference, at a significance level of 0.05
Does it have a hard primary **endpoint**?	+1		Grafts and patients survival
Is the endpoint surrogate?		0	
Is the follow-up appropriate?	+1		Average 3 years; up to 5 years follow-up
Was there a **Bias**?	−2		More second transplants, therefore higher risk, in the control group. Switching of patients between groups generates bias; 40 patients switched, after complications, from CyA to control group
Is the dropout >25 %?		+1	
Is the analysis **ITT**?	+3		Also switching between groups confounds such analysis
Utility/usefulness			
Can the findings be generalized?	+1		
Was the NNT <100?	N/A		Comparative study between two treatment regimens
Score	**46 %**		

Comments and Discussion

This pivotal trial comparing the impact of CyA versus azathioprine-based immunosuppressive regimens in renal cadaveric allograft recipients showed an advantage for those treated with CyA compared to controls in terms of graft and patient survival.

There was no difference in the incidence of graft rejection although the severity of allograft rejection episodes seemed more severe in the control group than in those treated with CyA. Renal function was lower in the CyA group.

This study has some limitations including:

1. Its unblinded nature, claimed by the investigators to be due in part to the necessity to monitor CyA blood levels and adjust treatment accordingly, is liable to generate an element of observer bias.
2. A bias in favor of the CyA arm may have been generated by having more recipients with second renal allografts, thus at a higher risk, in the control group. Also, patients who suffered CyA-induced side effects, mostly renal dysfunction, were allowed to switch to the control group, thus biasing the control group in a negative fashion. This may be compounded by the fact that the study was not blinded, thus raising concern over investigators' bias and decision-making.
3. Patients assumed to have acute rejection (AR) were not biopsied; this can create a diagnostic bias by unblinded investigators.
4. The severity of the graft rejection was based on changes in serum creatinine rather than confirmed by a renal biopsy in all cases.

Conclusion

The Canadian multicenter study confirmed earlier and shorter follow-up studies [9, 10] showing the superiority of CyA-steroids combination treatment over the conventional immunosuppressive regimen of azathioprine plus steroids in recipients of cadaveric renal allograft recipients. From the mid-1980s onward, calcineurin inhibitor (CNI)-based induction immunosuppression has become the cornerstone of renal transplantation.

Tacrolimus Versus Cyclosporine in Renal Transplantation

If the advent of cyclosporine in the area of transplantation had marked a revolution in terms of 1-year survival, then the arrival of tacrolimus represented a further step in the evolution of immunosuppression [11]. Registry data had suggested that tacrolimus was a more potent immunosuppressive agent and furthermore head-to-head studies had demonstrated that tacrolimus was associated with significantly reduced rates of acute cellular rejection (ACR) and also more severe rejection episodes requiring antibody therapy.

However, tacrolimus was associated with increased rates of neurotoxicity and new-onset diabetes after transplantation in these studies.

Lancet. 2002 Mar 2;359(9308):741–6.

Efficacy and safety of tacrolimus compared with cyclosporine microemulsion in renal transplantation: a randomized multicenter study.

Margreiter R; European tacrolimus vs Cyclosporine Microemulsion Renal Transplantation Study Group.

Abstract

Background: In previous comparative studies, tacrolimus was superior to the standard formulation of cyclosporine in preventing acute rejection after renal transplantation. We have compared the microemulsion formulation of cyclosporine with tacrolimus in a multicenter randomized trial.

Methods: The 6-month open study involved 560 patients in 50 European centers. Two hundred and eighty-seven patients were randomly assigned tacrolimus and 273 cyclosporine microemulsion plus azathioprine and corticosteroids. The initial oral daily doses were 0.30 mg/kg for tacrolimus and 8–10 mg/kg for cyclosporine. The primary endpoint was the proportion of patients with biopsy-proven acute rejection and the time to this event.

Findings: The two study groups were similar in terms of baseline characteristics. Three patients did not receive study treatment or did not undergo transplantation (one tacrolimus, two cyclosporine). The rate of biopsy-confirmed acute rejection was significantly lower with tacrolimus than with cyclosporine microemulsion (56 patients [19.6 %] vs 101 [37.3 %]; 17.7 % difference [95 % CI 10.3–25.1]; $p < 0.0001$). Biopsy-confirmed corticosteroid-resistant rejection was also significantly lower with tacrolimus (27 [9.4 %] vs 57 [21.0 %]; 11.6 % difference [5.7–17.5]; $p < 0.0001$). Crossover between therapies because of biopsy-proven rejection was judged necessary in one of 286 (0.3 %) tacrolimus-group patients and 27 of 271 (10.0 %) cyclosporine-group patients ($p < 0.0001$). There were no significant differences in survival of patients or grafts or in renal function. The overall frequency of adverse events was similar in the two groups, though hypertension and hypercholesterolemia were more common in the cyclosporine group and tremor and hypomagnesemia were more frequent in the tacrolimus group.

Interpretation: Tacrolimus was significantly more effective than cyclosporine microemulsion in preventing acute rejection after renal transplantation and had a superior cardiovascular risk profile.

Critical Appraisal

Parameters	Yes	No	Comment
Validity			
Is the **randomization** procedure well described?	+1		All eligible participants from each study center were randomized centrally in a one-to-one ratio to receive immunosuppressive therapy with tacrolimus (Prograf, Fujisawa GmbH, Munich, Germany) or cyclosporine microemulsion (Neoral, Novartis, Basel, Switzerland), with adjunctive azathioprine (Imuran, Glaxo Wellcome, Middlesex, UK) and corticosteroids
Double **blinded**?		−2	Open label, thus subject to investigator bias
Is the **sample size** calculation described/ adequate?	+3		The sample size estimate was based on the assumption that the rate of acute rejection in tacrolimus-treated patients during the first 6 months after transplantation would be 25 %. It was estimated that 450 patients would be required to give a statistical test on a 0.05 significance level (two-sided) the power of 80 % to detect a difference of 13 % in the rate of acute rejection
Does it have a hard primary **endpoint**?		−1	The primary endpoint of the study was the proportion of patients with a first biopsy-proven acute rejection (BPAR) within 6 months of transplantation and the time to onset of such a rejection episode
Is the endpoint surrogate?	−2		No
Is the follow-up appropriate?		−1	6 months
Was there a **Bias**?		+2	
Is the dropout >25 %?		+1	
Is the analysis **ITT**?	+3		
Utility/usefulness			
Can the findings be generalized?	+1		
Was the NNT <100?	N/A		Comparative study between two treatment regimens
Score	**33 %**		

Comments and Discussion

After a number of smaller studies implied superiority of tacrolimus (FK506) over cyclosporine (CyA) [12, 13], this European multicenter study showed that tacrolimus was more effective in preventing acute cadaveric allograft rejection. This larger European study was well powered to confirm previous observations. There was no difference in the secondary endpoints of graft and patients survival or renal function.

This study was confirmed by the US FK506 multicenter study that had a longer 12–18 months follow-up but smaller power and sample size [13]. The 5-year follow-up of the US multicenter study showed a favorable impact of tacrolimus on graft survival [14]. Of note, a meta-analysis performed in 2005 suggested that for every 100 patients treated with tacrolimus as opposed to cyclosporine, 12 patients would avoid an episode of rejection and 2 patients would keep their grafts 12 months after transplantation. However, five additional patients would have developed new-onset diabetes [15].

This study is not without limitations including:
1. Its open-label nature thus raising concern over potential observer bias.
2. Its soft primary endpoint of biopsy-proven acute rejection (BPAR) has become apparent since there is no strong correlation between BPAR and longer-term functional and graft-survival outcomes. There was no comment on the severity of the BPAR, but comments were made on a lower incidence of steroid-resistant AR episodes in patients treated with tacrolimus.
3. It is unclear whether the biopsy and histology evaluation of BPAR was blinded to the investigators.
4. The study follow-up of 6 months was too short as acute-rejection episodes continue to occur during the first 12 months after transplantation.

Conclusion

This study had a major impact on immunosuppression practice and induction therapy in recipients of cadaveric renal allograft recipients. Tacrolimus has since replaced CyA as the standard and preferred immunosuppressive agent.

Mycophenolate Mofetil in Renal Transplantation

Lancet. 1995 May 27;345(8961):1321–5.

Placebo-controlled study of mycophenolate mofetil combined with cyclosporine and corticosteroids for prevention of acute rejection. European Mycophenolate Mofetil Cooperative Study Group.

[No authors listed]

Abstract

Preliminary studies suggested that mycophenolate mofetil (MMF), which inhibits proliferation of T and B cells, may reduce the frequency of acute rejection after renal transplantation. Our randomized, double-blind, multicenter, placebo-controlled study compared the efficacy and safety of MMF with placebo for prevention of acute-rejection episodes after first or second cadaveric renal allograft transplantation. Four hundred and ninety-one patients were enrolled; 166 were assigned placebo, 165 MMF 2 g, and 160 MMF 3 g. Patients also received cyclosporine and corticosteroids. Significantly fewer ($p <$ or $= 0.001$) patients had biopsy-proven rejection or withdrew early from the trial (for any reason) during the first 6 months after transplantation with MMF 2 g (30.3 %) or 3 g (38.8 %) than with placebo (56.0 %). The corresponding percentages for biopsy-proven rejection were 17.0, 13.8, and 46.4 %. 28.5 % of MMF 2 g and 24.4 % of MMF 3 g patients needed full courses of corticosteroids or antilymphocyte agents for treatment of rejection episodes in the first 6 months, compared with 51.8 % of placebo recipients. By 6 months, 10.2, 6.7, and 8.8 % of the patients in the placebo, MMF 2 g and MMF 3 g groups, respectively, had died or lost the graft. Overall, the frequency of adverse events was similar in all treatment groups, although gastrointestinal problems, leukopenia, and opportunistic infections were more common in the MMF groups and there was a trend for more events in the 3 g than the 2 g group. MMF significantly reduced the rate of biopsy-proven rejection or other treatment failure during the first 6 months after transplantation and was well tolerated. The 3 g dose was somewhat less well tolerated.

Critical Appraisal

Parameters	Yes	No	Comment
Validity			
Is the **randomization** procedure well described?	+1		
Double **blinded**?	+2		
Is the **sample size** calculation described/ adequate?	+3		Comparative analysis between CyA + steroids + placebo (166 patients) versus CyA + steroids + MMF 2 g/day (165) versus CyA + steroids + MMF 3 g/day (160)

Parameters	Yes	No	Comment
Does it have a hard primary **endpoint**?		−1	Biopsy-proven acute rejection (BPAR)
			Also time to BPAR and treatment failure
Is the endpoint surrogate?	−2		Graft and patient survival were not primary endpoints
Is the follow-up appropriate?		−1	6 months
Was there a **Bias**?	−2		Absence of azathioprine as comparator
Is the dropout >25 %?		+1	Large withdrawal from the study ranging from 22 to 35 %
Is the analysis **ITT**?	+3		
Utility/usefulness			
Can the findings be generalized?		−1	Not in the absence of an adequate comparator group
Was the NNT <100?	N/A		
Score	**20 %**		

Comments and Discussion

The European Mycophenolate Mofetil (MMF) Cooperative Study showed the superiority of MMF over cyclosporine and steroid alone, in terms of biopsy-proven acute rejection (BPAR) for a regimen, in cadaveric renal transplantation. This was achieved by adding MMF to CyA and steroids compared to CyA and steroids alone. The percentage of those with BPAR on the CyA + steroids group was 46 %, compared to 17 % and 13.8 % in the MMF 2 and 3 g/day, respectively. The two MMF groups had comparable results up to 10 weeks; thereafter, the MMF 3 g/day had the higher cumulative rate of BPAR and treatment failure.

Of note, the dose of CyA and the blood levels achieved were not given and seemed to vary according to the clinical practice in the different European centers included in the study.

This study has the main limitation of not including a valid comparator to MMF using another antimetabolite such as azathioprine (Imuran), thus precluding any possible comparison with best practice at the time in cadaveric renal transplantation including CyA, azathioprine, and steroids. This was subsequently addressed by the US Renal Transplant Mycophenolate Mofetil Study Group that showed the superiority of MMF over azathioprine in terms of BPAR as well as graft loss at 6 months [16]. A systematic review undertaken in 2009, including 19 studies and 3,143 patients, confirmed the superiority of MMF-containing regimen over azathioprine [17]. This systematic review showed MMF used with a CNI conferred a benefit over azathioprine containing regimen as far as acute rejection, and "possibly" graft loss was concerned. Of interest, no difference was noted in terms of renal function [17].

Conclusion

A body of evidence has shown the superiority of MMF ove azathioprine containing immunosuppressive regimen i cadaveric renal transplantation.

ELITE-Symphony Trial

N Engl J Med. 2007 Dec 20;357(25):2562–75.

Reduced exposure to calcineurin inhibitors in rena transplantation.

Ekberg H, Tedesco-Silva H, Demirbas A, Vítko S, Nasha B, Gürkan A, Margreiter R, Hugo C, Grinyó JM, Frei U Vanrenterghem Y, Daloze P, Halloran PF; ELITE-Symphon Study.

Abstract

Background: Immunosuppressive regimens with the fewes possible toxic effects are desirable for transplant recipients This study evaluated the efficacy and relative toxic effects o four immunosuppressive regimens.

Methods: We randomly assigned 1,645 renal-transplan recipients to receive standard-dose cyclosporine, mycophe nolate mofetil, and corticosteroids or daclizumab induction mycophenolate mofetil, and corticosteroids in combination with low-dose cyclosporine, low-dose tacrolimus, or low dose sirolimus. The primary endpoint was the estimated glo merular filtration rate (GFR), as calculated by the Cockcroft-Gault formula, 12 months after transplantation Secondary endpoints included acute rejection and allograf survival.

Results: The mean calculated GFR was higher in patient receiving low-dose tacrolimus (65.4 mL/min) than in the other three groups (range, 56.7–59.4 mL/min). The rate o biopsy-proven acute rejection was lower in patients receiv ing low-dose tacrolimus (12.3 %) than in those receiving standard-dose cyclosporine (25.8 %), low-dose cyclospo rine (24.0 %), or low-dose sirolimus (37.2 %). Allograf survival differed significantly among the four groups ($P = 0.02$) and was highest in the low-dose tacrolimus grouj (94.2 %), followed by the low-dose cyclosporine grouj (93.1 %), the standard-dose cyclosporine group (89.3 %) and the low-dose sirolimus group (89.3 %). Serious advers events were more common in the low-dose sirolimus grouj than in the other groups (53.2 % vs. a range of 43.4– 44.3 %), although a similar proportion of patients in eacl group had at least one adverse event during treatmen (86.3–90.5 %).

Conclusions: A regimen of daclizumab, mycophenolate mofetil, and corticosteroids in combination with low-dose tacrolimus may be advantageous for renal function, allograft survival, and acute-rejection rates, as compared with regimens containing daclizumab induction plus either low-dose cyclosporine or low-dose sirolimus or with standard-dose cyclosporine without induction. (ClinicalTrials.gov number, NCT00231764 [ClinicalTrials.gov].)

Critical Appraisal

Parameters	Yes	No	Comment
Validity			
Is the **randomization** procedure described well?	+1		Patients were randomly assigned in a 1:1:1:1 ratio to receive one of four treatments
Was the study **double blinded**?		−2	Not investigators blinded
Was the **sample**-size calculation described/adequate?	+3		The initial protocol called for the enrolment of 1,300 patients. In an amendment to the protocol, the number was increased to 1,760 patients (440 per group) to provide a power of 80 % to detect a difference of 6.5 mL/min in GFR in one group with respect to the others in a global test, a value that was considered to be clinically relevant. To calculate GFR, a last-observation-carried-forward method was used for serum creatinine and weight, and 10 mL/min was imputed for missing values
Did the study have a hard primary **endpoint**?		−1	Estimated GFR by the Cockcroft-Gault method was used to evaluate renal function. True GFR was not measured
Was the endpoint surrogate?	−2		Same as above and somewhat unrelated to hard endpoints such as allograft and patient's survival
Was the follow-up appropriate?	+1		Yes for the surrogate endpoint, but not for the harder secondary endpoints
Was there any **Bias**?	−2		The low-cyclosporine and the low-sirolimus groups received subtherapeutic doses of immunosuppressants.
			Blood levels of cyclosporine, tacrolimus, and sirolimus were measured using locally available assays. Hence, in this protocol, because immunosuppressants were used at very low doses, this heterogeneity gives a huge bias because, for a given target, the result can be very different depending on the test used to measure it
Was the dropout rate >25 %?	−1		Withdrawal from an assigned treatment ranged from 20 % in the low-dose tacrolimus to 48.9 % in the low-sirolimus group. In all groups, treatment failure was the main reason for withdrawal
Was the analysis **ITT**?	+3		
Utility/usefulness			
Can the findings be generalized?	+1		
Was the NNT <100?	N/A		As comparative study between different drug regimens
Score	**6.5** %		

Comments and Discussion

This important study defined our current immunosuppression-preferred induction regimen, with emphasis on short-term renal functional preservation.

However, the study is not without its limitations:
1. Not double blinded, thus subject to investigator bias.
2. There was no comparison made between low and high tacrolimus dose but instead comparison between tacrolimus and CyA, with the former having a potential therapeutic advantage over the latter as discussed above [18].
3. The low-cyclosporine and the low-sirolimus groups received subtherapeutic doses of immunosuppressants.
4. In the absence of calcineurin inhibitors (i.e., cyclosporine or tacrolimus) and because of the half-life of sirolimus (~60 h, implying that its steady state is not achieved in less than 8 days), it could be anticipated that, in the low-sirolimus group, there would be more treatment failures. Thus, the low-cyclosporine as well as the low-sirolimus groups started the study with a handicap and an inherent bias.
5. eGFR is a soft endpoint as graft and patient survival are considered hard endpoints in renal transplantation.
6. eGFR was relied upon and true GFR was not measured (mGFR); patients with more frequent rejection episodes and higher cumulative dose of steroids may be confounded by weight loss/sarcopenia and/or the impact of steroid therapy on muscle/creatinine metabolism. eGFR

has also not been validated for the evaluation of renal function trajectories in renal transplantation.

7. Blood levels of cyclosporine, tacrolimus, and sirolimus were measured using locally available assays. Of the 83 participating sites, the reference tests were used in 33.3 % of sites for cyclosporine, in 61.7 % of site for sirolimus, and in 65 % of sites for tacrolimus. Hence, in this protocol, because immunosuppressants were used at very low doses, this heterogeneity gives a huge bias because, for a given target, the result can be very different depending on the test used to measure it.

8. Also, with issues with drug blood level measurements and the related bias, optimization of treatment in different groups is doubtful.

Conclusion

Major and pivotal study in renal transplantation that defined the current, preferred, immunosuppression/induction regimen.

However, the study is not without its serious limitations described above including potential observer bias, patient allocation bias, and issues related to drug blood level measurements as well as estimation of kidney function.

Monoclonal Antibodies in Renal Transplantation

Basiliximab (anti-IL-2 Receptor) in Renal Transplantation

Lancet. 1997 Oct 25;350(9086):1193–8.

Randomized trial of basiliximab versus placebo for control of acute cellular rejection in renal allograft recipients. CHIB 201 International Study Group.

Nashan B, Moore R, Amlot P, Schmidt AG, Abeywickrama K, Soulillou JP.

Abstract

Background: Currently available immunosuppressive regimens for cadaver kidney recipients are far from ideal because acute-rejection episodes occur in about 30–50 % of these patients. In the phase III study described here, we assessed the ability of basiliximab, a chimeric interleukin (IL)-2 receptor monoclonal antibody, to prevent acute-rejection episodes in renal allograft recipients.

Methods: Three hundred and eighty adult recipients of a primary cadaveric kidney transplant were randomly allocated, in this double-blind trial, to receive a 20 mg infusion of basiliximab on day 0 (day of surgery) and on day 4, to provide IL-2-receptor suppression for 4–6 week (n = 193), or to receive placebo (n = 187). Both group received baseline dual immunosuppressive therapy with cyclosporine and steroids throughout the study. The primary outcome measure was incidence of acute-rejection episodes during the 6 months after transplantation. Safety and tolerability were monitored over the 12 month of the study.

Findings: Three hundred and seventy-six patients were eligible for intention-to-treat analysis (basiliximab, n = 190 placebo, n = 186). No significant differences in patient characteristics were apparent. The incidence of biopsy-confirmed acute rejection 6 months after transplantation was 5 (29.8 %) of 171 in the basiliximab group compared with 7 (44.0 %) of 166 in the placebo group (32 % reduction 14.2 % difference [95 % Kaplan-Meier CIs 3–24 %] p = 0.012). The incidence of steroid-resistant first rejection episodes that required antibody therapy was significantly lower in the basiliximab group (10 % vs 23.1 %, 13.1 % difference [5.4–20.8 %], p < 0.001). At weeks 2 and 4 posttransplantation, the mean daily dose of steroids was significantly higher in the placebo group (p < 0.001 with one-way analysi of variance). The incidence of graft loss at 12 month posttransplantation was 23 (12.1 %) of 190 in the basilix imab group and 25 (13.4 %) of 186 in the placebo group (1.3 % difference [−5 to 9 %], p = 0.591). The incidence of infection and other adverse events was similar in the two treatment groups. The acute tolerability of basiliximab was excellent, with no evidence of cytokine-release syndrome Fourteen deaths (basiliximab n = 9; placebo n = 5; −2.0 % difference [−6 to 2 %], p = 0.293) occurred during the 12-month study and a further three deaths (basiliximab n = 1 placebo n = 2) occurred within the 380-day cutoff period One posttransplantation lymphoproliferative disorder was recorded in each group.

Interpretation: Prophylaxis with 40 mg basiliximab reduces the incidence of acute-rejection episodes significantly, with no clinically relevant safety or tolerability concerns.

Critical Appraisal

Parameters	Yes	No	Comment
Validity			
Is the **randomization** procedure well described?	+1		376 patients were eligible for intention-to-treat analysis (basiliximab, n = 190; placebo, n = 186).
			Basiliximab or placebo on a background of CyA + steroids-only therapy
Double **blinded**?	+2		

Parameters	Yes	No	Comment
Is the **sample size** calculation described/adequate?	+3		
Does it have a hard primary **endpoint**?		−1	The primary-efficacy assessment was a comparison of the proportion of patients in each group who experienced at least one acute-rejection episode during the first 6 months after transplantation, with follow-up data to 12 months. Biopsy-confirmed acute rejection was a secondary endpoint
Is the endpoint surrogate?	−2		
Is the follow-up appropriate?		−1	6 months, too short
Was there a **Bias**?		+2	
Is the dropout >25 %?		+1	
Is the analysis **ITT**?	+3		
Utility/usefulness			
Can the findings be generalized?	+1		European transplantation centers. As US practice often includes the addition of an ATG/ALG during induction
Was the NNT <100?	+1		
Score	62 %		

Comments and Discussion

The study showed clearly that the addition of basiliximab to baseline dual immunosuppression including CyA and steroids significantly decreased the number of rejection episodes and the number of BPAR including those that were steroids resistant. However, there was no difference in the severity of the AR episodes between the groups.

Graft and patient survival were comparable between the groups. Basiliximab was not associated with more side effects in the study's short observation period.

This study has some limitations:

1. Basiliximab was added to a dual therapy of CyA and steroids without the added benefit of an antimetabolite such as azathioprine, available at the time of the trial and considered a useful adjunct to dual therapy.
2. Basiliximab-enhanced induction was not compared to common practice in the USA of inclusion of an anti-lymphocyte or an antithymocyte globulin (ALG/ATG). In that respect, further studies (reviewed in [19]) and a systematic review showed no advantage of IL-2R

monoclonal antibodies over ATG in terms of graft and patient survival [20].

3. The use of the soft endpoint of acute rejection while showing a benefit does not always translate to improved graft function or survival at 12 months. Of relevance here is that basiliximab did not reduce the histological severity of BPAR, as severe AR may impact longer-term outcomes.

Conclusion

Compared with ATG (antithymocyte globulin), basiliximab, as with daclizumab, is generally associated with similar efficacy in standard/low-risk patients, but reduced efficacy in high-risk patients. It also appears to be less effective than alemtuzumab in low immunological risk patients [21]. Compared to other induction regimen, basiliximab has not demonstrated improved graft or patient survival over the long term. An advantage of basiliximab induction in low-risk patients is that it allows for reduced dosage of corticosteroids or calcineurin inhibitors, while maintaining adequate immunosuppression.

Alemtuzumab (Anti-CD52 Antibody) Induction in Renal Transplantation

Alemtuzumab was originally discovered by virtue of its ability to cause profound lymphodepletion, initially in rodents but later in humans. It is a humanized monoclonal IgG_1 antibody derived from rat antihuman CD52. It was originally used in renal transplantation by the Cambridge group who showed that in combination with cyclosporine monotherapy, it provided effective medium-term immunosuppression.

Interest intensified following the demonstration in animal models that profound lymphocyte depletion permitted the induction of tolerance and this prompted a number of trials in humans using alemtuzumab induction and then minimal single agent immunosuppression. However, these latter trials were blighted by unacceptably high acute-rejection rates in immunologically low-risk transplants (reviewed in [22]). However, a number of groups have demonstrated that alemtuzumab can be an effective induction agent if used as part of a more conventional multidrug regimen. Unfortunately, many of these studies were short term, underpowered, and very short term [22].

The INTAC Trial

N Engl J Med. 2011 May 19;364(20):1909–19. doi:10.1056/NEJMoa1009546.

Alemtuzumab induction in renal transplantation.

Hanaway MJ, Woodle ES, Mulgaonkar S, Peddi VR, Kaufman DB, First MR, Croy R, Holman J; INTAC Study Group.

Collaborators (28)

Abstract

Background: There are few comparisons of antibody induction therapy allowing early glucocorticoid withdrawal in renal-transplant recipients. The purpose of the present study was to compare induction therapy involving alemtuzumab with the most commonly used induction regimens in patient populations at either high immunological risk or low immunological risk.

Methods: In this prospective study, we randomly assigned patients to receive alemtuzumab or conventional induction therapy (basiliximab or rabbit antithymocyte globulin). Patients were stratified according to acute-rejection risk, with a high risk defined by a repeat transplant, a peak or current value of panel-reactive antibodies of 20 % or more, or black race. The 139 high-risk patients received alemtuzumab (one dose of 30 mg, in 70 patients) or rabbit antithymocyte globulin (a total of 6 mg per kilogram of body weight given over 4 days, in 69 patients). The 335 low-risk patients received alemtuzumab (one dose of 30 mg, in 164 patients) or basiliximab (a total of 40 mg over 4 days, in 171 patients). All patients received tacrolimus and mycophenolate mofetil and underwent a 5-day glucocorticoid taper in a regimen of early steroid withdrawal. The primary endpoint was biopsy-confirmed acute rejection at 6 and 12 months. Patients were followed for 3 years for safety and efficacy endpoints.

Results: The rate of biopsy-confirmed acute rejection was significantly lower in the alemtuzumab group than in the conventional-therapy group at both 6 months (3 % vs. 15 % $P < 0.001$) and 12 months (5 % vs. 17 %, $P < 0.001$). At 3 years the rate of biopsy-confirmed acute rejection in low-risk patients was lower with alemtuzumab than with basiliximab (10 % vs 22 %, $P = 0.003$), but among high-risk patients, no significant difference was seen between alemtuzumab and rabbit antithymocyte globulin (18 % vs. 15 %, $P = 0.63$). Adverse-event rates were similar among all four treatment groups.

Conclusions: By the first year after transplantation biopsy-confirmed acute rejection was less frequent with alemtuzumab than with conventional therapy. The apparent superiority of alemtuzumab with respect to early biopsy-confirmed acute rejection was restricted to patients at low risk for transplant rejection; among high-risk patients, alemtuzumab and rabbit antithymocyte globulin had similar efficacy. (Funded by Astellas Pharma Global Development INTAC ClinicalTrials.gov number, NCT00113269.)

Critical Appraisal

Parameters	Yes	No	Comment
Validity			
Is the **randomization** procedure well described?	+1		Block randomization was performed by the sponsor and concealed until intervention assignment
Double **blinded**?		−2	
Is the **sample size** calculation described/adequate?	+3		Assuming a difference of 9–11 percentage points in the rate of biopsy-confirmed acute rejection and a two-sided type I error rate of 5 %, the investigators calculated that a total sample of 500 patients would be needed to provide 85 % power to detect a significant difference between patients receiving alemtuzumab and patients receiving conventional therapy at months 6 and 12
Does it have a hard primary **endpoint**?		−1	The primary-efficacy endpoint was the rate of biopsy-confirmed acute rejection (defined as Banff grade I) at 6 and 12 months
Is the endpoint surrogate?	−2		
Is the follow-up appropriate?	+1		1 year for primary endpoint but 3 years for safety and other efficacy data
Was there a **Bias**?		+2	
Is the dropout >25 %?		+1	Not in low-risk arm but in high-risk arm
Is the analysis **ITT**?	+3		Analyses were performed on data from study patients who received at least one dose of tacrolimus and one dose of induction therapy
Utility/usefulness			
Can the findings be generalized?	+1		Yes but with caveats about the recruited population
Was the NNT <100?	N/A		
Score	**46 %**		

Comments and Discussion

The study clearly shows significantly lower rates of BPAR, in low immunological risk patients, treated with alemtuzumab compared to those treated with an anti-IL-2R. Lower incidence of BPAR correlated with the degree of lymphopenia induced by alemtuzumab; clearly, basiliximab, an anti-IL-2R antibody, did not deplete lymphocytes. Alemtuzumab had no advantage over ATG in high immunological risk patients. It was not compared to ATG in low-risk allograft recipients.

There were no significant differences in the hard endpoints of patient survival, graft function, or graft survival although these were not primary endpoints and the study was therefore not powered to detect differences.

The authors pointed out that lower acute-rejection rates in an earlier trial looking at induction with ATG versus basiliximab as induction agents after renal transplantation did translate into significantly better clinical outcomes after 5 years. Others might argue that the sort of mild acute cellular rejection that is prevented by alemtuzumab is not detrimental to long-term outcome. Only long-term follow-up of these patients can test this hypothesis.

In the meanwhile, a systematic review of 10 RCTs and 1,223 patients concluded that alemtuzumab induction reduces the risk of BPAR compared with IL-2RAs but not rATG. However, it reported that the incidence of other efficacy outcomes such as graft loss, DGF, and patient death was similar [23].

The INTAC study has limitations including:

1. No comparison was made with standard therapy in many US centers where ATG is an integral part of the standard induction protocol in cadaveric renal transplantation.
2. Criticisms of the study include those which can often be leveled at US studies, namely, the high proportion of living donors (60 % in the low risk, 40 % in the high-risk group) and poor HLA matching (c. 80 % patients ≥3 HLA antigen mismatch). The study also excluded all DCD kidneys and also DBD donors with extended criteria and those with cold ischemia times greater than 36 h.
3. Biopsy-proven acute rejection is a soft endpoint that does not necessarily inform long-term impact of therapies on graft and patient survival.
4. They also did describe the late occurrence of acute cellular rejection between 12 and 36 months, which was 8 % in the alemtuzumab arm versus 3 % in the basiliximab arm ($P=0.03$) in the low-risk patients. Although the incidence was low, there was no significant difference in the occurrence of more severe histological rejection and C4d-positive rejection rates were similar. This is in spite of expressions of concern by some of potential increased rate in the long run of antibody-mediated rejection (AMR) in patients treated initially with alemtuzumab [24]. A retrospective analysis of 1,687 adult renal transplants treated with either ATG, basiliximab or alemtuzumab, followed up for up to 5 years, revealed much worse graft survival in the alemtuzumab-treated patients possibly due to an increased rate of AMR and infectious complications [24].

Conclusion

This is a well-conducted study that demonstrates a lower risk of biopsy-proven acute cellular rejection in renal-transplant recipients induced with alemtuzumab compared to basiliximab. Alemtuzumab does not seem to confer any short-term advantage as far as graft and patient survivals are concerned. Concerns have been expressed in the long term about high incidence of infections and graft loss, due to increased rate of antibody-mediated rejection (AMR), in those treated by alemtuzumab [24].

Belatacept in Renal Transplantation

After kidney transplantation, maintenance immunosuppression mainly relies on calcineurin inhibitors (CNIs), which are thought to be nephrotoxic. However, since the SYMPHONY trial, it has been demonstrated that when the most potent CNI is used, i.e., tacrolimus, in a low-dose fashion and is aimed at trough levels of <7 ng/mL, it is almost non-nephrotoxic. Belatacept is a fusion protein that blocks the second signal within lymphocytes, whereas CNIs block the first signal, and so might be an alternative to the use of CNIs.

BENEFIT Trial

Am J Transplant. 2012 Jan;12(1):210–7. doi:10.1111/j.1600-6143.2011.03785.x. Epub 2011 Oct 12.

Three-year outcomes from BENEFIT, a randomized, active-controlled, parallel-group study in adult kidney-transplant recipients.

Vincenti F, Larsen CP, Alberu J, Bresnahan B, Garcia VD, Kothari J, Lang P, Urrea EM, Massari P, Mondragon-Ramirez G, Reyes-Acevedo R, Rice K, Rostaing L, Steinberg S, Xing J, Agarwal M, Harler MB, Charpentier B.

Abstract

The clinical profile of belatacept in kidney-transplant recipients was evaluated to determine if earlier results in the BENEFIT study were sustained at 3 years. BENEFIT is a randomized 3-year, phase III study in adults receiving a kidney transplant from a living-or standard-criteria deceased donor. Patients were randomized to a more (MI) or less intensive (LI) regimen of belatacept or cyclosporine. 471/666 patients completed ≥3 years of therapy. A total of 92 % (MI), 92 % (LI), and 89 % (cyclosporine) of patients survived with a functioning graft. The mean calculated GFR (cGFR) was ~21 mL/min/1.73 m(2) higher in the belatacept groups versus cyclosporine at year 3. From month 3 to month 36, the mean cGFR increased in the belatacept groups by +1.0 mL/min/1.73 m(2)/year (MI) and +1.2 mL/min/1.73 m(2)/year (LI) versus a decline of −2.0 mL/min/1.73 m(2)/year (cyclosporine). One cyclosporine-treated patient experienced acute rejection between year 2 and year 3. There were no new safety signals and no new posttransplant lymphoproliferative disorder (PTLD) cases after month 18. Belatacept-treated patients maintained a high rate of patient and graft survival that were comparable to cyclosporine-treated patients, despite an early increased occurrence of acute rejection and PTLD.

Critical Appraisal

Parameters	Yes	No	Comment
Validity			
Was the **randomization** procedure described well?	+1		The BENEFIT study (Belatacept Evaluation of Nephroprotection and Efficacy as First-line Immunosuppression Trial) was a 3-year, randomized, partially blinded, active-controlled, parallel-group study on adult patients. It included living-donor and deceased-donor kidney transplants that had an anticipated cold ischemia time of <24 h
Was the study **double blinded**?		−2	The study was partially blinded, i.e., only for the dose of belatacept
Was the **sample size** calculation described/adequate?	+3		
Did the study have a hard primary **endpoint**?	+1		The co-primary endpoints at 12 months were patient-/graft-survival rates, a composite renal-impairment endpoint (% of patients with a calculated glomerular filtration rate (cGFR) <60 mL/min/1.73 m^2 at month 12 or decreased mGFR of ≥10 mL/min/1.73 m^2 between months 3 and 12), or the incidence of an acute rejection
Was the endpoint surrogate?		0	
Was the follow-up period appropriate?	+1		This 3-year study had an appropriate follow-up period
Was there any **Bias**?	−2		Yes, in the way that the control arm, i.e., the calcineurin inhibitor (CNI) arm, relied on CsA and not on tacrolimus.
Was the dropout rate >25 %?	−1		A total of 666 patients ($n=219$ MI; $n=226$ LI; $n=221$ cyclosporine) were randomized and received a transplant. Of these, 471 (70.7 %) completed the 3 years of study therapy, i.e., 72 % of MIs, 75 % of LIs, and 67 % of CsA
Was the analysis **ITT**?	+3		
Utility/usefulness			
Can the findings be generalized?		−1	No, because the control arm relied on CsA, which is very rarely used nowadays. It has been replaced in daily practice by tacrolimus
Was the NNT <100?	N/A		Comparative drug regimen
Score	**20 %**		

Comments and Discussion

Cytotoxic T-lymphocyte-associated antigen 4 (CTLA4)-Ig is a fusion protein that is prepared as abatacept, which conserves the natural structure of CTLA4, and as belatacept, which has enhanced activity because of two amino acid substitutions. Abatacept and belatacept block the interaction between CD86 and CD28, but belatacept blocks this more powerfully [25]. Abatacept is approved for the treatment of rheumatoid arthritis and is marketed as Orencia(®) (Bristol-Myers Squibb, Princeton, NJ, USA), whereas belatacept is approved for maintenance immunosuppression in de novo kidney-transplant recipients and is marketed as Nulojix(®) (Bristol-Myers Squibb, Princeton, NJ, USA).

In the BENEFIT study, both belatacept regimens had similar patient-/graft-survival rates compared to cyclosporine and were associated with superior renal function, as measured by the composite renal-impairment endpoint and by cGFR. Patients receiving belatacept had a higher incidence and grade of acute-rejection episodes. Safety was generally similar between groups, but posttransplant lymphoproliferative disorders were more common in the belatacept groups [26].

Further analysis showed that the benefits to renal function and the safety profiles observed within the belatacept-treated groups in the early posttransplant period were sustained through 5 years [27].

The BENEFIT study had some limitations:

1. Unblinded to the investigator, thus generating the potential for observer bias.
2. But mostly, a patient's bias in the way that the control arm, i.e., the calcineurin inhibitor (CNI) arm, relied on CsA and not on tacrolimus. After kidney transplantation, the most preferred and most efficient CNI for both the short- and long-term periods has been shown to be tacrolimus (see results from the SYMPHONY trial [28]). Thus, the observed results in this BENEFIT trial with regard to the control arm may have been different had tacrolimus been used instead of CsA.
3. Changes in renal function may solely reflect the reversible and well-known hemodynamic effects of CNI on renal allografts and may therefore not represent a long-term graft or patient's survival advantage. This was also shown in another study when patients where switched from cyclosporine to belatacept [28].
4. The use of composite endpoint may somewhat diminish the clarity of the impact of belatacept as its functional benefit may be due to CNI avoidance.

Conclusion

The use of belatacept in renal transplantation has to be tempered by the fact that data is not available of any therapeutic advantage over currently used induction regimen including tacrolimus and the potential higher risk of malignancy, in particular PTLD, as well as the increased risk of infection, in particular tuberculosis. The effect on improved renal function may merely be the result of CNI avoidance or withdrawal.

BENEFIT-EXT Trial

Am J Transplant. 2012 Mar;12(3):630–9. doi:10.1111/j.1600-6143.2011.03914.x. Epub 2012 Feb 2.

Three-year outcomes from BENEFIT-EXT: a phase III study of belatacept versus cyclosporine in recipients of extended-criteria donor kidneys.

Pestana JO, Grinyo JM, Vanrenterghem Y, Becker T, Campistol JM, Florman S, Garcia VD, Kamar N, Lang P, Manfro RC, Massari P, Rial MD, Schnitzler MA, Vitko S, Duan T, Block A, Harler MB, Durrbach A.

Abstract

Recipients of extended-criteria donor (ECD) kidneys have poorer long-term outcomes compared to standard-criteria donor kidney recipients. We report 3-year outcomes from a randomized, phase III study in recipients of de novo ECD kidneys ($n = 543$) assigned (1:1:1) to either a more intensive (MI) or less intensive (LI) belatacept regimen or cyclosporine. Three hundred and twenty-three patients completed treatment by year 3. Patient survival with a functioning graft was comparable between groups (80 % in MI, 82 % in LI, 80 % in cyclosporine). Mean calculated GFR (cGFR) was 11 mL/min higher in belatacept-treated versus cyclosporine-treated patients (42.7 in MI, 42.2 in LI, 31.5 mL/min in cyclosporine). More cyclosporine-treated patients (44 %) progressed to GFR <30 mL/min (chronic kidney disease [CKD] stage 4/5) than belatacept-treated patients (27–30 %). Acute-rejection rates were similar between groups. Posttransplant lymphoproliferative disorder (PTLD) occurrence was higher in belatacept-treated patients (two in MI, three in LI), most of which occurred during the first 18 months; four additional cases (3 in LI, 1 in cyclosporine) occurred after 3 years. Tuberculosis was reported in two MI, four LI, and no cyclosporine patients. In conclusion, at 3 years after transplantation, immunosuppression with belatacept resulted in similar patient survival, graft survival, and acute rejection, with better renal function compared with cyclosporine. As previously reported, PTLD and tuberculosis were the principal safety findings associated with belatacept in this study population.

Critical Appraisal

Parameters	Yes	No	Comment
Validity			
Was the **randomization** procedure described well?	+1		BENEFIT-EXT (Belatacept Evaluation of Nephroprotection and Efficacy as First-line Immunosuppression Trial-EXTended-criteria donors) is a 3-year, phase III study that assessed a more (MI) or less intensive (LI) regimen of belatacept versus cyclosporine (CsA) in adult extended-criteria donor (ECD) kidney-transplant recipients. The ECD was either a donor aged ≥60 years or a donor aged 50–59 years with at least two other risk factors, i.e., a cardiovascular incident, hypertension, or terminal serum creatinine >1.5 mg/dL (UNOS definition), plus patients with an anticipated cold ischemia time of ≥24 h or donation after cardiac death
Was the study **double blinded**?		−2	It was partially blinded, i.e., only for the dose of belatacept
Was the **sample size** calculation described/adequate?	+3		
Did the study have a hard primary **endpoint**?	+1		The co-primary endpoints at 12 months were composite patient-/graft-survival rates and a composite renal-impairment endpoint
Was the endpoint surrogate?		0	
Was the follow-up period appropriate?	+1		This 3-year study had an appropriate follow-up period
Was there any **Bias**?		−2	Yes, in the way that the control arm, i.e., the calcineurin inhibitor (CNI) arm relied on CsA and not on tacrolimus long term after kidney transplantation. The most preferred and most efficient CNI in both the short- and long-term periods is tacrolimus (see results from the SYMPHONY trial). Thus, the observed results in this BENEFIT-EXT trial with regard to the control arm may have been different had tacrolimus been used instead of CsA
Was the dropout rate >25 %?		−1	A total of 543 randomly assigned patients received an ECD kidney transplant ($n = 184$ MI; $n = 175$ LI; $n = 184$ CsA). At 3 years posttransplant, 323 patients (59.5 %) remained within the study and receiving treatment
Was the analysis **ITT**?	+3		
Utility/usefulness			
Can the findings be generalized?		−1	No, because the control arm relied on CsA, which is used very rarely nowadays. It has been replaced in daily practice by tacrolimus
Was the NNT <100?	N/A		
Score	**20** %		

At month 12 posttransplant, patient-/graft-survival rates with belatacept were similar to those with CsA (86 % MI, 89 % LI, 85 % CsA). Fewer belatacept patients reached the endpoint of composite renal impairment versus the CsA group (71 % MI, 77 % LI, 85 % CsA; p=0.002 for MI vs. CsA; p=0.06 for LI vs. CsA). The mean measured glomerular filtration rate was 4–7 mL/min higher in the belatacept compared to the CsA group (p=0.008 for MI vs. CsA; p=0.1039 for LI vs. CsA), and the overall cardiovascular/metabolic profile was better in the belatacept group compared to the CsA group. The incidence of acute rejection was similar across all three groups (18 % MI, 18 % LI, 14 % CsA). Overall rates of infection and malignancy were similar between the groups; however, more cases of posttransplant lymphoproliferative disorder (PTLD) occurred in the central nervous system (CNS) within the belatacept group (Durrbach A et al., *Am J Transplant.* 2010 Mar; 10(3):547–57). At 3 years posttransplant, survival of patients with a functioning graft was comparable between groups (80 % in MI, 82 % in LI, 80 % in CsA). Mean calculated GFR (cGFR) was 11 mL/min higher in the belatacept-treated versus the CsA-treated group (42.7 in MI, 42.2 in LI, 31.5 mL/min in CsA). More patients treated with CsA (44 %) progressed to GFR <30 mL/min (chronic kidney disease stage 4/5) compared to belatacept-treated patients (27–30 %). Acute-rejection rates were similar between groups. PTLD occurred more frequently in belatacept-treated patients (two in MI, three in LI), with most occurring within the first 18 months; four additional cases (3 in LI, 1 in CsA) occurred after 3 years. Tuberculosis was reported in two MI, four LI, and no CsA patients.

Comments and Discussion

The two BENEFIT studies have clearly demonstrated that, in both the setting of standard donors (living or deceased) and extended-criteria donors, compared to cyclosporine, belatacept is associated in the long term (i.e., 5 years posttransplant) with significantly better renal function, which could be also translated into prolonged kidney half-life.

The BENEFIT-EXT study had the same limitations of BENEFIT, namely:

1. Unblinded to the investigator thus generating the potential for observer bias.
2. But mostly, a patient's bias in the way that the control arm, i.e., the calcineurin inhibitor (CNI) arm, relied on CsA and not on tacrolimus. After kidney transplantation, the most preferred and most efficient CNI for both the short- and long-term periods has been shown to be tacrolimus (see results from the SYMPHONY trial [29]. Thus, the observed results in this BENEFIT-EXT trial with regard to the control arm may have been different had tacrolimus been used instead of CsA.
3. Changes in renal function may solely reflect the reversible and well-known hemodynamic effects of CNI on renal

allografts and may therefore not represent a long-term graft or patient's survival advantage. This was also shown in another study when patients where switched from cyclosporine to belatacept [30].

4. The use of composite endpoint may somewhat diminish the clarity of the impact of belatacept as its functional benefit may be due to CNI avoidance, while the use of composite endpoint suggests patients' survival advantage.

Conclusion

The use of belatacept in renal transplantation has to be tempered by the fact that data is not available of any therapeutic advantage over currently used induction regimen including tacrolimus and the potential higher risk of malignancy, in particular PTLD, as well as the increased risk of infection, in particular tuberculosis. The effect on improved renal function may merely be the result of CNI avoidance or withdrawal.

Corticosteroid Withdrawal Study

Ann Surg. 2008 Oct;248(4):564–77.

A prospective, randomized, double-blind, placebo-controlled multicenter trial comparing early (7 day) corticosteroid cessation versus long-term, low-dose corticosteroid therapy.

Woodle ES, First MR, Pirsch J, Shihab F, Gaber AO, Van Veldhuisen P; Astellas Corticosteroid Withdrawal Study Group.

Collaborators (39)

Chan L, Stegall M, Stevens B, Bromberg J, Ojogho O, Washburn K, Gugliuzza K, Parasuraman R, Pankewycz O, Schweitzer E, Van der Werf W, Johnson C, Loss G, Francos G, Morrisey P, Mendez R, Shaffer D, Kapur S, Thistlethwaite R, Freeman R, Laskow D, Johnston T, Matas A, Hricik D, Abul-Ezz S, Alloway R, Moore LW, Nezakatgoo N, Gao J, Henning A, Lu L, Miller R, Holman J, Barge K, Fallon L, Reisfield R, Salm K, Tolzman D, Fitzsimmons W.

Abstract

Objective: To compare outcomes with early corticosteroid withdrawal (CSWD) and chronic low-dose corticosteroid therapy (CCS).

Summary Background Data: Final 5-year results from the first randomized, double-blind, placebo-controlled trial of early CSWD (at 7 days posttransplant) are presented.

Methods: Adult recipients of deceased- and living-donor kidney transplants without delayed graft function were randomized to receive prednisone (5 mg/day after 6 months posttransplant) or CSWD. Blinding was maintained for 5 years. This clinical trial is registered at www.clinicaltrials. gov (NCT00650468).

Results: Results in 386 patients CSWD ($n = 191$) and CCS ($n = 195$) are presented (CSWD; CCS). No differences were observed at 5 years in the proportion of patients experiencing primary endpoint (composite of death, graft loss, or moderate/severe acute rejection) (30/191 (15.7 %); 28/195 (14.4 %)), patient death (11/191(5.8 %);13/195 (6.7 %)), death-censored graft loss (11/191 (5.8 %); 7/195(3.6 %)), biopsy-confirmed acute rejection (BCAR) (34/191 (17.8 %); 21/195 (10.8 %), $P = 0.058$), and moderate/severe acute rejection (15/191 (7.9 %); 12/195 (6.2 %)). Kaplan-Meier analyses of the primary endpoint and its components also showed no differences; but BCAR was higher with CSWD ($P = 0.04$). Increased BCAR episodes were primarily corticosteroid-sensitive Banff 1A rejections: the incidence of antibody-treated BCAR was similar between groups (11/191 (5.8 %); 13/195 (6.7 %)). No differences in renal function were observed at 5 years: mean serum creatinine (1.5 ± 0.6;

1.5 ± 0.7 mg/dL) or Cockroft-Gault calculated creatinine clearance (58.6 ± 19.7; 59.8 ± 20.5 mL/min). CSWD was associated with improved serum triglycerides (evaluated by mean and median change from baseline) at all time points (except at 5 years measured by mean change). Weight change also demonstrated changes favoring CSWD (median change from baseline at 5 years: 5.1 vs. 7.7 kg, $P = 0.05$). New-onset diabetes after transplant (NODAT) was similar with respect to proportions who required treatment (23/107 (21.5 %)); 18/86 (20.9 %); however, fewer CSWD patients required insulin for NODAT at 5 years (4/107 (3.7 %)); 10/86 (11.6 %), $P = 0.049$). Changes in HgA1c values (from baseline) were lower in CSWD patients at all time points except 4 years.

Conclusions: Early CSWD, compared with CCS, is associated with an increase in BCAR primarily because of mild, Banff 1A, steroid-sensitive rejection, yet provides similar long-term renal allograft survival and function. CSWD provides improvements in cardiovascular risk factors (triglycerides, NODAT requiring insulin, weight gain). Tacrolimus/MMF/antibody induction therapy allows early CSWD with results comparable to long-term low-dose (5 mg/day) prednisone therapy.

Critical Appraisal

Parameters	Yes	No	Comment
Validity			
Is the **randomization** procedure described well?	+1		Patients were randomized in a 1:1 ratio according to being African-American or not and according to donor type (living vs. deceased)
Was the study **double blinded**?	+2		Over a 5-year period
Was the **sample size** calculation described/adequate?	+3		Assuming a rate of 10 % in the primary endpoint for the chronic corticosteroid therapy (CCS), 312 patients were required to detect a 10 % increase in the corticosteroid therapy withdrawal group (CSWD at 7 days posttransplant) to achieve an alpha error of 5 % (one-tailed) and a statistical power of 80 %
Did the study have a specific primary **endpoint**?	+1		Primary endpoint: death, graft loss, or moderate/severe acute rejection (Banff grades 95 ≥ 2B or 97 ≥ 2A) or acute rejection that required antilymphocyte antibodies
Was the endpoint surrogate?		0	
Was the follow-up appropriate?	+1		5 years
Was there any **Bias**?	−2		Mycophenolate mofetil exposure was significantly lower in the CSWD group from week 4 until year 3
Was the dropout rate >25 %?	−1		Blinded drug discontinuation of 35.1 % in the CSWD group vs. 37.4 % in the CSS group
Was the analysis **ITT**?	+3		
Utility/usefulness			
Can the findings be generalized?	+1		
Was the **NNT** < 100?	N/A		
Score	**60 %**		

Comments and Discussion

The above study concluded that in this selected population of kidney-transplant candidates (first transplant, non-sensitized patients, male, Caucasians), embarking on steroid-free immunosuppression resulted in very good long-term

graft survival and allograft function and avoided the side effects of steroids. Conversely, in the population at medium and high immunological risk, steroid-based therapy was preferable.

Whether or not steroid-avoidance protocols in the setting of kidney transplantation are appropriate is still debated within the era of powerful immunosuppression therapies based on tacrolimus and mycophenolate mofetil (MMF). A recent meta-analysis [31] reported that corticosteroid withdrawal (CSWD) protocols, as compared to corticosteroid maintenance protocols (CCS), resulted in the same long-term patient- and graft-survival rates, although there were significantly more episodes of acute rejection in the CSWD group, although with a marginal effect on allograft function.

Current ongoing trials are further investigating alternative immunosuppression induction protocols to accommodate CSWD, including the use of alemtuzumab (an anti-CD52 monoclonal antibody) [32].

The study has some limitations:

1. Mycophenolate mofetil exposure was significantly lower in the CSWD group from week 4 until year 3, thus potentially generating a bias against the CSWD group.
2. Beneficial effects on secondary endpoints such as cardiovascular complications are at best hypothesis generating and should not be considered conclusive as the study was not powered to detect them.

Conclusion

While there is little doubt that long-term steroid treatment is associated with numerous complications and cessation of treatment is preferable when possible, the impact of complete corticosteroid withdrawal protocols and the timing of such intervention remain to be clarified in renal allograft recipients.

Transplantation Complications

DIRECT Study

Am J Transplant. 2007 Jun;7(6):1506–14. Epub 2007 Mar 12.

Results of an international, randomized trial comparing glucose metabolism disorders and outcome with cyclosporine versus tacrolimus.

Vincenti F, Friman S, Scheuermann E, Rostaing L, Jenssen T, Campistol JM, Uchida K, Pescovitz MD, Marchetti P, Tuncer M, Citterio F, Wiecek A, Chadban S, El-Shahawy M, Budde K, Goto N; DIRECT (Diabetes Incidence after Renal Transplantation: Neoral C Monitoring Versus tacrolimus) Investigators.

Abstract

DIRECT (Diabetes Incidence after Renal Transplantation: Neoral C(2) Monitoring Versus tacrolimus) was a 6-month, open-label, randomized, multicenter study which used American Diabetes Association/World Health Organization criteria to define glucose abnormalities. De novo renal-transplant patients were randomized to cyclosporine microemulsion (CsA-ME, using C(2) monitoring) or tacrolimus, with mycophenolic acid, steroids, and basiliximab. The intent-to-treat population comprised 682 patients (336 CsA-ME, 346 tacrolimus): 567 were nondiabetic at baseline. Demographics, diabetes risk factors, and steroid doses were similar between treatment groups. The primary-safety endpoint, new-onset diabetes after transplant (NODAT) or impaired fasting glucose (IFG) at 6 months, occurred in 73 CsA-ME patients (26.0 %) and 96 tacrolimus patients (33.6 %, $p = 0.046$). The primary-efficacy endpoint, biopsy-proven acute rejection, and graft loss or death at 6 months occurred in 43 CsA-ME patients (12.8 %) and 34 tacrolimus patients (9.8 %, $p = 0.211$). Mean glomerular filtration rate (Cockcroft-Gault) was 63.6 ± 20.7 mL/min/1.73 m(2) in the CsA-ME cohort and 65.9 ± 23.1 mL/min/1.73 m(2) with tacrolimus ($p = 0.285$); mean serum creatinine was 139 ± 58 and 133 ± 57 mumol/L, respectively ($p = 0.005$). Blood pressure was similar between treatment groups at month 6, but total cholesterol, LDL cholesterol, and triglyceride levels were significantly higher with CsA than with tacrolimus (total cholesterol:HDL remained unchanged). The profile and incidence of adverse events were similar between treatments. The incidence of NODAT or IFG at 6 months posttransplant is significantly lower with CsA-ME than with tacrolimus without a significant difference in short-term outcome.

Critical Appraisal

Parameters	Yes	No	Comment
Validity			
Was the **randomization** procedure described well?	+1		The DIRECT study was a 6-month, open-label, randomized, multicenter study on de novo kidney-transplant recipients. Adult recipients of a first or second renal transplant from a deceased, living-related, or living-unrelated donor were randomized in a 1:1 ratio to receive either cyclosporine as a microemulsion or tacrolimus
Was the study **double blinded**?		−2	
Was the **sample size** calculation described/adequate?	+3		A sequentially ordered testing strategy was defined a priori such that the primary-safety endpoint (NODAT or IFG) was tested first. Because the result was statistically significant, the primary-efficacy endpoint was also tested in a confirmative way without further adjustment of the significance level. The primary-safety analysis was based on a superiority null hypothesis and the primary-efficacy analysis was based on a non-inferiority null hypothesis, whereby cyclosporine microemulsion was inferred as being non-inferior to tacrolimus if the upper limit of the 95 % confidence interval for the difference observed was less than the non-inferiority margin of 10 %

Parameters	Yes	No	Comment
Did the study have a hard primary **endpoint**?	+1		There were two primary endpoints. The primary-safety endpoint was a composite of new-onset diabetes after transplant (NODAT) or IFG (impaired fasting glucose) within the first 6 months posttransplantation among patients classified as nondiabetic at the time of transplantation.
			The primary-efficacy endpoint was a composite of biopsy-proven acute rejection and graft loss or death at 6 months posttransplant for all patients
Was the endpoint surrogate?		0	
Was the follow-up period appropriate?		−1	The 6-month follow-up period was too short. In such a study, a 1-year period should be a minimum
Was there any **Bias**?		−2	Open-label and unblinding generate the potential for an observer bias
Was the dropout rate >25 %?		−1	In the cyclosporine microemulsion arm, 21 % of patients discontinued therapy, whereas only 11 % discontinued within the tacrolimus arm
Was the analysis **ITT**?	+1		
Utility/usefulness			
Can the findings be generalized?	+1		
Was the **NNT** < 100?	N/A		Comparative study between different drug regimens
Score	**6 %**		

Comments and Discussion

The conclusion of this randomized controlled study is that the incidence of NODAT or IFG in de novo kidney-transplant recipients at 6 months posttransplant was significantly lower in those that received cyclosporine microemulsion compared to tacrolimus, but there were no significant differences in short-term outcomes, e.g., BPAR and kidney-allograft function.

Since the DIRECT study, the NODAT-inducing effect of tacrolimus has been confirmed in a number of studies [33], with suggestions of increased susceptibility in patients with preoperative high FPG level, age, high body mass index, hepatitis C virus infection, and recipients of cadaveric donor kidney [34].

Other longer-term studies showed a therapeutic advantage of tacrolimus over Cyclosporine in relation to BPAR and allograft survival [35].

The study has some limitations:

1. It is open label and unblinded, thus potentially generating observer/investigator's bias.
2. The 6-month follow-up period was too short. In such a study, a 1-year period should be a minimum.
3. Composite endpoints such as death and graft loss along with BCAR raise concern in view of the difference weighting and likelihood of these events, especially over a 6-month period [36].

Conclusion

The study has highlighted the potential higher diabetogenic effect of tacrolimus compared to cyclosporine.

IMPACT (Improved Protection Against CMV in Transplantation) Study

Transplantation. 2010 Dec 27;90(12):1427–31.

Extended valganciclovir prophylaxis in D+/R− kidney-transplant recipients is associated with long-term reduction in cytomegalovirus disease: Two-year results of the IMPACT study.

Humar A, Limaye AP, Blumberg EA, Hauser IA, Vincenti F, Jardine AG, Abramowicz D, Ives JA, Farhan M, Peeters P.

Abstract

Background: Whether the early reduction in cytomegalovirus (CMV) disease seen at 1 year with prolongation of antiviral prophylaxis (up to 200 days) persists in the long term is unknown.

Methods: This international, randomized, prospective, double-blind study compared 318 CMV D+/R− kidney-transplant recipients receiving valganciclovir (900 mg) once daily for up to 200 days vs. 100 days. Long-term outcomes including CMV disease, acute rejection, graft loss, patient survival, and seroconversion were assessed.

Results: At 2 years posttransplant, CMV disease occurred in significantly less patients in the 200- vs. the 100-day group: 21.3 % vs. 38.7 %, respectively ($P < 0.001$). Between year 1 and 2, there were only 10 new cases of CMV disease; 7 in the 200-day group and 3 in the 100-day group. Patient survival was 100 % in the 200-day group and 97 % in the 100-day group ($p =$ not significant). Biopsy-proven acute-rejection and graft loss rates were comparable in both groups (11.6 % vs. 17.2 %, $P = 0.16$, and 1.9 % vs. 4.3 %, $P = 0.22$, in the 200-day vs. 100-day groups, respectively). Seroconversion was delayed in the 200-day group but was similar to the 100-day group by 2 years post-transplant (IgM or IgG seroconversion; 55.5 % in the 200-day group vs. 62.0 % in the 100-day group at 2 years;

$P=0.26$). Assessment of seroconversion at the end of prophylaxis was of limited utility for predicting late-onset CMV disease.

Conclusion: Extending valganciclovir prophylaxis from 100 to 200 days is associated with a sustained reduction in CMV disease up to 2 years posttransplant.

Critical Appraisal

Parameters	Yes	No	Comment
Validity			
Was the **randomization** procedure described well?	+1		There was 1:1 randomization to receive valganciclovir 900 mg daily either for 200 days or for 100 days followed by 100 days of a placebo.
			318 patients were randomized to receive either 100 days of valganciclovir prophylaxis ($n=163$) or 200 days of valganciclovir prophylaxis ($n=155$)
Was the study **double blinded**?	+2		
Was the **sample size** calculation described/adequate?	+3		A two-group continuity-corrected chi-square test with a 0.05 two-sided significance level had 80 % power to detect a difference between the two groups if the CMV disease rate in the 200-day valganciclovir prophylaxis groups was 15 % and that in the 100-day valganciclovir prophylaxis group was 30 % (odds ratio 0.412) if the sample size in each group was 134 patients. Assuming a premature termination rate of ~15 %, 158 patients per arm would be required to ensure 134 patients per arm completed the full course of treatment plus a 52-week follow-up or reached the primary endpoint
Did the study have a hard primary **endpoint**?	+1		The primary-efficacy parameter was the proportion of D+/R− patients who developed CMV disease (CMV syndrome or tissue-invasive CMV) within the first 52 weeks. CMV syndrome was defined by CMV viremia plus at least one of the following: a fever, new-onset severe malaise, leukopenia, atypical lymphocytosis, thrombocytopenia, or elevated hepatic transaminase. Tissue-invasive CMV was defined as evidence of localized CMV infection in a biopsy plus symptoms of organ dysfunction. This definition of CMV disease is consistent with current international consensus guidelines for CMV
Was the endpoint surrogate?		0	
Was the follow-up period appropriate?		−1	A 2-year follow-up is an ideal time period, although follow-up was shorter (by 100 days) in the longer vangancyclovir treatment group
Was there any **Bias**?	−2		Different follow-up duration between the two groups
Was the dropout rate >25 %?		+1	21.1 % of patients in the 200-day arm and 42.7 % in the 100-day arm withdrew from treatment
Was the analysis **ITT**?	+3		
Utility/usefulness			
Can the findings be generalized?	+1		
Was the **NNT** < 100?	+1		The number of patients that needed to be treated (NNT) with extended valganciclovir prophylaxis (for up to 2 years posttransplant) to prevent one additional patient developing CMV disease (compared to 100 days of prophylaxis) was 5.7
Score	**62 %**		

Comments and Discussion

The 1-year results of the IMPACT study have been already published showing a prophylaxis advantage of longer valganciclovir treatment (200 days) over shorter prophylaxis (9,100 days) [37].

The above multicenter, double-blind, randomized, controlled trial compared the efficacy and safety of 200 days versus 100 days of valganciclovir prophylaxis (900 mg once daily) given to 326 high-risk (D+/R−) kidney-allograft recipients. Significantly fewer patients in the 200-day group versus the 100-day group developed confirmed CMV disease posttransplant. No difference in patients' survival was noted.

The conclusion of this study is that extending valganciclovir prophylaxis (900 mg once daily) to 200 days significantly reduced the development of CMV disease and viremia until at least 24 months when compared to 100 days of prophylaxis. In addition, the 200-day treatment had no significant additional safety concerns.

The IMPACT study has some limitations:

1. The difference in follow-up time between the groups may account for some of the differences in CMV infection/viremia rates.

2. Comparison between long-term prophylaxis versus closer CMV PCR monitoring has not been undertaken, to fully justify long-term treatment of valganciclovir.
3. A pharmacoeconomics evaluation of long- versus short-term prophylaxis has not been conducted; this is of particular relevance to emerging low- and middle-economy countries where the cost of long-term prophylaxis may reduce its cost-effectiveness.

Conclusion

Long-term ganciclovir prophylaxis may offer a long-term advantage in significantly reducing the incidence of serious CMV infections in renal allograft recipients.

Machine Perfusion or Cold Storage in Deceased-Donor Kidney Transplantation

N Engl J Med. 2009 Jan 1;360(1):7–19. doi:10.1056/NEJMoa0802289.

Machine perfusion or cold storage in deceased-donor kidney transplantation.

Moers C, Smits JM, Maathuis MH, Treckmann J, van Gelder F, Napieralski BP, van Kasterop-Kutz M, van der Heide JJ, Squifflet JP, van Heurn E, Kirste GR, Rahmel A, Leuvenink HG, Paul A, Pirenne J, Ploeg RJ.

Abstract

Background: Static cold storage is generally used to preserve kidney allografts from deceased donors. Hypothermic machine perfusion may improve outcomes after transplantation, but few sufficiently powered prospective studies have addressed this possibility.

Methods: In this international randomized, controlled trial, we randomly assigned one kidney from 336 consecutive deceased donors to machine perfusion and the other to cold storage. All 672 recipients were followed for 1 year. The primary endpoint was delayed graft function (requiring dialysis in the first week after transplantation). Secondary endpoints were the duration of delayed graft function, delayed graft function defined by the rate of the decrease in the serum creatinine level, primary nonfunction, the serum creatinine level and clearance, acute rejection, toxicity of the calcineurin inhibitor, the length of hospital stay, and allograft and patient survival.

Results: Machine perfusion significantly reduced the risk of delayed graft function. Delayed graft function developed in 70 patients in the machine-perfusion group versus 89 in the cold-storage group (adjusted odds ratio, 0.57; $P=0.01$). Machine perfusion also significantly improved the rate of the decrease in the serum creatinine level and reduced the duration of delayed graft function. Machine perfusion was associated with lower serum creatinine levels during the first 2 weeks after transplantation and a reduced risk of graft failure (hazard ratio, 0.52; $P=0.03$). One-year allograft survival was superior in the machine-perfusion group (94 % vs. 90 %, $P=0.04$). No significant differences were observed for the other secondary endpoints. No serious adverse events were directly attributable to machine perfusion.

Conclusions: Hypothermic machine perfusion was associated with a reduced risk of delayed graft function and improved graft survival in the first year after transplantation. (Current Controlled Trials number, ISRCTN83876362.)

Critical Appraisal

Parameters	Yes	No	Comment
Validity			
Is the **randomization** procedure well described?	+1		A randomization scheme based on permuted blocks within regions was used with separate randomization lists for each trial region
Double **blinded**?			Not applicable
Is the **sample size** calculation described/adequate?	+3		This study was powered to detect a reduction in delayed graft function of at least 10 %, based on a presumed incidence of 35 % among recipients of kidneys that had been preserved by means of cold storage. With a statistical power of 0.8 and a one-sided type I error of 0.05, the minimum required sample size was 300 kidney pairs.
			336 kidney pairs were used.
Does it have a hard primary **endpoint**?		−1	The primary analysis of the primary endpoint – delayed graft function requiring dialysis during the first posttransplant week
			Secondary endpoints were the duration of delayed graft function, delayed graft function defined by the rate of the decrease in the serum creatinine level, primary nonfunction, the serum creatinine level and clearance, acute rejection, toxicity of the calcineurin inhibitor, the length of hospital stay, and allograft and patient survival

Parameters	Yes	No	Comment
Is the endpoint surrogate?	−2		
Is the follow-up appropriate?	+1		
Was there a **Bias**?	+2	+2	
Is the dropout >25 %?		+1	
Is the analysis **ITT**?	+3		
Utility/usefulness			
Can the findings be generalized?	+1		To allografts from deceased donors
Was the NNT <100?			
Score	**60 %**		

Comments and Discussion

This study showed the advantage of hypothermic machine perfusion of renal allografts compared to cold storage in terms of decreased incidence of delayed graft function (DGF).

There were no significant differences between the study groups in creatinine clearance at 14 days after transplantation, length of hospital stay of recipients, the incidence of toxicity of the calcineurin inhibitor, and acute-rejection rate in the first 14 days. However, 1-year graft survival was higher in the machine-perfusion group than in the cold-storage group (94 % vs. 90 %, $P=0.04$), a finding difficult to explain in view of the comparable renal function of the two groups at 14 days. Of relevance, it is surprising that such RCT did not report on the impact of decreased DGF on the incidence of acute cellular rejection.

Also, the study takes little count of modulation of immunosuppression to prevent DGF in those considered at higher risk (older donor kidneys, longer cold ischemia time, etc.). However, it is apparent that most confounders were equally distributed between the two groups; this may suggest comparable exposure to potentially nephrotoxic agents such as CNI.

Conclusion

Hypothermic machine perfusion of cadaveric renal allografts seems to confer some advantage over conventional cold storage. Whether this translates in the long term in better patients and graft survival warrants confirmation.

TUMORAPA Study

N Engl J Med. 2012 Jul 26;367(4):329–39. doi:10.1056/ NEJMoa1204166.

Sirolimus and secondary skin cancer prevention in kidney transplantation.

Euvrard S, Morelon E, Rostaing L, Goffin E, Brocard A, Tromme I, Broeders N, del Marmol V, Chatelet V, Dompmartin A, Kessler M, Serra AL, Hofbauer GF, Pouteil-Noble C, Campistol JM, Kanitakis J, Roux AS, Decullier E Dantal J; TUMORAPA Study Group.
Collaborators (59)

Abstract

Background: Transplant recipients in whom cutaneous squamous cell carcinomas develop are at high risk for multiple subsequent skin cancers. Whether sirolimus is useful in the prevention of secondary skin cancer has not been assessed.

Methods: In this multicenter trial, we randomly assigned transplant recipients who were taking calcineurin inhibitors and had at least one cutaneous squamous cell carcinoma either to receive sirolimus as a substitute for calcineurin inhibitors (in 64 patients) or to maintain their initial treatment (in 56). The primary endpoint was survival-free of squamous cell carcinoma at 2 years. Secondary endpoints included the time until the onset of new squamous cell carcinomas, occurrence of other skin tumors, graft function, and problems with sirolimus.

Results: Survival-free of cutaneous squamous cell carcinoma was significantly longer in the sirolimus group than in the calcineurin inhibitor group. Overall, new squamous cell carcinomas developed in 14 patients (22 %) in the sirolimus group (6 after withdrawal of sirolimus) and in 22 (39 %) in the calcineurin inhibitor group (median time until onset, 15 vs. 7 months; $P=0.02$), with a relative risk in the sirolimus group of 0.56 (95 % confidence interval, 0.32–0.98). There were 60 serious adverse events in the sirolimus group, as compared with 14 such events in the calcineurin inhibitor group (average, 0.938 vs. 0.250). There were twice as many serious adverse events in patients who had been converted to sirolimus with rapid protocols as in those with progressive protocols. In the sirolimus group, 23 % of patients discontinued the drug because of adverse events. Graft function remained stable in the two study groups.

Conclusions: Switching from calcineurin inhibitors to sirolimus had an antitumoral effect among kidney-transplant recipients with previous squamous cell carcinoma. These observations may have implications concerning immunosuppressive treatment of patients with cutaneous squamous cell carcinomas. (Funded by Hospices Civils de Lyon and others; TUMORAPA ClinicalTrials.gov number, NCT00133887.)

Critical Appraisal

Parameters	Yes	No	Comment
Validity			
Is the **randomization** procedure well described?	+1		
Double **blinded**?		−2	
Is the **sample size** calculation described/adequate?		−3	Pooling data of two studies
			No calculation of sample size
Does it have a hard primary **endpoint**?	+1		Survival-free of new SCC at 2 years
Is the endpoint surrogate?		0	
Is the follow-up appropriate?	+1		
Was there a **Bias**?		+2	
Is the dropout >25 %?		+1	23 % in the sirolimus group
Is the analysis **ITT**?	+3		
Utility/usefulness			
Can the findings be generalized?	+1		
Was the NNT <100?	N/A		
Score	**31** %		

Comments and Discussion

Skin cancer is the most prevalent solid cancer after organ transplantation, particularly after kidney transplantation. This can be either basal cell carcinoma or squamous cell carcinoma (SCC) [38]. In the setting of organ transplantation, both BCC and SCC can metastasize. In addition, the prevalence of skin cancers after kidney transplantation increased as compared to the dialysis treatment period. This increase is related to the potency of chronic immunosuppression.

For the first time, it has been shown that after an SCC has occurred in a kidney-transplant patient on calcineurin-inhibitor (CNI)-based immunosuppression, the modification of immunosuppressive from CNI to sirolimus-based immunosuppression was able to significantly decrease the recurrence of SCC. Sirolimus belongs to the m-TOR inhibitors family which has the potential of antineoplastic effects. This was demonstrated in this study.

Moreover, in another randomized, controlled study in maintenance kidney-transplant patients presenting with chronic allograft dysfunction and in whom CNI was replaced by sirolimus, 2 years later, there were significantly less de novo skin cancers in those that had been converted to sirolimus [39].

The TUMORAPA study has some limitations:

1. It was unblinded and raised concern about potential observer bias.
2. It is the pooled analysis of two studies, raising concern about the heterogeneity of the patients studied and the power of the study.
3. The study protocol does not allow to determine whether it is the discontinuation of the CNI or the specific antiproliferative, and weaker immunosuppressive, effects of sirolimus that confer benefit.

4. The power of the study and sample size is small thus raising concern about the possibility of a statistical bias and type1 (alpha), false positive, error.

Conclusion

There is growing evidence that CNI-based immunosuppression withdrawal and/or rapamycin addition (sirolimus) has the capacity for primary and secondary prevention of skin cancers in renal allograft recipients.

General Discussion

Renal transplantation is most probably an area of nephrology where most advances have taken place over the last quarter of a century. Also, it is probably the field of nephrology where the largest number of RCT has taken place. Many of these have been discussed above and raise a number of issues:

1. How to evaluate drug/immunosuppressive regimen superiority, initially for induction therapy. It is clear from the many RCTs reviewed in this chapter that the success and superiority of most new regimens have initially relied on the incidence of acute rejection as primary endpoint, mostly biopsy-confirmed acute rejection (BCAR). In that respect, very few have bothered to define the type of acute rejection or its severity based on Banff criteria. Clearly, not all acute rejection have the same clinical significance or prognosis in terms of renal dysfunction and ultimately graft loss.

2. Estimated GFR has been used to evaluate renal dysfunction in many instances, in spite of the absence of

validation of this parameter in renal transplantation, especially in the follow-up of renal functional trajectories after renal transplantation. GFR is never measured, in spite of the risk of confounders such as illness, rejection, and steroid therapy on serum creatinine estimation and derived estimated GFR.

3. Very few studies have published hard primary endpoints such as graft and/or patient survival. When published, this has been over too short an observation time such as 12 months or in a post hoc fashion when the rigor of the RCT follow-up no longer apply.

4. Few, if any, studies focused on a given and well-defined group of allograft recipients. Published literature emanates mostly from high-economy countries, USA/Canada, EU, and Australasia, where cadaveric renal transplantation has been the most prevalent for therapy. Very few large RCT address issues related to living-related transplantation, the most prevalent modality in low and middle economies.

5. Few trials have distinguished and stratified for low- and high-risk allograft recipients, choosing instead to include all comers thus confounding outcomes and response to treatment.

6. The best comparator has not always been chosen, raising concern of bias from the investigators or sponsors.

Recommendations

It would be advisable that future RCTs in renal transplantation have:

1. Hard and well-defined endpoints, with an appropriate follow-up to establish their therapeutic worth. Surrogate endpoints such as changes in serum creatinine, eGFR, or BCAR are at best hypothesis generating but not conclusive of intervention true value in terms of long-term graft or patient survival.

2. Focus on well-defined allograft recipient populations may help addressing more specific questions including the management of those at higher risk of rejection, graft and patient loss, as well as complications such as CVD, infections, and cancer.

3. Focus of chronic allograft loss. While huge progress has been made in the short (1–3 years) graft survival in recent years, the field is marred by the chronic and relentless loss of most allograft after 5 years. This needs to be addressed with protocols aimed at optimization of maintenance immunosuppression therapies.

References

1. Nankivell BJ, Borrows RJ, Fung CL, et al. Calcineurin inhibitor nephrotoxicity: longitudinal assessment by protocol histology. Transplant. 2004;27;78(4):557–65.

2. Loupy A, Lefaucheur C, Vernerey D, et al. Complement-binding anti-HLA antibodies and kidney-allograft survival. N Engl J Med 2013;369(13):1215–26.

3. Hirai T, Furusawa M, Omoto K, Ishida H, Tanabe K. Analysis of Predictive and Preventive Factors for De Novo DSA in Kidney Transplant Recipients. Transplantation. 2014 Apr 7. [Epub ahead of print].

4. Stegall MD, Chedid MF, Cornell LD. The role of complement in antibody-mediated rejection in kidney transplantation. Nat Rev Nephrol. 2012;8(11):670–8.

5. Hirsch HH, Brennan DC, Drachenberg CB, et al. Polyomavirus-associated nephropathy in renal transplantation: interdisciplinary analyses and recommendations. Transplantation. 2005;79(10):1277–86.

6. Suwelack B, Malyar V, Koch M, Sester M, Sommerer C. The influence of immunosuppressive agents on BK virus risk following kidney transplantation, and implications for choice of regimen. Transplant Rev (Orlando). 2012;26(3):201–11.

7. Dantal J, Pohanka E. Malignancies in renal transplantation: an unmet medical need. Nephrol Dial Transplant. 2007 May;22 Suppl 1:i4–10.

8. Borel JF. Comparative study of in vitro and in vivo drug effect on cell-mediated cytotoxicity. Immunology. 1976;31:631–41.

9. Calne RY, Rolles K, White DJ, Thiru S, Evans DB, McMaster P, Dunn DC, Craddock GN, Henderson RG, Aziz S, Lewis P. Cyclosporin A initially as the only immunosuppressant in 34 recipients of cadaveric organs: 32 kidneys, 2 pancreases, and 2 livers. Lancet. 1979;2(8151):1033–6.

10. Cyclosporin in cadaveric renal transplantation: one-year follow-up of a multicenter trial. Lancet. 1983;2(8357):986–9.

11. Murase N, Starzl TE, Demetris AJ, Valdivia L, Tanabe M, Cramer D, Makowka L. Hamster-to-rat heart and liver xenotransplantation with FK506 plus antiproliferative drugs. Transplantation. 1993;55(4): 701–7; discussion 707–8.

12. Mayer AD, Dmitrewski J, Squifflet JP, et al. Multicenter randomized trial comparing tacrolimus (FK506) and cyclosporine in the prevention of renal allograft rejection: a report of the European Tacrolimus Multicenter Renal Study Group. Transplantation. 1997;64:436–43.

13. Pirsch JD, Miller J, Deierhoi MH, Vincenti F, Filo RS. A comparison of tacrolimus (FK506) and cyclosporine for immunosuppression after cadaveric renal transplantation. FK506 Kidney Transplant Study Group. Transplantation. 1997;63(7):977–83.

14. Vincenti F, Jensik SC, Filo RS, Miller J, Pirsch J. A long-term comparison of tacrolimus (FK506) and cyclosporine in kidney transplantation: evidence for improved allograft survival at five years. Transplantation. 2002;73(5):775–82.

15. Webster A, Woodroffe RC, Taylor RS, Chapman JR, Craig JC. Tacrolimus versus cyclosporine as primary immunosuppression for kidney transplant recipients. Cochrane Database Syst Rev. 2005;(4):CD003961.

16. Sollinger HW. Mycophenolate mofetil for the prevention of acute rejection in primary cadaveric renal allograft recipients. US Renal Transplant Mycophenolate Mofetil Study Group. Transplantation. 1995;60(3):225–32.

17. Knight SR, Russell NK, Barcena L, Morris PJ. Mycophenolate mofetil decreases acute rejection and may improve graft survival in renal transplant recipients when compared with azathioprine: a systematic review. Transplantation. 2009;87(6):785–94.

18. Webster AC, Woodroffe RC, Taylor RS, Chapman JR, Craig JC. Tacrolimus versus cyclosporine as primary immunosuppression for kidney transplant recipients: meta-analysis and meta-regression of randomized trial data. BMJ. 2005;331(7520):810.

19. Boggi U, Danesi R, Vistoli F, et al. A benefit-risk assessment of basiliximab in renal transplantation. Drug Saf. 2004;27:91–106.

20. Hao WJ, Zong HT, Cui YS, Zhang Y. The efficacy and safety of alemtuzumab and daclizumab versus antithymocyte globulin during organ transplantation: a meta-analysis. Transplant Proc. 2012;44(10):2955–60.

21. Hanaway MJ, Woodle ES, Mulgaonkar S, et al. Alemtuzumab induction in renal transplantation. N Engl J Med. 2011;364:1909–19.

22. Cianco G, Burke 3rd GW. Alemtuzumab (Campath-1H) in kidney transplantation. Am J Transplant. 2008;8:15–20.

23. Morgan RD, O'Callaghan JM, Knight SR, Morris PJ. Alemtuzumab induction therapy in kidney transplantation. Transplantation. 2012;93:1179–88.

24. LaMattina JC, Mezrich JD, Hofmann RM, et al. Alemtuzumab as compared to alternative contemporary induction regimens. Transpl Int. 2012;25:518–26.

25. Kirk AD, Tadaki DK, Celniker A, et al. Induction therapy with monoclonal antibodies specific for CD80 and CD86 delays the onset of acute renal allograft rejection in non-human primates. Transplantation. 2001;72(3):377–84.

26. Vincenti F, Charpentier B, Vanrenterghem Y, et al. A phase III study of belatacept-based immunosuppression regimens versus cyclosporine in renal transplant recipients (BENEFIT study). Am J Transplant. 2010;10(3):535–46. doi:10.1111/j.1600-6143.2009.03005.x.

27. Rostaing L, Vincenti F, Grinyó J, et al. Long-term belatacept exposure maintains efficacy and safety at 5 years: results from the long-term extension of the BENEFIT study. Am J Transplant. 2013;13(11):2875–83. doi:10.1111/ajt.12460. Epub 2013 Sep 18.

28. Rostaing L, Massari P, Garcia VD, Mancilla-Urrea E, Nainan G, del Carmen Rial M, Steinberg S, Vincenti F, Shi R, Di Russo G, Thomas D, Grinyó J. Clin J Am Soc Nephrol. 2011;6(2):430–9.

29. Ekberg H, Tedesco-Silva H, Demirbas A, Vítko S, Nashan B, Gürkan A, Margreiter R, Hugo C, Grinyó JM, Frei U, Vanrenterghem Y, Daloze P, Halloran PF, ELITE-Symphony Study. N Engl J Med. 2007;357(25):2562–75.

30. Rostaing L, Massari P, Garcia VD, Mancilla-Urrea E, Nainan G, del Carmen Rial M, Steinberg S, Vincenti F, Shi R, Di Russo G, Thomas D, Grinyó J. Clin J Am Soc Nephrol. 2011;6(2):430–9.

31. Knight SR, Morris PJ. Steroid avoidance or withdrawal after renal transplantation increases the risk of acute rejection but decreases cardiovascular risk. A meta-analysis. Transplantation. 2010;89(1):1–14. doi:10.1097/TP.0b013e3181c518cc.

32. Supe-Markovina K, Melquist JJ, Connolly D, DiCarlo HN, Waltzer WC, Fine RN, Darras FS. Alemtuzumab with corticosteroid minimization for pediatric deceased donor renal transplantation: a seven-yr experience. Pediatr Transplant. 2014;18(4):363–8.

33. Porrini E, Moreno JM, Osuna A, Benitez R, Lampreabe I, Diaz JM, Silva I, Domínguez R, Gonzalez-Cotorruelo J, Bayes B, Lauzurica R, Ibernon M, Moreso F, Delgado P, Torres A. Prediabetes in patients receiving tacrolimus in the first year after kidney transplantation: a prospective and multicenter study. Transplantation. 2008;85(8):1133–8.

34. Guitard J, Rostaing L, Kamar N. New-onset diabetes and nephropathy after renal transplantation. Contrib Nephrol. 2011;170:247–55.

35. Webster A, Woodroffe RC, Taylor RS, Chapman JR, Craig JC. Tacrolimus versus cyclosporine as primary immunosuppression for kidney transplant recipients. Cochrane Database Syst Rev. 2005;(4):CD003961.

36. Montori VM, Permanyer-Miralda G, Ferreira-González I, et al. Validity of composite end points in clinical trials. BMJ. 2005;12;330(7491):594–6.

37. Humar A, Lebranchu Y, Vincenti F, et al. The efficacy and safety of 200 days valganciclovir cytomegalovirus prophylaxis in high-risk kidney transplant recipients. Am J Transplant. 2010;10(5):1228–37.

38. Euvrard S, Kanitakis J, Pouteil-Noble C, Claudy A, Touraine JL. Ann Transplant. 1997;2(4):28–32.

39. Alberú J1, Pascoe MD, Campistol JM, et al. Lower malignancy rates in renal allograft recipients converted to sirolimus-based, calcineurin inhibitor-free immunotherapy: 24-month results from the CONVERT trial. Transplantation. 2011;92(3):303–10. doi:10.1097/TP.0b013e3182247ae2.

General Conclusions

The chapters included in this monograph have highlighted the strengths and weaknesses of the published literature and RCT upon which we base our daily clinical nephrology practice.

In general and across the different chapters covering most aspects of clinical nephrology, the review and critical appraisal of RCT undertook by experts in the filed has revealed the following:

1. A large number of poorly randomized studies not devoid of bias
2. A large number of open label studies open to observer selection and management biases
3. A large number of underpowered studies with a sample size too small to be conclusive
4. A large number of studies with surrogate primary endpoints that bear little direct impact on harder endpoint such as ESRD, morbidity or mortality
5. A large number of studies with composite and unrelated endpoints with different clinical significance, questioning the validity of such combination of endpoints
6. A large number of studies with poor experimental design including a number of confounders making the interpretation of the results at best challenging and at worst impossible
7. A large number of studies with such a short observation time to preclude any meaningful clinical outcome
8. A large number of studies that based their conclusions on secondary endpoints for which the original study was not powered to evaluate
9. A large number of studies that based their conclusions on posthoc or subgroup analyses, for which the original design was not powered to evaluate and that would be at best hypothesis generating
10. A large number of studies with misleading conclusions not supported by the RCT findings, interpretation or thorough appraisal

We therefore hope that this monograph will draw the nephrology community's attention to the issues listed above and improve in the long term the conduct, analysis, and interpretation of RCT. This will ultimately provide nephrologists worldwide with a stronger and more sound basis upon which to build their daily clinical practice.

Printed in the United States
By Bookmasters